W0106353

The Future of Predictive Safety Evaluation

The Future of Predictive Safety Evaluation

In Two Volumes
Volume 2

Edited by

A.N. Worden
Cantab Group, Cambridge, England

D.V. Parke
Department of Biochemistry, University of Surrey, Guildford, England

J. Marks
Director of Medical Studies, Girton College, Cambridge, England

ERRATUM
The Future of Predictive Safety Evaluation Vol. 2
The correct ISBN is 0-85200-694-2

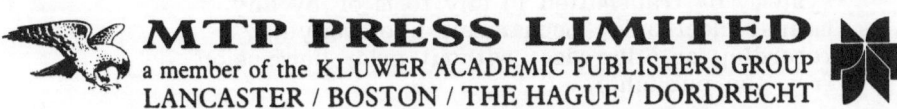

MTP PRESS LIMITED
a member of the KLUWER ACADEMIC PUBLISHERS GROUP
LANCASTER / BOSTON / THE HAGUE / DORDRECHT

Published in the UK and Europe by
MTP Press Limited
Falcon House
Lancaster, England

British Library Cataloguing in Publication Data

The Future of predictive safety evaluation.
    Vol. 2
1. Toxicology---Technique   2.   Laboratory
animals
I. Worden, Alastair N.   II. Parke, Dennis, V.
III. Marks, John
615.9'00724   RA1199

Published in the USA by
MTP Press
A division of Kluwer Academic Publishers
101 Philip Drive
Norwell, MA 02061, USA

Library of Congress Cataloging-in-Publication Data

The Future of predictive safety evaluation

Includes bibliographies and index
    1. Toxicity testing--Evaluation.   2. Health risk
    assessment--Evaluation.   I. Worden, Alastair N.
    II. Parke, Dennis V.   III. Marks, John, 1924-
    [DNLM: 1. Drugs--standards.   2. Drugs--toxicity.
    3. Environmental Monitoring--trends.   4. Environmental
    Pollutants--toxicity.   5. Environmental Pollution--
    prevention & control.   WA 670 F996]
    RA1199.F87   1986   363.1'79   86-10269
    ISBN-13: 978-94-010-7936-5   e-ISBN-13: 978-94-009-3201-2
    DOI: 10.1007/978-94-009-3201-2

Copyright 1987 MTP Press Limited
Softcover reprint of the hardcover 1st edition 1987

iv

Contents

CONTENTS

[*]Based in part on information from various, including industrial,
sources.

List of Contributors

Dr JE Blundell
Department of Psychology
University of Leeds
Leeds, England

Dr VK Brown
Maidstone
Kent, England

Dr DG Clark
Sittingbourne Research Centre
Sittingbourne
Kent, England

Dr AJ Dewar
Chemicals Planning
Shell International Chemical
  Company Limited
Shell Centre
London SE1, England

Dr DL Frape
CANTAB Group
Alexandra House
Hinchingbrooke Hospital
Huntingdon, England

Dr WM Galbraith
Assistant Director for
  Pharmacology and Toxicology
Office for Biologics Research
  and Review
Center for Drugs and Biologics
Food and Drug Administration
Rockville, Maryland, USA

Dr AJ Hill
Department of Psychology
University of Leeds
Leeds, England

Dr ABG Lansdown
Charing Cross and Westminster
  Medical School
St Dunstan's Road
London W6 8RP, England

Dr J Marks
Fellow, Tutor, and Director of
  Medical Studies
Girton College
Cambridge, England

Professor DV Parke
Professor and Head of the
  Department of Biochemistry
University of Surrey, England

Dr NW Shephard
Director, Medical Science
  Research
Beaconsfield, England

Professor SR Walker
Centre for Medicines Research
12 Whitehall
London SW1, England

Dr JH Weisburger
Vice President for Research
  and Director
Naylor Dana Institute for
  Disease Prevention
American Health Foundation
320 East 43rd Street
New York, USA

Professor AN Worden
Hon. Professor of Toxicology
University of Surrey
Emeritus Fellow of Wolfson
  College Cambridge, and
Chairman CANTAB Group,
Hinchingbrooke Hospital
Cambridge, England

ATTRIBUTION

Several authors have asked us to state that the opinions expressed in their articles are personal and do not necessarily represent the official policy of their organizations. Rather than repeat this statement many times throughout the book, it should be regarded as applying to all the material submitted for publication.

ERRATUM AND APOLOGY

The authors of the Introduction to Volume 1 should read: A.N Worden, A.J Dewar, D.V Parke and J. Marks. The Editors wish to acknowledge the substantial contribution which Dr Dewar made to this chapter.

PART 1
Molecular Aspects of Toxicology

1

Molecular Aspects of Toxicology

D. V. PARKE

INTRODUCTION

Chemical toxicity is essentially a molecular process in which a drug, or another environmental chemical (xenobiotic), interacts reversibly or irreversibly with chemical components of the biological system, thereby disturbing the normal metabolic and physiological homeostasis resulting in cell death (acute lethal injury), cellular oxidations, mutations and malignancy (autoxidative injury), or allergies and inflammatory conditions (immunological injury). Chemical toxicity has, at various times, been considered to be due to (1) interaction of the chemical with vital cellular constituents or (2) activating metabolism of the chemical to reactive intermediates, but these are essentially in vitro concepts derived from the study of isolated systems, including enzyme inhibition kinetics, metabolism studies with microsomal tissue preparations, and cell culture and organ perfusion studies. Although such studies considerably advance our knowledge of the molecular mechanisms of chemical toxicity and give useful information concerning receptors they may yield quite misleading perspectives of potential toxicity in that they largely remove and disregard the various biological defence mechanisms which protect against chemical toxicity, and hence such studies alone are inappropriate for making risk assessments. A more realistic definition, therefore, of the cause of chemical toxicity, is that this results from an inability of the chemicals to be detoxicated. This may be due to a variety of reasons, including:

1. species differences in enzyme activities or in the predominant pathways of metabolism (e.g. malathion is toxic to insects because it is metabolically activated to the cholinesterase inhibitor malaxon, whereas mammalia detoxicate the pesticide by hydrolysis to malathion diacid, catalysed by the carboxylesterases);
2. inhibition of the detoxicating enzymes by the presence of another chemical or impurity (e.g. the greatly enhanced

3

toxicity of malathion in mammalia by isomalathion);

3. genetic differences in the rates of metabolic detoxication and clearance (e.g. the drug perhexiline, which shows marked individual differences in toxicity[1]);
4. saturation of the detoxication pathways (e.g. the toxic oxidation of paracetamol at high dosage, when the conjugation pathways are saturated); and
5. nutritional deprivation (e.g. the toxicity of bromobenzene in isolated hepatocytes or starved animals, due to deficient liver glutathione[2]).

Chemical toxicity may therefore be considered to result from:

1. Interaction of the chemical or its metabolites with vital biological constituents (glutathione, proteins, enzymes, DNA, etc.).
2. Metabolism of the chemical to reactive intermediates, electrophiles which can interact non-enzymically, and often irreversibly, with vital biological constituents.
3. Inability of the body's defence enzymes to detoxicate the chemical and its metabolites or to effect their clearance from the animal organism, because of species or genetic characteristics, enzyme inhibitors, nutritional deficiencies, or saturation of detoxication pathways through high dosage.

The safety evaluation of drugs, food additives, pesticides, and other environmental chemicals is usually undertaken to determine risk assessment for human exposure, or for the various aquatic species whose ecology may be disturbed by the release of these xenobiotic chemicals into the environment. Alternative approaches have developed over the past 40 years that safety evaluation studies have been undertaken, from the "empirical" approach based largely on lethality and morphological studies, to the "current good practice" of today, based on the scientific validation of the animal species selected for toxicological studies, to the "ideal" approach advocated some 10 years ago by the eminent Soviet toxicologist, Sanockji, and the "quantitative-structure-activity (QSAR)" approach used by the Environmental Protection Agency, U.S.A. for the safety evaluation of new industrial chemicals (see Table 1.1).

Safety evaluation studies of new chemicals should therefore be carried out in laboratory animal species scientifically selected as appropriate models for man. Contrary to certain naive assumptions, convenience of handling, short life-span, cost, and known history of pathology are not the principal factors involved in the selection of animal species for safety evaluation studies. Instead, the selection of species as appropriate models for human risk assessment should be based on similarities to man in (1) the metabolic pathways of the chemical being evaluated, (2) the rates of its metabolism, (3) the mechanisms of its toxicity, and (4) receptor interactions. Failure to make this scientific selection of animal models before undertaking animal toxicity studies degrades these activities to expensive but largely meaningless rituals which, as a consequence, could fail to satisfy regulatory authorities, with loss of potential markets.

4

Table 1.1 Alternative approaches to safety evaluation of chemicals

Empirical	Current good practice	Ideal	QSAR
Lethality and morphological studies, mostly on rodents, with emphasis on statistics.	Limited but adequate animal studies. Species and doses chosen from metabolic and toxicokinetic studies.	Progressive development of safety evaluation from QSAR and in vitro tests to three-generation studies, neurotoxicology and behavioural toxicology, linked to scale of production and nature of usage.	log P and physicochemical parameters. Structure/activity relationships with chemicals of known toxicity and known metabolism and toxicokinetics.
Little or no concern with mechanisms, metabolism or toxicokinetics.	Human risk assessments made on scientific basis from animal experiments and human studies, including mechanisms of toxicity and comparative receptor studies.	Choice of animal species and human risk assessment based on mechanisms, metabolism, toxicokinetic and receptor studies.	Discard chemical if toxic and redesign rather than conduct animal studies.
		(Sanockji, USSR)	(Environmental Protection Agency - USA)

Comparative studies of the metabolism of the chemical are essential in the initial selection of the animal species to be used as models for man. Comparative toxicokinetics are necessary for setting the doses to be used in long-term toxicological studies, and also for interpretation of the animal toxicity data. Similarly, studies of the mechanism(s) of toxicity in the experimental animals, and wherever possible in man, not only give validity to the whole concept of toxicological studies in animal models, but also enable the animal studies to be appropriately designed to accord with the established mechanism. Mechanistic studies also enable receptors to be identified, so that quantitative receptor studies may subsequently be undertaken. Where receptors for toxicity are identified, e.g. intracellular glutathione, cholinesterases, DNA, steroid receptors, it may be possible to select an animal species that will behave in a similar manner to man or, alternatively, to use this information in the interpretation of toxicity data for risk assessment estimations for humans (see Figure 1.1).

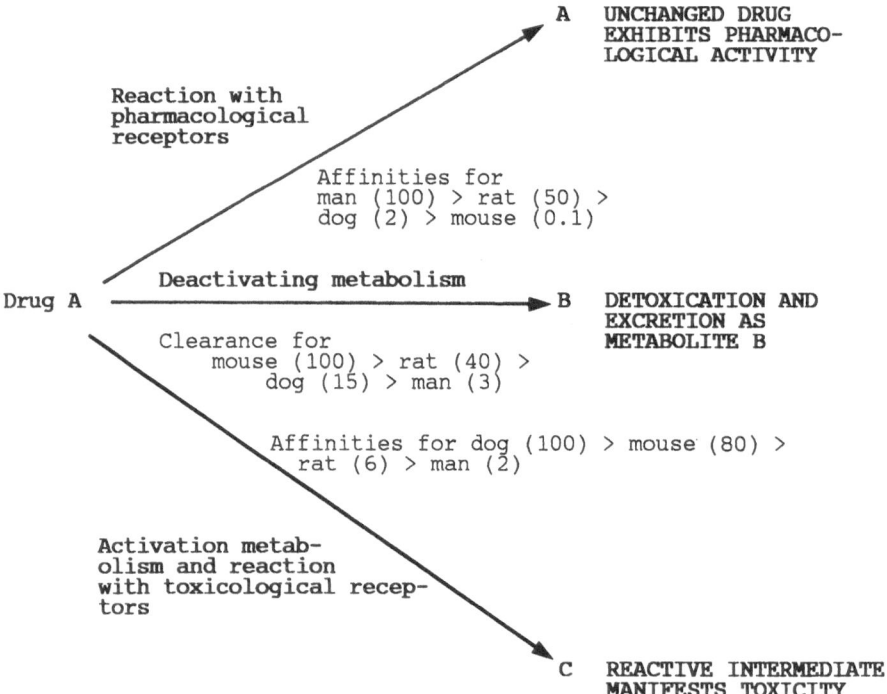

Figure 1.1   Hypothetical scheme for species differences in the pharmacological activity, detoxication and toxicity of a drug. Drug A exhibits pharmacological activity, is detoxicated by metabolism to B, and activated by metabolism to C. Hypothetical species differences in rates of metabolism, clearance and receptor affinities indicate that rat, but not mouse, is a suitable species as a model for man

METABOLISM

Most exogenous chemicals, unless they are highly hydrophilic or contain many substituents such as halogens that deactivate the molecule, are metabolized by enzymes of the mammalian tissues and gastrointestinal microflora (Table 1.2), to render lipophilic molecules more polar and more water-soluble, and thus to expedite their elimination from the body. These processes which are involved in the metabolism of drugs, pesticides and other environmental chemicals have been extensively studied during the past half-century and are fully reviewed in "Introduction to Drug Metabolism", by Gibson and Skett[3].

Table 1.2 Metabolic reactions in the biotransformation and conjugation of drugs and xenobiotic chemicals

Chemical reaction	Mammalian microsomal enzymes	Mammalian non-microsomal enzymes	Enzymes of the intestinal microflora
Phase 1 Metabolism - Biotransformation			
Oxidation (oxygenation)	Aromatic hydroxylation Acyclic hydroxylation Alicyclic hydroxylation Epoxidation N-Oxidation S-Oxidation Desulphuration Dealkylation Deamination	Alcohol oxidation (cytoplasm) Aldehyde oxidation (cytoplasm) Alicyclic aromatization (mitochondria) Deamination (mitochondria and blood plasma)	
Reduction	Nitro reduction Azo reduction Dehalogenation	Reduction of sulphoxides and N-oxides (cytoplasm) Reduction of disulphides	Reduction of N-oxides Azoreduction Dehydroxylation
Hydrolysis	Epoxide hydrolysis Hydrolysis of esters	Hydrolysis of esters and amides (blood plasma) Hydrolytic ring scission Dehalogenation (cytoplasm)	Hydrolysis of esters Hydrolytic ring scission
Phase 2 Metabolism - Conjugation			
Glucuronylation	UDP-glucuronyl transfer		

(Table 1.2 continued)

Chemical reaction	Mammalian microsomal enzymes	Mammalian non-microsomal enzymes	Enzymes of the intestinal microflora
Sulphation		PAPS-sulphotransfer (cytoplasm)	
Glutathione conjugation (mercapturate formation)	GSH-transfer	GSH-transfer	
Peptide conjugations		Acyl CoA conjugation (mitochondria)	
Methylation		S-adenosylmethionine methyltransfer	

The major role of metabolism studies in chemical safety evaluation programmes is to identify the principal metabolic routes of the chemical in animals and man so as to ascertain that the species of experimental animals chosen for the various toxicology studies are scientifically appropriate models for human risk assessment. For example, the drug carbenoxolone is metabolized in man, dog and monkeys by pathways completely different from those seen in rodents and lagomorphs[4], so that it became necessary to repeat in dogs and monkeys the earlier toxicology studies conducted in rodents. A further role of metabolism studies is the identification of individual metabolites for their quantitative determination in disposition and pharmacokinetic/toxicokinetic studies, and their further study in the elucidation of mechanisms of toxicity and the identification of receptors. The Committee on Safety of Medicines and other regulatory agencies are progressing to the acceptance of toxicity data from a **single** animal species, when validated as a suitable model for man by metabolism and toxicokinetic studies, in preference to data from **two** different species chosen empirically.

Enzymic mechanisms

These processes of the metabolism of drugs and xenobiotic chemicals have been classified appropriately into Phase I reactions, or "biotransformations", and Phase II reactions, or "conjugations" (see Table 1.2). Phase I metabolism, or biotransformations, include oxygenations, oxidations, reductions of nitro groups and azo groups, and hydrolysis of esters and amides, catalysed by mammalian enzymes. They are mostly reductions and hydrolyses where enzymes of the gastrointestinal microflora are concerned. The enzymes of Phase II reactions, or conjugations, which involve the transfer of small molecular moieties to existing functional groups, or to new functional groups introduced by Phase I biotransformations, include the glucuronyl transferases, sulphotransferases, epoxide hydrolases, glutathione S-transferases, methyl transferases, and amino-acyl transferases.

The mammalian enzymes concerned with the metabolism of exogenous chemicals, or xenobiotics, are found mostly in the liver and in the gastrointestinal tract, although both Phase I and Phase II enzymes are found in many other tissues. Chemicals that are metabolized by the enzymes of the gastrointestinal tract, or are absorbed by the portal system and then rapidly metabolized by enzymes of the liver, may present little of the original unchanged chemical in the systemic circulation or tissues, such metabolism being known as "first-pass" metabolism.

The routes of excretion of metabolites are determined by their molecular weight and lipophilicity; lipophilic metabolites and conjugates of molecular weight > 300 are excreted via the bile, whereas more polar metabolites of molecular weight < 300 are preferentially excreted in the urine. Metabolites that are excreted via the bile may undergo further metabolism in the gut, by the enzymes of the gastrointestinal microflora, followed by reabsorption of the products of this metabolism; this may often be the original ingested drug or chemical, subsequently released in the intestines by microbial hydrolysis of a biliary-excreted conjugate. This process of biliary excretion, metabolism, and reabsorption, is known as enterohepatic circulation, and for highly lipophilic compounds such as the polychlorinated biphenyls or the drug carbenoxolone, may lead to repeated circulation of the chemical resulting in a long biological half-life and high biological persistence.

Drugs and other environmental chemicals may be classified broadly into four groups according to their metabolic fate, namely, (1) hydrophilic, polar compounds which if absorbed, are readily excreted, generally without metabolism; (2) lipophilic compounds of small molecular weight, which are readily absorbed, readily metabolized and readily excreted, mostly via the kidneys; (3) highly lipophilic compounds, generally of higher molecular weight, which are fairly readily absorbed, are metabolized slowly, excreted mostly in the bile, often undergoing enterohepatic circulation, have long biological half-lives, and are known as "persistent chemicals"; and (4) highly lipophilic chemicals of high molecular weight containing numerous halogen atoms or other substituents that inhibit metabolism, which are only very slowly metabolized (< 10% per annum), are excreted via the bile, have half-lives measured in years, and are known as "non-metabolisable chemicals"[5]. Toxicity is often determined by clearance, which for chemicals of classes (2) and (3) depends on metabolism. Target organ toxicity is often determined by a specific form of metabolism associated with the

Table 1.3 Activation of chemicals to toxic entities

Chemical class	Example	Metabolic reaction	Toxic metabolites	Toxic effects
Alkanes	n-Hexane	ω-1 C-oxygenation by microsomal cytochromes	Hexan-2,5-dione	Neurotoxicity and encephalopathy
Haloalkanes	Carbon tetrachloride	Reductive dehalogenation by microsomal cytochromes	Trichloromethyl radical, and active oxygen	Hepatotoxicity
Olefines	Styrene	Epoxidation by microsomal cytochromes	Styrene epoxide	Carcinogenicity
Haloalkenes	Trichloro-ethylene	Epoxidation by microsomal cytochromes	Epoxide	Toxicity, carcinogenicity
Aromatic hydrocarbons	Benzene	Oxygenation by microsomal cytochromes, redox cycling involving flavoprotein mono-oxygenase	Benzoquinones and active oxygen	Aplastic anaemia, carcinogenicity
Polycyclic aromatic hydrocarbons	Benzo(a)pyrene	Oxygenation by microsomal cytochromes, epoxide hydrolase	Benzo(a)pyrene-7,8-dihydrodiol-9,10-epoxide	Carcinogenicity
Aromatic amines	2-Naphthylamine	N-Oxygenation by microsomal cytochromes and flavoprotein mono-oxygenases	2-Naphthyl-hydroxylamine	Carcinogenicity

Class	Compound	Process	Product	Toxicity
Acetanilides	Paracetamol	N-Oxygenation by microsomal cytochromes	Quinoneimine and active oxygen	Hepatotoxicity
Aromatic amides	2-Acetamidofluorene	N-Oxygenation by microsomal cytochromes	N-Hydroxy-acetamidofluorene	Carcinogenicity
Azo compounds	N,N-Dimethyl-aminoazobenzene	N-Oxygenation by microsomal cytochromes and flavoprotein mono-oxygenases	N-Hydroxymethyl N-methylaminoazo-benzene	Carcinogenicity
Nitro compounds	Nitrofurantoin	Reduction by cytochrome P-450 reductase and other reductases; redox cycling	Hydroxylamine analogue and reactive oxygen	Toxicity
Thiocarbonyl compounds	Carbon disulphide	S-Replacement by microsomal cytochromes	Carbonyl sulphide and sulphene derivative of cytochrome P-450	Neurotoxicity and hepatotoxicity
Thiophosphonate compounds	Parathion	S-Replacement by microsomal cytochromes and flavoprotein mono-oxygenases	Paraoxon	Neurotoxicity

target tissue (e.g. the nephrotoxicity of S-(1,2-dichlorovinyl)-L-cysteine, the conjugate of trichloroethylene, is attributed to the action of the renal enzyme, cysteine conjugate β-lyase, forming the highly toxic, reactive intermediate, 1,2-dichlorothioethylene during renal excretion[7].

Many enzymes responsible for the metabolism of drugs and other chemicals are poorly developed at birth, making neonates particularly susceptible to the toxicity of drugs and other chemicals. Similarly, for the activation of carcinogens, the slow development of the activating enzymes in the fetus results in the delayed activation of carcinogens, so that chemical carcinogenicity is often associated with the development of the activating enzymes.

Activation and detoxication

Although at first it was assumed that metabolism of drugs and toxic chemicals by the enzymes of the body would invariably lead to the detoxication of these chemicals, this is not always the case. Indeed, drugs are generally deactivated by metabolism, and are eventually detoxicated, but many chemicals, especially chemical carcinogens, may be activated by this metabolism[7] (see Table 1.3). This paradox by which the body's enzymes may either detoxicate or activate chemicals is one of the major problems of toxicology and oncogenesis. However, recent studies have clarified this problem, and it would appear that the alternative pathways of detoxication and activation depend greatly on the nature of the enzymes involved. The activation of chemicals to toxic entities, or ultimate carcinogens, may initially involve reduction or hydrolysis, but ultimately oxygenation (epoxidation and N-oxidation) appears to be the major activating process. Oxygenation of chemicals in Phase I reactions is effected mostly by the cytochromes P-450 and may involve insertion of oxygen into different positions of the molecule, namely, (1) at carbon groups which are spatially unhindered, allowing the oxygen function subsequently to be conjugated by Phase II reactions, and (2) at carbon and nitrogen groups that are spatially hindered, so that the oxygen functions are not subsequently readily detoxicated[8]. Thus, oxygenation at "unhindered" positions of the molecule is followed by Phase II conjugation reactions with the consequent detoxication of the chemical. Alternatively, oxygenation which occurs at "hindered" positions and which is not followed by conjugation, results in the formation of reactive intermediates, electrophilic products which react non-enzymically with tissue constituents such as glutathione, sulphydryl enzymes, DNA or proteins (Figure 1.2). In this way ultimate carcinogens can result in the alkylation of DNA, and reactive intermediates of toxic chemicals may covalently bind to proteins forming neoantigens, or to thiol enzymes, resulting in tissue necrosis.

The predominance of activation or detoxication pathways depends both on the chemical structure of the drug or environmental chemical, and on the nature of the enzymes in the animal species ingesting the chemical. Large planar molecules, such as polycyclic hydrocarbons and amines, offer the greatest possibility of "hindered" positions and, consequently, for Phase I oxygena-

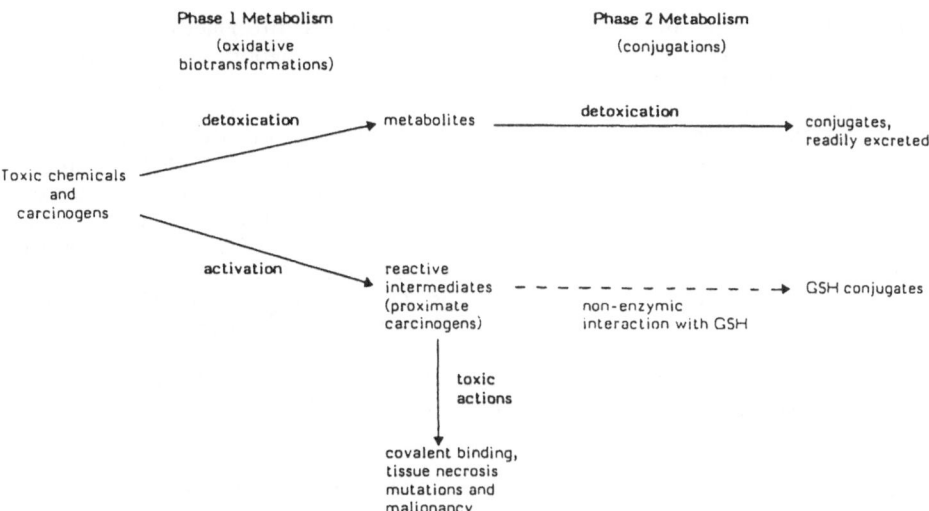

Figure 1.2 The alternative pathways of detoxication and activation of toxic chemicals. Reactive intermediates are generally poor substrates for conjugation by epoxide hydrolases and GSH S-transferase(s) and react non-enzymically with vital cellular macromolecules

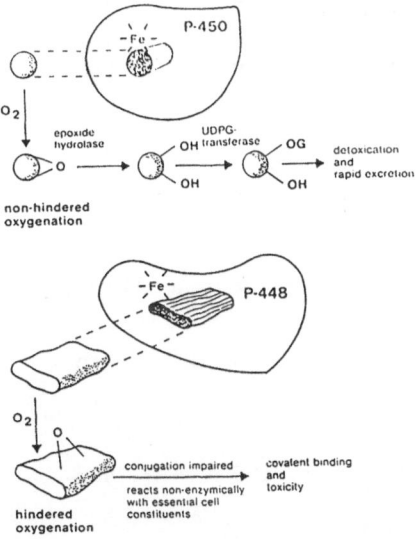

Figure 1.3 "Hindered" and "non-hindered" oxygenations of xenobiotics by cytochromes P-448 and P-450 due to different spatial dimensions of the enzyme active sites. Cytochrome P-450 oxygenates globular molecules, usually leading to subsequent conjugation and detoxication. Cytochrome P-448 oxygenates planar molecules, generally resulting in their activation

tions which lead to the formation of reactive intermediates. It is also now realized that there are at least two major families in the super-family of microsomal mixed-function oxidase enzymes. These are the cytochromes P-450 which usually result in "unhindered" oxygenations, leading to Phase II conjugations and the detoxication of chemicals and carcinogens, and the cytochromes P-448 which usually activate chemical molecules metabolizing them into ultimate carcinogens and reactive intermediates[9] (Figure 1.3). Furthermore, planar, highly lipophilic molecules (area/depth^2 of > 4) appear to be the preferred substrates for cytochrome P-448, whereas smaller, globular, more hydrophilic molecules (area/depth^2 of < 4) are the preferred substrates for the cytochromes P-450[10] (Table 1.4).

Table 1.4 The molecular dimensions of carcinogens and toxic chemicals and their activation by cytochrome P-448

Chemical	Molecular dimension (area/depth^2)	Preferred cytochrome	Toxicity
Dibenz(a,h)anthracene	14.4	448	Carcinogen
Benzo(a)pyrene	12.0	448	Carcinogen
Dimethylaminoazobenzene	9.7	448	Carcinogen
9-Hydroxyellipticine	7.0	448	Cytotoxin + carcinogen
2-Acetamidofluorene	5.0	448	Carcinogen
Paracetamol	4.8	448	Hepatotoxin at high dosage
Aflatoxin	3.2	448,450	Hepatotoxin, hepatocarcinogen
Metyrapone	2.0	450	Adrenal suppression, non-carcinogen
DDT	1.9	450	Cholinesterase inhibition, non-carcinogen
Phenobarbitone	1.1	450	Hypnotic, non-carcinogen

There is much to indicate that the preferred cytochrome P-448 substrates have similar spatial conformations and lipophilicity to cholesterol and the steroids, and the physiological role of this family of cytochromes may be associated with the biogenesis of the steroid hormones. It is believed that the modern cytochromes P-450 evolved from a primitive type of cytochrome many millions of years ago, probably around the time of the evolution of amphibia. In general, fish tend to have a greater abundance of the cytochrome P-448 family than of cytochrome P-450, and consequently tend to activate toxic chemicals more readily and extensively than do mammalia; fish are also more prone to the tumorigenic action of chemical carcinogens[11].

Chemicals and carcinogens may also be activated by oxygenations not involving the cytochromes P-448. The alternative mechanisms of oxygenation at "hindered" positions of the chemical molecule involve the action of hydroxyl radicals produced by (1) conversion of HPETE to HETE in prostaglandin synthesis, (2) redox cycling procedures involving quinone/semiquinone and other coupled one-electron reductions of tissue oxygen, (3) ionizing radiation and lipid peroxides, and (4) superoxide and peroxide production resulting from uncoupling of cytochrome P-450 from its reductase.

Species and genetic differences

Many species differences in chemical toxicity, attributable to differences in metabolism, are known (Table 1.5). For example, the mouse and hamster are much more susceptible to the hepatotoxic action of paracetamol than is the rat, due to the high cytochrome P-448 concentrations in mouse and hamster liver. Similarly, TCDD is much less toxic to the hamster than it is to the rat or guinea pig, and the hamster but not the rat is able to metabolize this "non-metabolizable" chemical, albeit very slowly. Species differences in chemical toxicity may therefore often be the consequences of differences in tissue concentrations of the enzymes involved in detoxication or activation. The most important of these differences would appear to be the ratio of the cytochromes P-450 to P-448 activities, especially as these two families of Phase I enzymes may lead, respectively, to detoxication on the one hand (cytochrome P-450) and activation, toxicity and carcinogenesis on the other (cytochrome P-448). Much research has therefore been devoted to identifying the different tissue activities of these enzymes in various species, and it is known that, in general, mice have high levels of the cytochromes P-448 in their livers, as do hamsters, whereas rat has low levels, even lower than those found in man. Many other species differences in chemical toxicity may be related to different activities of other Phase I enzymes, and also to differences in the activities of Phase II enzymes.

As man is genetically so heterogeneous, it is not surprising that one sees a much wider variety of differences in metabolism in man than is commonly seen in inbred laboratory animals. Furthermore, pharmacokinetic and pharmacogenetic studies have revealed that the metabolism of many drugs and chemicals in humans is polymorphic, resulting in idiosyncratic adverse reactions and

Table 1.5 Species differences in chemical toxicity due to differences in metabolism

Chemical	Sensitive species	Resistant species	Mechanism
Malathion	Insects	Mammals	Insects activate by oxidative metabolism, mammals detoxicate by carboxylesterase-mediated hydrolysis
Paracetamol	Hamster, mouse	Rat	Hamster and mouse have high concentrations of the activating cytochrome P-448
Acetanilide	Dog	Rat	Dog more extensively deacetylates and N-hydroxylates to the hydroxylamine
2-Acetamidofluorene	Dog, hamster	Guinea pig	Guinea pig does not N-hydroxylate 2-AAF to yield the proximate carcinogen
DDT	Insects, birds	Mammals	Is metabolized in insects and birds to DDE which accumulates in tissues, but in mammalia is metabolized to polar DDA which is excreted
Phenol	Cat	Rat, rabbit	Cat has impaired glucuronide conjugation
2,3,7,8-Tetrachlorodibenzodioxin (TCDD)	Guinea pig (LD_{50}= 1 µg/kg)	Hamster (LD_{50}=2500 µg/kg)	Hamster, but not guinea pig, metabolizes TCDD[21]

toxicity. Recent studies have focused attention on a number of polymorphic drug oxidations, including the metabolic detoxication of debrisoquine, sparteine, desmethylimipramine, and perhexiline, many of which have been related to particular forms of cytochromes P-450[12]. Similarly, certain isozymes of cytochrome P-450, particularly the cytochromes P-448, have been associated with a high spontaneous incidence of cancer, in both experimental animals and man.

Environmental factors

The activities of many drug-metabolizing enzymes may be increased, inhibited, or destroyed, by the actions of other environmental chemicals (Table 1.6). Many drugs and chemicals lead to the induction of new enzyme proteins, particularly the cytochromes P-450 which are induced by phenobarbital, DDT, and many similar small globular molecules, and the cytochromes P-448 which are induced by carcinogenic polycyclic aromatic hydrocarbons, polycyclic amines and other highly lipophilic planar molecules. Repeated dosage of these chemicals, especially drugs which are inducers of

Table 1.6 Some inductive and inhibiting effects of environmental chemicals on the drug-metabolizing enzymes

Environmental chemicals	Enzymic effect
Induction	
DDT, dieldrin, phenobarbitone	Cytochrome P-450, P-450 reductase, and various conjugases are enhanced
Polycyclic carcinogenic hydrocarbons, halogenated polycyclics, TCDD	Cytochrome P-448 and selected conjugases enhanced
Alcohol	A novel cytochrome P-450 is enhanced
Inhibitors	
Metyrapone, safrole, ketoconazole	Cytochromes P-450 are inhibited
9-Hydroxyellipticine, 7,8-benzo-flavone, cimetidine	Cytochromes P-448 are selectively inhibited
Destruction of enzymes	
Carbon disulphide, carbon tetrachloride, allylisopropyl-acetamide	Loss of microsomal cytochromes due to initiation of autoxidation

cytochrome P-450, may lead to marked enzyme induction over very long periods of time, resulting in high levels of the enzyme activity, more rapid metabolism of drugs, with consequently lowered pharmacological activity and shorter biological half-lives. Where this increase of enzymic activity (cytochromes P-450) results in detoxication, induction of the enzymes by the chemical itself, or by some other chemical present in the food or environment, may lead to an erroneously low assessment of the toxicity of a chemical under study for safety evaluation. Similarly, if the chemical, or some other chemical in the environment, induces the cytochromes P-448 which can lead to the activation of chemicals, the enzyme induction may considerably increase the toxicity/carcinogenicity of the chemical under consideration. For example, the potent carcinogen, 2-acetamidofluorene, is readily activated in the mouse, by N-hydroxylation, and this animal exhibits a high carcinogenic response; in contrast, the rat, which has little hepatic cytochrome P-448, does not initially activate 2-acetamidofluorene, but repeated administration of this chemical results in the induction of enzymes which N-hydroxylate the amide, so that on repeated administration carcinogenicity is evident also in the rat.

Similarly, chemicals may result in the inhibition of enzymes, and the product of an initial metabolic reaction may subsequently inhibit this reaction, or the enzymes catalysing a subsequent metabolic pathway. The drugs ketoconazole and cimetidine are well-known inhibitors of the microsomal mixed-function oxidase cytochromes, resulting in impaired oxidative metabolism of simultaneously administered drugs and other chemicals. Ketoconazole, a relatively non-specific inhibitor of the cytochromes P-450, is one of many chemicals that have been specifically devised to inhibit mixed-function oxidations and thereby to inhibit the biogenesis of sterols for the treatment of fungal infections, but its lack of specificity also results in inhibition of the biogenesis of steroid hormones, and selected members of the eicosanoid cascade. Cimetidine appears to be more specific in its inhibition of the cytochromes P-448, and drugs of this class could well have a role in the prevention of tumorigenicity.

Other chemicals may interact with the drug-metabolizing enzymes leading to their suicidal destruction. Many chemicals of this type are olefinic or acetylenic compounds, such as allobarbital and ethinyloestradiol, which bind to cytochrome P-450 and thereby result in its destruction, sometimes resulting in denaturation of the cytochrome and sometimes in the complete breakdown of the haem moiety. Such chemicals, known as "suicide substrates", result in a new phenomenon of toxicity, in which the chemical defence system of the body is selectively destroyed.

Another phenomenon of enzyme inhibition is seen with certain pesticide analogues. For example, malathion is selectively activated to the more toxic malaoxon by a cytochrome P-450 oxygenase, which results in replacement of the sulphur atom by oxygen. In contrast, mammalia preferentially metabolize malathion by the carboxyl esterases, which hydrolyse the ester moieties to form the non-toxic malathion diacid (Figure 1.4). These two pathways are so disparate and characteristic of insecta and mammalia respectively, that concentrations of malathion, and other organophosphate insecticides which are lethal to many insects, have little or no effect on man, so that malathion is used as an additive to grain in storage silos to prevent consumption by grain weevils. However, an impure form of malathion, containing isomalathion and a number of analogues and isomers as impurities, has been found to be many times more toxic to mammals because of the selective inhibition of carboxyl esterases by the impurities. This example, one of several in the field of pesticide toxicology, illustrates unequivocally the importance of studying the potential impurities of a chemical being evaluated for safety, and the need to ensure that the chemical which is marketed has the same purity specification as that tested for toxicity.

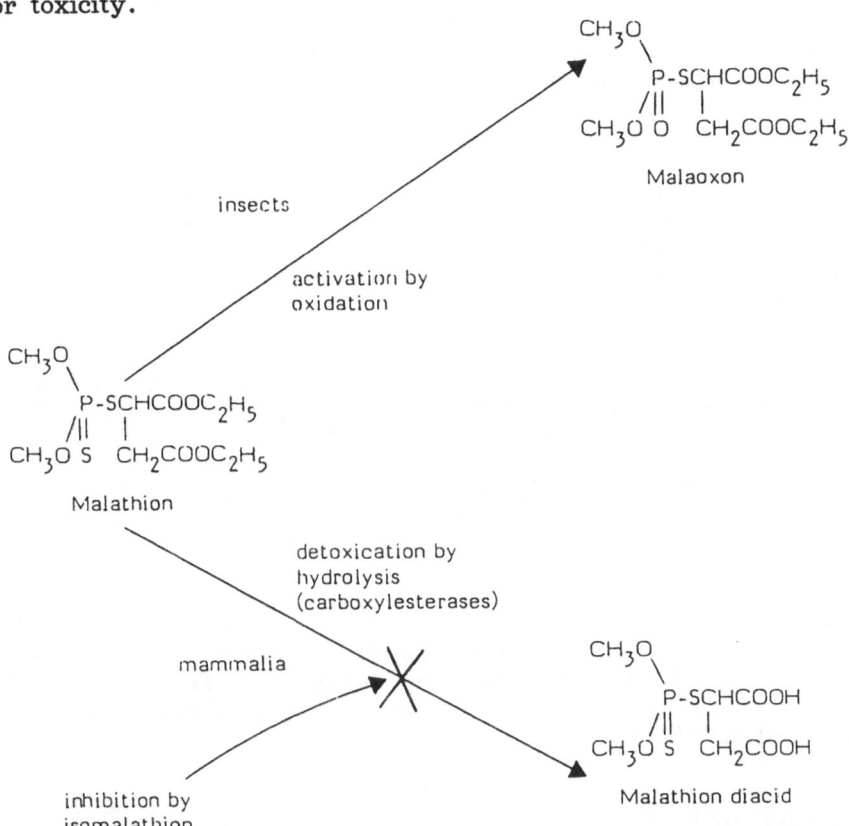

Figure 1.4 Species differences in the metabolism, detoxication and activation of malathion. Isomalathion inhibits the detoxicating enzyme, carboxylesterase, and markedly increases the toxicity of malathion to human subjects

Other environmental factors, especially nutrition and diet, can have a marked effect on the metabolism of drugs and toxic chemicals. This is especially true where large doses of chemicals are being administered, as occurs in the administration of "maximal tolerated doses" in chronic toxicity studies; such large amounts of

toxic chemicals can lead to selective depletion of various intermediates required for chemical detoxication pathways. For example,
many carcinogens and toxic chemicals which are oxidants, or
oxygen radical generators, make high demands on tissue
glutathione, and depletion of this material may quickly lead to cell
death or to the interaction of the electrophilic reactive intermediates with tissue proteins, nucleotides, and DNA, with consequent toxicity and carcinogenicity. Similarly, enzyme induction
may result in a deficiency of folate, which will then lead to an arrest of the enzyme induction, as folate is essential for the synthesis of the microsomal cytochromes; this depletion of folate by
enzyme induction has been proposed as the cause of the macrocytic
anaemia and teratogenicity seen in epileptic patients on long-term
administration of phenobarbitone and diphenylhydantoin. Continuous administration of toxic chemicals and drugs may also lead
to depletion of vitamin C, which seems to be necessary for the
detoxication of xenobiotic chemicals. Furthermore, it is now known
that a number of enzymes concerned in the metabolic detoxication
and activation of chemicals may be impaired or augmented by diet,
and induced or inhibited by other chemicals present in the environment. Among the most prominent of these enzymes is
cytochrome P-450, which initiates the detoxication of drugs and
chemicals, and appears to be enhanced by diets rich in fresh fruit
and vegetables; and cytochrome P-448, which tends to activate
toxic chemicals and carcinogens, and is known to be induced by
charcoal-broiled steaks and other cooked meats, by cigarette smoking, and by persistent halogenated chemicals such as TCDD,
polychlorinated biphenyls, etc. It is therefore obvious that the
toxicity of chemicals both in man and experimental animals can be
profoundly affected by diet and by previous and simultaneous exposure to environmental chemicals.

For further reading the following are recommended:
"Introduction to Drug Metabolism" by Gibson and Skett[3]; "Drug
Metabolism and Drug Toxicity", by Mitchell and Horning;
"Development of detoxication mechanisms in the neonate" by Parke;
"The role of nutrition in toxicology", by Parke and Ioannides;
"Concepts in Drug Metabolism" by Jenner and Testa; "Molecular
Aspects of Toxicology", by Hathaway; and "Cytochrome P-450", by
Ruckpaul and Rein.

TOXICOKINETICS

In the safety evaluation of drugs and toxic chemicals it is also
very important to know the extent and rate of absorption of the
compound, the rates of its metabolism, and the extents and rates
of excretion, by all routes. If the chemical is extensively and
rapidly excreted - that is, has a high rate of clearance - it is unlikely to exhibit chronic toxicity, whereas if the chemical has a low
clearance - that is, it is excreted only partially over a long period
of time, say 50% excreted in 7 days - it is most likely retained in
the animal organism by (1) reversible binding to tissue lipids and
tissue proteins, (2) enterohepatic recirculation, or (3) irreversible
interactions of reactive intermediates with vital tissue components,

the latter being indicative of chronic toxicity and possible tumorigenicity. It is also important to know if any tissues have high affinities for the chemical or any of its metabolites, which might be associated with specific organ toxicity (e.g. paraquat is selectively taken up by the lung). This can be achieved by routine analysis of the isolated tissues for the drug and its metabolites, at different intervals after dosing, or by using autoradiography when labelled chemicals are used. Simple, non-mathematical approaches to basic pharmacokinetics may be found in the review by Levy and Bauer[13].

With drugs, food additives and other chemicals which are likely to be administered orally, it is essential to have information concerning the plasma AUC values (area under the curve of plasma concentration/time after dosing) of the unchanged chemical, and also the chemical together with all of its metabolites. These may be obtained by quantification procedures using high-performance liquid chromatography, gas chromatography, or immunoassay procedures, or by radiometric assays using radiolabelled chemicals, after both oral and intravenous administration. If the AUC values of the unchanged chemical are very similar after both oral and intravenous administration, this is indicative that the orally administered chemical is readily absorbed, but not rapidly metabolized. If the AUC value of the unchanged drug and of the total drug products are much greater after intravenous administrations than after oral administration, this is indicative of poor gastrointestinal absorption. Similarly, if the AUC values of the total drug products are similar after oral and intravenous administration, but the AUC value of unchanged drug is much greater after intravenous administration, this is indicative of good absorption from the gastrointestinal tract, accompanied by a high degree of first-pass metabolism (metabolism in the gastrointestinal tract or liver). Determination of AUC values at different doses is necessary to check compliance of dosing, and that absorption increases with dosage.

From the determination of the plasma concentration of the unchanged chemical, and of its various metabolites, together with the rates of the urinary and biliary excretion of these compounds, it is possible to calculate a number of toxicokinetic parameters, including the volume of distribution (V_d), the systemic clearance (Cl) and the biological half-life ($t_{\frac{1}{2}}$). These three parameters are related
as follows:

$$t_{\frac{1}{2}} = \frac{0.693 \; V_d}{Cl}$$

which indicates that the larger the volume of distribution the longer the half-life, and the larger the clearance the shorter the half-life. The half-life is dependent both on the volume of distribution and the systemic clearance. The plasma drug concentration/time profiles and the plasma half-life may therefore vary greatly in different animal species, and such data are of paramount importance in the selection of suitable animal models for safety evaluation studies (Figure 1.5).

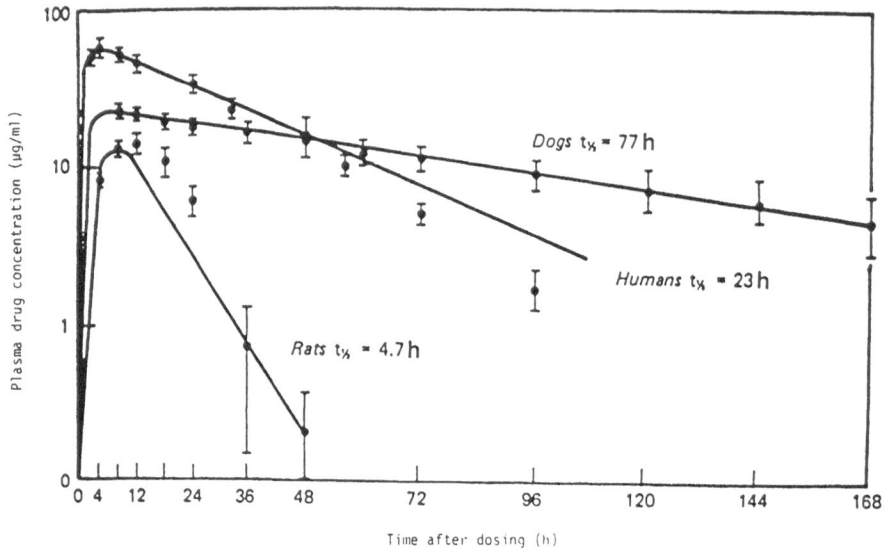

Figure 1.5 Species differences in the plasma pharmacokinetics of a hypothetical drug. The rate of elimination of the drug from the blood plasma, and the plasma half-lives ($t_{\frac{1}{2}}$), show marked species differences

Compounds with long biological half-lives are retained in the body for long periods, either by sequestration in the lipid depots, enterohepatic circulation, or by covalent binding to tissue proteins, DNA, etc. Low $t_{\frac{1}{2}}$ values (0.5 to 6 hours) are an assurance of the ready elimination of the chemical with little probability of chronic toxicity; higher values of $t_{\frac{1}{2}}$ on the other hand, may be indicative of tissue interaction and some degree of chronic toxicity. One toxicokinetic parameter, namely the clearance (Cl), of the chemical, is of especial value in assessing its overall potential toxicity, and in some instances it has been found to be a much more reliable parameter than extensive long-term animal toxicology studies (Table 1.7). It is essential to determine the clearance and other toxicokinetic parameters at different dose levels to ascertain if variation occurs with increasing dose, and if linear or non-linear.

For chemicals that are likely to be ingested daily over long periods, such as drugs, food additives and environmental chemicals, it is essential to undertake repeat-dose kinetic studies, in which the various toxicokinetic parameters are determined after a single dose of the chemical and then after repeated daily doses for at least 30 days. Comparison of single- and repeat-dose kinetics enables the detection of accumulation of the chemical or its metabolites, the induction or inhibition of the drug-metabolizing enzymes, and the extent of enterohepatic circulation of the drug. The theoretical extrapolation of single-dose toxicokinetic data to the repeat-dose situation is not acceptable, since various biological phenomena, such as enzyme induction and enzyme inhibition, can interfere markedly with such predictions leading to erroneous and dangerous conclusions.

Table 1.7 Relationship of toxicity of a chromone anti-asthma drug to its systemic clearance

Species	Dose (mg/kg)	Clearance (mg/kg per h)	Hepatotoxicity
Rat	10	138	none (400 mg/kg per day)
Rabbit	10	44	none (100 mg/kg per day)
Squirrel monkey	10	59	none (300 mg/kg per day)
Dog	1	20	
	5	12	
	10	13	
	50	13	Extensive centrilobular necrosis and fatalities after six doses at 40 mg/kg per day
Man	1	15	Raised plasma aminotransferase levels (4 mg/kg per day)

Data from refs 22 and 23

Often, on increasing the dose of the drug or toxic chemical, the toxicokinetic parameters may undergo change, indicating "nonlinear toxicokinetics". For example, increasing the dose of a chemical from 1 to 10 mg/kg may have no effect on the clearance and $t_{\frac{1}{2}}$ values, but progressive increases from 10 to 100 mg/kg may change both of these toxicokinetic parameters several-fold (see Figure 1.6). This is indicative of toxicokinetic and/or metabolic changes occurring at doses between 10 and 100 mg/kg, possibly because of the saturation of mechanisms of excretion or pathways of metabolism, or the involvement of new mechanisms of metabolism, activation or toxicity. A comprehensive study of the impact of nonlinear toxicokinetics on toxicology, with reference to the industrial chemical, dioxane, illustrates the importance of determining rates of metabolic detoxication at different doses before undertaking chronic toxicity studies[15].

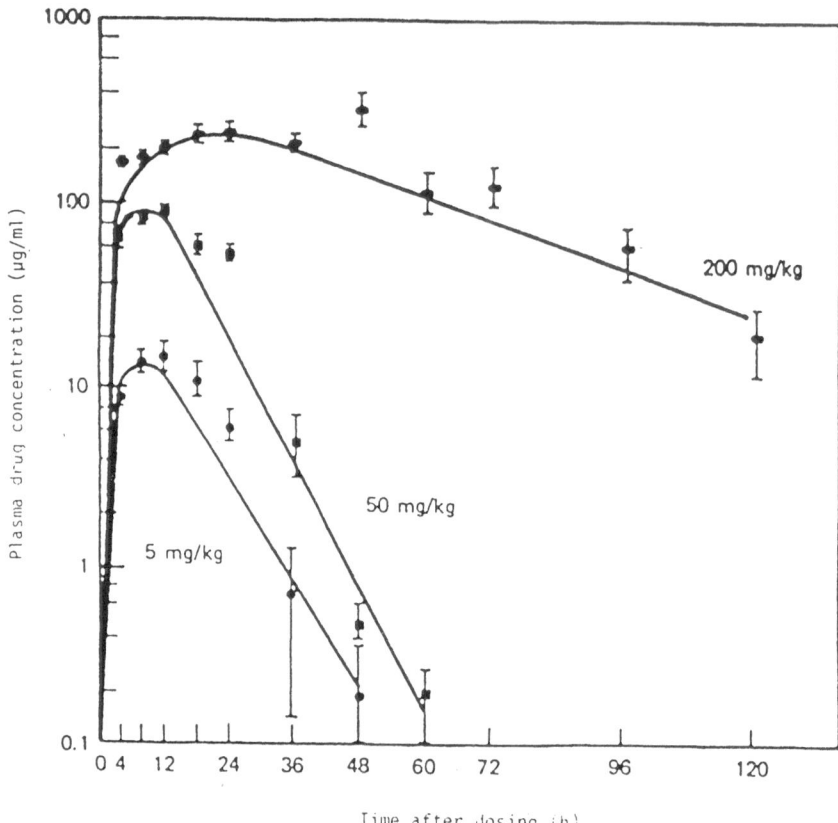

Figure 1.6 The effects of increased dosage of a hypothetical drug on plasma pharmacokinetics. The $t_{\frac{1}{2}}$ is markedly increased from 5 h at 5 and 50 mg/kg to 36 h at 200 mg/kg, probably because of saturation of a metabolic or excretory process essential to the plasma clearance of the drug

In the design of chronic toxicity studies it is especially important to have available data from toxicokinetic studies at increasing doses, to be able to detect dose-related changes in these parameters, especially clearance, and hopefully to correlate any changes in clearance with changes in the pathways of metabolic detoxication and activation, or with the appearance of toxic phenomena. This enables non-linear clearance/dose, or toxicity/dose plots to be established, which facilitate the allocation of doses to particular metabolic pathways of the chemical. The intersections of different slopes of the curve, commonly known as "breakpoints", identify changes in excretion or metabolism, and in chronic toxicity/carcinogenicity studies doses should be selected to monitor these changes of metabolic pathways, i.e. doses should bracket the breakpoints. This enables the pathways of detoxication or activation of the drug or chemical to be correlated with dose and with chronic toxicity/carcinogenicity, which is essential in the scientific approach to safety evaluation and risk assessment procedures (see Figure 1.7).

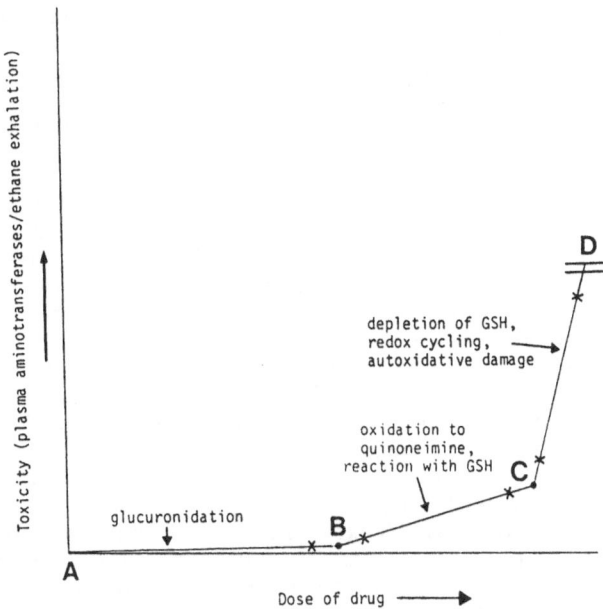

Figure 1.7 Correlation of dose-dependent toxicity of paracetamol with changes in metabolic detoxication and activation. Detoxication of the drug by glucuronide conjugation occurs at doses A to B, oxidation to the reactive intermediate with glutathione depletion occurs at doses from B to C, and redox cycling with progressive autoxidative tissue damage occur at doses beyond C, with death intervening at D. Suitable doses for chronic toxicity/carcinogenicity studies to monitor these changes in metabolic detoxication/activation are indicated by the points X

It is also highly desirable, in calculating doses for chronic toxicity/carcinogenicity studies, to use the toxicokinetically equivalent doses for the given species under study. For example it is well known that, where chemicals are extensively metabolized by oxidative pathways, small animals such as rats and mice will metabolize the chemicals at 20 to 50 times the rate observed in man. Toxicokinetically equivalent doses are calculated from comparative pharmacokinetic studies in man and in the animal models selected, but if these are not available it is common practice, where oxidative metabolism predominates, to consider that appropriate doses for mice, rats, rabbits and dogs are approximately 50, 25, 10 and 5 times the human doses. This practice is essential in designing chronic toxicity/carcinogenicity studies, as many safety evaluation submissions for new drugs, pesticides and other chemicals are invalidated because of the selection of inappropriately low doses.

Toxicokinetic studies are similarly important in the validation of reproduction and teratology studies, to determine to what extent, and at what rates, the drug or chemical and which of its metabolites, cross the placenta and are metabolized by, or retained

25

in, the tissues of the fetus. The rate of administration of the chemical to the dam in teratology studies is highly critical, for the same dose of a chemical administered at different rates may exert markedly different effects, and bolus injection of a chemical may result in teratogenicity because of exceedingly high plasma concentrations, whereas slow infusion of the same dose would have no adverse effect[15]. Also, in neonatal studies it is desirable to know the concentration of the drug and its metabolites in the maternal milk, since highly lipophilic, non-metabolized chemicals are extensively secreted in milk and substantial amounts may be ingested by suckling mammalian neonates. The high concentrations of TCDD (2,3,7,8-tetrachlorodibenzodioxin) and chlorinated biphenyls present in human milk are a major health problem.

For pesticides and industrial chemicals that are likely to be extensively released into the environment, it is also essential to determine their environmental persistence. Many chemicals may only be slowly metabolized in mammals, and therefore tend to accumulate, whereas, in contrast, these chemicals may be quite rapidly degraded in environmental systems, either by micro-organisms or by ultraviolet irradiation. Toxicokinetics of aquatic species are relatively more simple than those of mammalia, and the absorption of a chemical substance from water by an aquatic species may reasonably be predicted from its lipophilicity (log P values); moderately lipophilic chemicals are readily absorbed, whereas highly hydrophilic molecules are poorly absorbed, and highly lipophilic molecules are so insoluble in water that, again, little is absorbed by aquatic species. In detailed studies of the toxicokinetics of distribution of an environmental chemical between various microbiological, aquatic and terrestrial systems, as is needed for the marketing of certain pesticides in Japan and other countries, it is highly desirable to study the toxicokinetics of these chemicals in small isolated ecosystems.

For further reading the following texts and reviews are recommended: "Basic pharmacokinetics", by Levy and Bauer[13]; "Pharmacokinetics", by Gibaldi and Perrier; "Introduction to Drug Metabolism", by Gibson and Skett[3]; "Drug Metabolism and Drug Toxicity", by Mitchell and Horning.

MECHANISMS OF TOXICITY

It has been suggested that before any appropriate animal toxicology is undertaken for the evaluation for human risk assessment, at least the predominant mechanisms of toxicity of the chemical should be known. Only when the mechanism(s) of toxicity is understood can experiments be appropriately designed to quantify the toxicity, establish a dose response, or enable risk assessments to be made from chronic toxicity studies in animal models. In the selection of the animal model it is essential to demonstrate that the animal species will exhibit the same mechanisms of toxicity as are seen in man, and that these occur to similar extents, or can be quantified if they occur to different extents. Accordingly, considerable effort has been expended in the past few decades to elucidate the basic mechanisms of chemical toxicity.

MOLECULAR ASPECTS OF TOXICOLOGY

Three major pathobiological phenomena of chemical toxicity have been identified and characterized, and these are: "acute lethal injury", "autoxidative injury", and "inflammatory injury", and the mechanisms involved in each of these are briefly described in Table 1.8. All mechanisms of chemical toxicity appear to involve chemical interactions of the toxicant with vital biological entities, e.g. (1) the interaction of cyanide with the haem iron of cytochrome a_3 disrupting mitochondrial oxidation, (2) the phosphorylation of neurotoxic esterase in the delayed neurotoxicity of organophosphates, (3) the inhibition of cytosolic thiol enzymes by iodoacetate, preventing glycolysis, (4) the liganding of the sulphene sulphur of carbon disulphide to cytochrome P-450 resulting in the suicidal destruction of the latter, (5) the toxic depletion of intracellular glutathione by bromobenzene or paracetamol, and (6) the alkylation of DNA and the generation of genotoxic oxygen radicals by the polycyclic aromatic hydrocarbons.

Table 1.8 The major patho-biological phenomena resulting from chemical toxicity

Acute lethal injury	Damage to thiol enzymes, inhibition of mitochondrial electron transfer, inhibition of ATP biosynthesis, energy metabolism and ATP-ase cationic pumps
Autoxidative injury	Lipid peroxidation, membrane disruption, destruction of nicotinamide nucleotides, DNA damage and mutations, acute lethal injury
Immunological injury	Neoantigen formation, inflammation, oxygen radical production, autoxidative injury

However, relatively few chemicals are toxic per se, and these generally manifest acute toxicity, i.e. directly react with tissues or cause tissue reactions, such as narcosis (e.g. alcohols), acetylcholinesterase-induced paralysis (e.g. organophosphates), or "acute lethal injury" (e.g. fluoroacetate, barbiturates), or otherwise undergo aqueous hydrolysis in the biological system (e.g. nitrogen mustards) with consequent loss of chemical toxicity. Many other chemicals show little toxicity per se, but are metabolized into reactive intermediates which can react directly with tissue proteins, enzymes, nucleotides, or DNA to result in acute lethal injury, or chronic toxicity such as reproductive effects and tumorigenicity (see Table 1.3). These reactive intermediates may also exist in free radical forms, that can interact with tissue oxygen to form reactive oxygen radicals, which then interact with tissue components resulting in "autoxidative injury". Similarly, reactive intermediates may form neoantigens by covalent interactions with tissue protein, which can initiate "immunological injury", often leading subsequently to "autoxidative injury" and "acute lethal injury".

27

For further reading on the subject of mechanisms of toxicity, the following texts and reviews are recommended: "Enzymatic activation of chemicals to toxic metabolites", by Guengerich and Liebler; "Selective Toxicity", by Albert; and "Drug Metabolism and Drug Toxicity", by Mitchell and Horning.

RECEPTOR STUDIES

When the mechanisms of chemical toxicity have been elucidated, it is often possible to identify specific receptors, such as tissue glutathione, the various cholinesterase enzymes, steroid hormone cytosolic receptors, etc. Recent developments in molecular toxicology have enabled the isolation and characterization of some of these receptors, so that interactions with toxic chemicals, and specific inhibitors, can be studied in vitro. Furthermore, studies of the species differences in these receptors can similarly be undertaken in vitro, with studies of the species differences in tissue receptor concentration, and their comparative affinities for the chemicals under study, being made where necessary.

For example, organophosphates, carbamates and other pesticides interacting with acetylcholinesterase, also interact in varying degrees with a number of other cholinesterases, leading to different types of peripheral and central nervous system toxicity, including delayed neurotoxicity associated with the enzyme neurotoxic esterase. As these different cholinesterases are found in erythrocytes, it is now becoming common practice to determine the inhibitory characteristics of new pesticides and their metabolites with the different erythrocyte cholinesterases, in different animal species, including man, so that comparative toxicities may be determined. This quantification of the comparative toxicities of the chemical at the receptor site can be used in the setting of suitable doses in chronic toxicity studies, or in the final safety assessments of these pesticides for man. Similarly, the new anti-cancer hormone antagonists (e.g. tamoxifen) have been studied in respect of the cytosolic steroid receptors; furthermore, as these drugs may also act as inhibitors of the cytochrome P-450/448 enzymes concerned with the biogenesis of the steroid hormones, studies are now being made of the comparative interactions of the anti-cancer drugs with these enzymes.

Perhaps the most notable example of the use of receptor studies in the safety evaluation of chemicals was the risk assessment of carcinogenicity in humans from the use of the progestational agent, lynestrenol, from 6-year carcinogenicity studies in the beagle dog. Administration of lynestrenol alone, at very high doses, over long periods of time, resulted in production of breast tumours in beagle dogs that were ultimately considered to be malignant, but of little significance to humans. Elegant receptor studies showed that the concentration of progestational receptors, and their affinity for the lynestrenol metabolite, were several orders of magnitude greater in dogs than in humans. From these comparative receptor studies a fairly precise, scientifically based, risk assessment was evaluated for this drug, and at the doses prescribed for humans the drug was considered to present a very minimal risk for lifetime exposure. This highly esoteric approach was substantiated by studies with the natural progestational hormone, progesterone, which, as might have been predicted, also resulted in carcinoma of the breast of the beagle dog at doses similar to those that gave rise to tumours with lynestrenol.

For further reading the following review is recommended: "Biochemical pharmacology of anti-oestrogen action", by Jordan.

OXYGEN TOXICITY

During the past decade or so it has become increasingly realized that oxygen and iron, two essential elements of life, are also two of the most toxic chemicals. The reason for this is that oxygen is readily reduced first to superoxide anion then to peroxide, both of which are toxic to biological systems, but are produced naturally by leucocytes for protection against microbial infections. Similarly, ferrous iron is readily oxidized to ferric, a reaction that can be coupled in aqueous media with the reduction of molecular oxygen to superoxide and peroxide; equally facile is the reduction of ferric iron to ferrous, so that very low concentrations of inorganic iron in the presence of water and molecular oxygen can cyclically generate superoxide. Furthermore, inorganic iron is capable of catalysing the conversion of superoxide anion and peroxide into the more highly toxic hydroxyl radical and singlet oxygen. Another well-known mechanism for the generation of hydroxyl radicals is ionizing radiation, which results in a homolytic scission of H_2O to $OH\cdot$ and $H\cdot$ radicals. In biological systems, therefore, inorganic iron in the presence of oxygen acts in a very similar way to ionizing radiation, and hydroxyl radicals derived from both these sources are capable of peroxidizing unsaturated lipids, disrupting lipoprotein biological membranes, oxidatively disrupting nicotinamide nucleotides, and cross-linking DNA, all of which are characteristic of "autoxidative injury".

Although the term lipid peroxidation is used, it should be realized that reactive oxygen radicals, and especially hydroxyl radicals, are also capable of causing autoxidative damage to structural and functional proteins, carbohydrates, nucleotides, RNA and DNA. Nevertheless, lipid peroxides, formed from unsaturated fatty acids by autoxidation, have longer half-lives than that of the hydroxyl radical, and are able to act in a similar manner but with greater toxic effect than hydroxyl radicals because of their greater stability. Indeed, animals exposed to ionizing radiation have high circulating levels of lipid peroxides, which can reach parts of the body far removed from the site of the ionizing radiation, producing cytotoxic and genotoxic damage, and resulting in the formation of reactive intermediates from toxic chemicals and carcinogens.

This spontaneous activation of oxygen, with the formation of free hydroxyl radicals, can be markedly exacerbated by toxic chemicals. Among the known mechanisms by which toxic chemicals are known to manifest oxygen toxicity are the following:

1. activation by oxidative metabolism to ortho- or para-quinones or quinoneimines, which are then reduced by flavoprotein

29

oxidoreductases to semi-quinones, which catalyse redox cycling with molecular oxygen, to generate superoxide anions and ultimately hydroxyl radicals (see Figure 1.8);

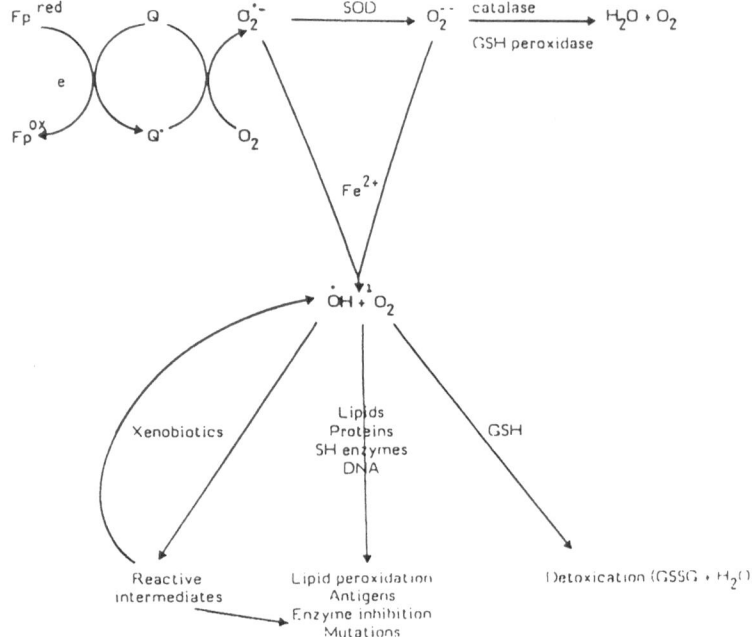

Figure 1.8 Redox cycling mediated by quinone reactive intermediates. This is shown to result in oxygen radical generation, lipid peroxidation, autoxidative tissue injury, and further activation of toxic chemicals and carcinogens to reactive intermediates

2. nitro compounds may be similarly reduced to nitroso radical reactive intermediates, or amines may be oxidatively metabolized to nitroso radicals, which may then catalyse redox cycling;
3. free radical chemicals, e.g. paraquat, can interact directly with molecular oxygen to produce the superoxide anion and hydroxyl radicals;
4. reactive intermediates of polycyclic aromatic hydrocarbons, such as benzo(a)pyrene 7,8-dihydrodiol-9,10-epoxide, may exist in tautomeric free radical forms, which are also capable of generating hydroxyl radicals with consequent cytotoxicity and genotoxicity;
5. highly lipophilic chemicals may become incorporated into the endoplasmic reticulum of cells resulting in major changes of the lipid milieu of the cytochrome P-450/cytochrome P-450 reductase system, leading to uncoupling of the cytochrome from its reductase and leakage of electrons, with consequent

generation of superoxide and hydroxyl radicals.

Not only can toxic chemicals produce oxygen free radicals and manifest toxicity by "autoxidative injury", but they can also be activated by interaction with oxygen free radicals, similar to the activation by cytochrome P-448 or flavoprotein oxido-reductases. Polycyclic aromatic hydrocarbons have been shown to be oxidatively converted into their reactive intermediate ultimate carcinogens by: cytochrome P-448, and hydroxyl free radicals produced by redox cycling, coupled prostaglandin synthesis, ioniz-ing radiation, or by lipid peroxides.

Production of reactive oxygen free radicals, and autoxidative injury, may be quantified in vitro by the determination of malon-dialdehyde, a decomposition product of lipid peroxides, by high-performance liquid chromatography or by colorimetric reaction with thiobarbituric acid. Other in vitro methods include determination of chemiluminescence, spectrophotometric determination of alkenals, and histological detection of lipofuscin formation and of autophagic vacuolation. Methods for the determination of autoxidation in vivo include the determination of malondialdehyde excreted in urine or present in blood, chemiluminescence of whole tissues or limbs or, preferably, determination of ethane or pentane, which are autoxidative decomposition products exhaled in the expired air of the intact animal. The most sensitive methods are the chemilumines-cence and alkane quantifications.

As in the detoxication of drugs and chemicals, the body has a very effective defence mechanism against reactive oxygen radi-cals, which comprises the enzymes superoxide dismutase and catalase, that catalyse the conversion of superoxide anion to peroxide and of peroxide to water and oxygen. Other components of this defence mechanism include the antioxidants, vitamin E, vitamin C and ubiquinone; the free radical scavengers, the retinoids and flavanoids; and glutathione (GSH). The final defence against oxygen free radicals is GSH, which may be oxidized to GSSG by oxygen radicals or by peroxides in the presence of glutathione peroxidase (see Table 1.9). Reduced glutathione is regenerated from GSSG by glutathione reductase and NADPH. Adequate nutrition is therefore an essential protection against autoxidative injury, and dietary deficiencies of sulphur amino acids, methyl donors, vitamins C, E, and other lipotropes, will tend to exacerbate autoxidative injury.

As autoxidative injury can manifest itself naturally as car-diovascular disease, leading ultimately to atherosclerosis, myocar-dial infarction and cerebrovascular accidents, and is also associated with diabetes, cataract, male sterility, nephrotoxicity, arthro-pathies, and malignancy, it is difficult to distinguish autoxidative-induced lesions from natural degenerative diseases. Autoxidative in-jury is therefore a particularly difficult form of chemical toxicity to detect and quantify, although all of its possible manifestations have been seen with various drugs and pesticides submitted for safety evaluation studies. In particular, many cytotoxic drugs, which act by promoting redox cycling, have long been known to manifest all of these toxic effects, together with several others, such as neurotoxicity and cardiotoxicity, which are probably the consequence of oxygen radical-induced acute lethal injury.

Table 1.9 Natural antioxidants protecting against active oxygen species

Reactive oxygen species		Antioxidants
Superoxide anion radical	$O_2^{-\bullet}$	Superoxide dismutases ascorbic acid reduced glutathione (GSH)
Hydrogen peroxide	H_2O_2	Catalase glutathione peroxidase
Hydroxyl radical	$\bullet OH$	Ascorbic acid polyunsaturated fatty acids methionine
Singlet oxygen	$^1O_2$	GSH α-tocopherol β-carotene polyunsaturated fatty acids histidine
Polyunsaturated fatty acid radicals	PUFA•	α-tocopherol β-carotene
Fatty acid hydroperoxides	ROOH	Glutathione peroxidase
Oxidized proteins	Pr-S-S-Pr	GSH
Oxidized glutathione	G-S-S-G	Glutathione reductase

In chronic inflammation, oxygen free radicals are released from invading leucocytes, resulting in lipid peroxidation, the release of arachidonate from phospholipids, and the excessive formation of the leukotrienes LTB_4 and LTC_4. Consequently, chemical toxicity mediated through the production of reactive intermediates, with the subsequent covalent binding to proteins and the formation of neoantigens, may result in immunological injury, leading to chronic inflammation, with the production of free radicals, and consequent autoxidative injury. The production of reactive oxygen radicals, and the manifestation of oxygen toxicity, is thus now recognized as a major mechanism of chemical toxicity and an important aspect of the toxicity of drugs and environmental chemicals.

For a comprehensive account of all aspects of oxygen toxicity, readers are referred to the works by Halliwell and Gutteridge[16], Balentine[17] and Yagi[18].

SPECIES AND GENETIC DIFFERENCES AND RISK ASSESSMENT

The major problem in the safety evaluation of chemicals for man is the great difficulty of extrapolating animal toxicity data for human risk assessment. Species differences in the routes and rates of metabolism, in the toxicokinetics of absorption, disposition and excretion, and in receptor concentration and receptor affinities, are the very fundamentals of selective toxicity, and the basis of the present ubiquitous application of drugs, pesticides and other selectively toxic chemicals for the benefit of man. Hence we are faced with the paradox that the fundamental basis for the use of these chemicals, namely their species differences in toxicity, constitutes the major obstacle in their safety evaluation from studies of toxicity in experimental animals. Even when the mechanism of toxicity is known and comparative metabolism, toxicokinetics and receptor studies have been undertaken, and suitable animal species selected as being appropriate models for man, one is confronted with genetic differences in toxicity in both laboratory animals and man, which has become one of the present major problems in the safety evaluation of chemicals. For experimental animals these genetic differences in toxicity, particularly rodent carcinogenicity, are often overcome by reference to historical pathological data, or by further studies in other species, but for human subjects such experimentation is not feasible.

For, unlike the inbred strains of rats and mice, man is genetically very heterogeneous, and a large enough population presents most of the variations in toxicity, metabolism etc., that one would see in a wide diversity of animal species. For this reason these xenobiotic chemicals ingested by man, such as drugs, pesticides and food additives, can never be absolutely safe and the degree of risk of toxic manifestations must be offset against the benefits to the individual and to society, by safety assessments. Indeed, the pharmacokinetics of most drugs show a twenty-fold variation or more in man, as evidenced by the wide individual differences in pharmacokinetic constants, plasma concentrations of the unchanged drug, plasma AUC values, etc. Because of this broad genetic heterogeneity of man, many genetic polymorphisms of the drug-metabolizing enzymes are known, including: (1) acetylations as in isoniazid toxicity; (2) hydrolysis of esters, as in suxamethonium toxicity; (3) activities of glucose-6-phosphate dehydrogenase, giving rise to methaemoglobinaemia and other toxic manifestations following the ingestion of various oxidants; and (4) cytochrome P-450 isoenzymes associated with polymorphic drug oxidations, and the consequent adverse reactions and toxicity of perhexiline, debrisoquine, mephenytoin, demethylimipramine, nor triptyline, sparteine, etc.[19].

Perhaps the most important aspect of species differences in chemical toxicity is attributable to the differences in the rates of oxidative metabolism, and differences in tissue oxygen uptake, which varies inversely with the body weight of the animal species concerned. The results of such a study with ^{14}C-aminopyrine are shown in Figure 1.9, and similar findings have been described for species differences in the rates of oxidative metabolism of caffeine[20]

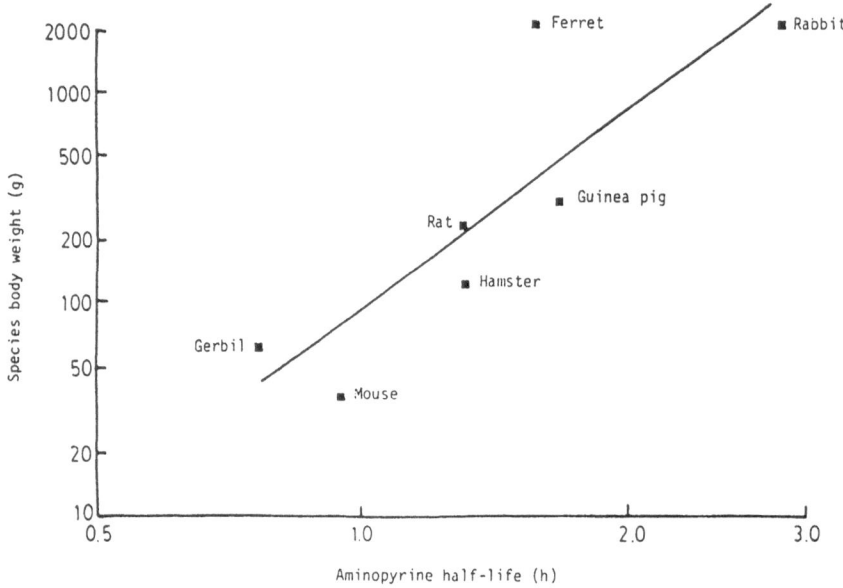

Figure 1.9 Dependence of aminopyrine oxidative metabolism on species body weight. The aminopyrine half-life determined in vivo by oxidative demethylation of ^{14}C-aminopyrine to $^{14}CO_2$ is shown to be inversely proportional to the body weight of the animal species studied

This is because basal metabolism and therefore tissue oxygen consumption, varies inversely with the size of the animal species, at least within the various species of mammalia. As oxygenation reactions are of paramount importance in the detoxication and activation of chemicals and the activation of oxygen to highly toxic free radical species can also be a major cause of chemical toxicity, this species difference in tissue oxygen uptake becomes fundamental to all safety evaluation procedures and is vital to risk assessment for human exposure to chemicals. Where the oxygenation procedure leads ultimately to detoxication, the chemical will be more rapidly and often more extensively, detoxicated in small rodents than in larger species such as dog and man (e.g. hexobarbitone to hydroxyhexobarbitone). Conversely, where the oxygenation procedure leads to activation and toxicity, small rodents may exhibit greater toxicity than dog or man. Similarly, where the chemical is volatile and may be cleared by exhalation unchanged or, alternatively, activated by oxidative metabolism, such as chloroform which is oxidatively metabolized to the toxic/tumorigenic carbonyl chloride and thence to CO_2, toxicity is directly related to oxidative metabolism and consequently occurs most extensively in small rodent species (see Table 1.10). An appreciation of these fundamentals by the toxicologists and regulatory agencies concerned would possibly have deterred some of them from considering chloroform to be potentially tumorigenic in man.

Table 1.10 Species differences in the rates of oxidative metabolism of chloroform and its dependence on body weight

Species	Body wt. (g)	% dose excreted in 2 days as		
		$^{14}CO_2$	$^{14}CHCl_3$	Total recovered %
Mouse CBA	20-30	76±5	7±2	83
C57	20-30	79	5	84
CF/LP		76	6	82
Rat (Sprague-Dawley)	200-300	66±4	20±5	86
Monkey (Squirrel)	500-1000	18±2	79±3	97

Dose of chloroform was 60 mg/kg (from ref. 24)

This species difference in oxygen uptake becomes even more important, where more than one oxygenation is involved in the metabolism of the chemicals and where oxygen activation by redox cycling occurs, as with bleomycin and other quinonoid cytotoxic drugs. Similarly, in the toxicity and tumorigenicity of benzene, several oxygenations and oxidations occur, resulting in both detoxication and activation, although the ultimate mechanism of toxicity and tumorigenicity probably involves the generation of hydroxyl radicals from redox cycling of the semi-quinones of ortho- and para-benzoquinones (see Figure 1.10). These marked species differences in oxygen metabolism, in the oxidative detoxication/activation of chemicals, and in oxygen toxicity, further illustrate the uniqueness of man, and the difficulties in making human risk assessments of chemicals from toxicological studies in experimental animals. Only by the most detailed consideration of the scientific principles involved can these inherent difficulties be surmounted.

$$C_6H_6 + \overset{\cdot}{O}_2 + NADPH_2 \longrightarrow C_6H_5OH + H_2O + NADP$$

$$\text{rate of reaction} = k_1 \, [C_6H_6] \, [O_2]^{1.5}$$

$$C_6H_5OH + O_2 + NADPH_2 \longrightarrow C_6H_4(OH)_2 + H_2O + NADP$$

$$\text{rate of reaction} = k_2 \, [C_6H_6] \, [O_2]^{3}$$

$$C_6H_5(OH_2) \longrightarrow C_6H_4{\overset{\text{O}}{{<}}}_{\text{O}} \xrightarrow{e} C_6H_4{\overset{\text{O}^-}{{<}}}_{\text{O}^\cdot} \xrightarrow[\text{redox cycling}]{O_2} O_2^{-\cdot}$$

$$\text{rate of reaction} = k_3 \, [C_6H_6] \, [O_2]^{\infty}$$

Figure 1.10 Dependence of the toxicity and metabolism of benzene on tissue oxygen. In the redox cycling of benzoquinone the generation of reactive oxygen is more dependent on tissue oxygen concentration than on the concentration of benzene

REFERENCES

1. Gould, BJ, Amoah, AGB and Parke, DV (1986). Stereoselective pharmacokinetics of perhexiline. Xenobiotica, 16, 491-502
2. Pessayre, D, Dolder, A and Artigou, J-V (1979). Effect of fasting on metabolite-mediated hepatotoxicity in the rat. Gastroenterology, 77, 264-71
3. Gibson, GG and Skett, P (1986). Introduction to Drug Metabolism. (London: Chapman & Hall)
4. Iveson, P, Lindup, WE, Parke, DV and Williams, RT (1971). The metabolism of carbenoxolone in the rat. Xenobiotica, 1, 79-95
5. Bickel, MH and Muehlebach, S (1980). Pharmacokinetics and ecodisposition of polyhalogenated hydrocarbons: aspects and concepts. Drug Metab Rev, 11, 149-90
6. Elfarra, AA, Jakobson, I and Anders, MW (1986). Mechanism of S-(1,2-dichlorovinyl)glutathione-induced nephrotoxicity. Biochem Pharmacol, 35, 283-8
7. Guengerich, FP and Liebler, DC (1985). Enzymatic activation of chemicals to toxic metabolites, CRC Crit Rev Toxicol, 14, 259-307
8. Parke, DV (1986). Activation mechanisms to chemical toxicity. Arch Toxicol, (In press)

9.   Ioannides, C, Lum, PY and Parke, DV (1984). Cytochrome P-448 and the activation of toxic chemicals and carcinogens. Xenobiotica, 14, 119-38

10.   Lewis, DFV, Ioannides, C and Parke, DV (1986). Molecular dimensions of the substrate binding site of cytochrome P-448. Biochem Pharmacol, 35, 2179-85

11.   Parke, DV (1985). The role of cytochrome P-450 in the metabolism of pollutants. Marine Environ Res, 17, 97-101

12.   Guengerich, FP, Distlerath, LM, Reilly, PEB, Wolff, T, Shimada, T, Umbenhauer, DR and Martin, MV (1986). Human-liver cytochromes P-450 involved in polymorphisms of drug oxidation. Xenobiotica, 16, 367-78

13.   Levy, RH and Bauer, CA (1986). Basic pharmacokinetics. Therapeutic Drug Monitoring, 8, 47-58

14.   Dietz, FK, Stott, WT and Ramsey, JC (1982). Non-linear pharmacokinetics and their impact on toxicology: Illustrated with dioxane. Drug Metab Rev, 13, 963-81

15.   Nau, H (1985). Improvement of testing for teratogenicity by pharmacokinetics. In Homburger, F (ed.), Concepts in Toxicology, pp. 130-137. (Basel: Karger)

16.   Halliwell, B and Gutteridge, JMC (1985). Free Radicals in Biology and Medicine. (Oxford: Clarendon Press)

17.   Balentine, JD (1985). Pathology of Oxygen Toxicity. (New York: Academic Press)

19.   Franklin, RA and Parke, DV (1986). Human genetic variations in oxidative drug metabolism. Xenobiotica, 16, 359-509

18.   Yagi, K (1982). Lipid Peroxides in Biology and Medicine. (New York: Academic Press)

20.   Bonati, M, Latini, R, Tognoni, G, Young, JF and Garattini, S (1984-85). Interspecies comparison of in vivo caffeine pharmacokinetics in man, monkey, rabbit, rat and mouse. Drug Metab Rev, 15, 1355-83

21.   Kociba, RJ and Schwetz, BA (1982). Toxicity of 2,3,7,8-tetrachlorodibenzo-p-dioxin (TCDD). Drug Metab Rev, 13, 387-406

22.   Clark, B, Smith, DA, Eason, CT and Parke, DV (1982). Metabolism and excretion of a chromone carboxylic acid (FPL 52757) in various animal species. Xenobiotica, 12, 147-53

23.   Clarke, AJ, Clark, B, Eason, CT and Parke, DV (1985). An assessment of a toxicological incident in a drug development program and its implications. Reg Toxicol Pharmacol, 5, 109-19

24.   Brown, DM, Langley, PF, Smith, D and Taylor, DC (1974). Metabolism of chloroform - I. The metabolism of ^{14}C-chloroform by different species. Xenobiotica, 4, 151-63

FURTHER READING

Albert, A (1985). Selective Toxicity: The Physico-chemical Basis of Therapy, 7th edition. (London and New York: Chapman & Hall)

Gibaldi, M and Perrier, D (1982). Pharmacokinetics, 2nd edn. (New York: Marcel Dekker)

Guengerich, FP and Liebler, DC (1985). Enzymatic activation of chemicals to toxic metabolites, CRC Crit Rev Toxicol, 14, 259-307

Hathway, DE (1984). Molecular Aspects of Toxicology. (London: The Royal Society of Chemistry)

Jenner, P and Testa, B (1980). Concepts in Drug Metabolism, Parts A and B. (New York: Dekker)

Jordan, VC (1984). Biochemical pharmacology of anti-oestrogen action. Pharmacol Rev, 36, 245-75

Mason, RP (ed.) (1985). Monograph on free radical metabolites of toxic chemicals. Environ Health Perspect, 64, 1-342

Mitchell, JR and Horning, MG (1984). Drug Metabolism and Drug Toxicity. (New York: Raven)

Parke, DV (1984). Development of detoxication mechanisms in the neonate. In: Kacew, S and Reasor, MJ (eds), Toxicology and the Newborn, pp. 1-31. (Amsterdam: Elsevier)

Parke, DV and Ioannides, C (1981). The role of nutrition in toxicology. Ann Rev Nutr, 1, 207-34

Ruckpaul, K and Rein, H (1984). Cytochrome P-450. (Berlin: Akademie-Verlag)

PART 2
Preclinical:
in Vivo and Combined Approaches

2

The Organization of Preclinical and Premarketing Toxicity Testing

A. N. WORDEN

As indicated elsewhere in this book[1], the first substantial official or quasi-official pronouncement on the conduct and interpretation of toxicity tests - of the kind relevant to safety evaluation - was made in 1955 by the staff of the US Food and Drug Administration[2]. With the thalidomide episode, legislation and codes of practice were introduced into or expanded by many countries, with in many instances the issue of guidelines for the type of testing regarded as necessary.

Fortunately the scientific judgement of the individual toxicologist has not been entirely discounted by the increased trend towards formal testing procedures. Nevertheless there has been expectation of the presentation to the regulatory authority of a basal package of tests. The quasi-routine nature of toxicity tests was not diminished by the introduction of Good Laboratory Practice, which has done much to improve the quality or checking of the conduct of test procedures - but not of its "science"[3].

The pattern of testing anticipated by the regulatory authorities has not been the same for different categories of material or compound. In the UK, for example, there are separate authorities, and differing requirements, for medicines or drugs[4], food additives[5], pesticides and other agricultural chemicals[6] and industrial chemicals[7], and until recently some of these involved voluntary as distinct from statutory notification. It is of interest that the use of an "expert" system, in vogue in France for some years[8], was applied in another form in the UK in 1983 to the Clinical Trial Exemption Certificate procedure[9] and - more recently - to all submissions involving medicines, which include a summary appraisal of the pharmacological and toxicological data[10]. In this respect the UK became the first country to adopt the recommendations that followed from the European Community (EC) Directive 75/319, which established a Committee on Proprietary Medicinal Products. Under the same directive the Committee established in 1977 a working party to produce guidelines on the various aspects of the preclinical safety evaluation of medicinal products.

Toxicity tests, whether for submission to regulatory

41

authorities or not, were at first conducted by those who had developed the new compound, or by their colleagues within the same academic institution or manufacturing company. Shortly after World War II some existing independent laboratories, and others formed for the purpose, undertook contract testing. These included the Food and Drug Research Laboratories in New York, the Hazleton Laboratories in Virginia, Industrial BioTest in Illinois, what is now the Bio-Research Division of CDC Life Sciences in Canada and the Huntingdon Research Centre in England. Such organizations undertook to conduct the various animal toxicity tests and some others of the required preclinical or premarketing studies. Their independence was an advantage in the preparation of reports and in dealings with the regulatory authorities, while their relevant experience rapidly surpassed that of even the largest academic or commercial "in-house" facility. Moreover their use was, in most instances, more economical than the provision of staff and of laboratory space by the sponsor. A pharmaceutical company, for example, would need to set aside considerable space - with accompanying staff - that otherwise would have been allocated to the more basic aspects of research and development.

The trend towards use of contract laboratories developed rapidly. When the writer first visited the United States in 1960 there were in existence the contract houses of any size already indicated, and a few smaller organizations that offered to undertake one or more aspects of the studies required in connection with registration. By 1969 there were no fewer than 114 laboratories on the North American continent alone. Many of these were ill-equipped and inadequately staffed. Unfortunately, there was a temptation even to some well-established contract houses to react to this increasing competition by indulging in a price war - with the almost inevitable consequence that standards would also be lowered. By the mid-1970s one of the established houses was deemed to be guilty of serious errors in the conduct and reporting of toxicity studies, many of which had to be repeated elsewhere at great expense and with considerable loss of time.

The writer visited the contract house concerned a week after officials of the US Food and Drug Administration had made their memorable inspection: he was rapidly convinced that, whatever sins of commission might or might not have been committed, there had been ample scope for many of omission.

At about the same time there were serious questions asked by the US Food and Drug Administration of another established contract house that had conducted toxicity studies for a pharmaceutical company, while a small independent group was found to have reported the results of clinical trials that had apparently never been carried out.

The impact of these unfortunate happenings was considerable. Soon afterwards the Food and Drug Administration established the requirements of Good Laboratory Practice[3], with an inspectorate, while some of the larger pharmaceutical and chemical corporations established or re-created extensive "in-house" facilities.

Within a few years, however, the better contract houses, which had in any event avoided the temptation to lower standards, recovered their momentum and by the mid-1980s they had largely regained their share of the total market. This market is indeed expanding.

The degree to which contract organizations will participate in future may to a degree depend upon the modification of existing test procedures and their supplementation with - or, as many would wish, replacement of - animal models by in vitro procedures. The likely pattern of change has been indicated at the meetings held at the Royal Society in November 1982 to discuss the FRAME Toxicity Committee report[11] and in the chapter in this work on long-term tests. At present, the most sensible forecast would seem to consist of a combination of refined and sophisticated tests on animals with so-called "alternatives" being used as adjunct measures and in their own right - and with early and more extensive use of man himself.

The potential geographical markets for which a new compound or material is intended has hitherto influenced the scope of toxicity testing. In the case of medicines or drugs, the guidelines from different national regulatory authorities have often shown variations. Griffin[12] has compared the guidelines on preclinical safety evaluation of medicinal products of the EC, the Nordic countries and Japan, concluding that the EC and Nordic guidelines, while not differing markedly from the Japanese, have the clear advantage over the latter in their flexibility and their requirement for somewhat fewer animals: they also render it possible to get therapeutically important drugs into man more expeditiously.

The future pattern of toxicity testing should most certainly include flexibility[13,14], always provided that this is combined with an informed scientific approach and with quality assurance procedures. It should always be possible to discuss a toxicity programme with the relevant regulatory authorities, either in advance or at an early stage of the conduct of the actual test procedures. This has not always proved feasible, although during the early 1960s it was a straightforward matter - at least for the head of a contract house - to hold detailed discussions with the then Director of Pharmacology at the US Food and Drug Administration[15], not only prior to definitive toxicity studies but also during their progress - a happy situation that altered considerably with the internal reconstruction of the relevant FDA bureaux and with the growing vulnerability of physicians, scientists, regulators and commercial houses to legal prosecution. There were also opportunities for informal discussions with the medical advisers to - and even with the Chairman himself of - the UK Committee on Safety of Drugs, set up after the thalidomide episode, but the situation tended to change with the implementation of the 1968 Medicines Act[15].

As is made evident elsewhere in this book, safety evaluation requires far more than an assessment of the inherent toxicity of a substance. It is the **circumstances** in which a given substance could prove toxic - or carcinogenic, or teratogenic - that need to be assessed or predicted. This makes it all the more important that the design, conduct, interim results, positive findings and evaluation of a toxicity study should be subject to collective assessment involving not only the scientists - and in appropriate instances clinicians or engineers from the fields of application - but also the regulators and their advisers. Conning[14], in his summary of papers presented at the Royal Society meetings[1], referred to:

> the difficulty of achieving specialist contribution, when a regulatory system is designed to be administered by those untutored in toxicology (and in some countries untutored in science). On the other hand it is quite clear that many industrial concerns, which need regulatory clearance in order to market their products, are anxious to provide the information that the system demands rather than the information that the science requires.

Parke[16] has cited excellent examples of substances for which appraisal before and during the course of toxicity studies would have been likely to eliminate unnecessary work and also to focus attention upon findings of practical significance - the nonsteroidal anti-inflammatory drug benoxaprofen being one such case[17].

Refinement of animal - and of in vitro - models will almost certainly require the specific input of those who, whether in academia or attached to a commercial house, have been responsible for the design and early pharmacological and biochemical assessment of the test substance. Always provided that problems associated with confidentiality may be overcome, as indeed they should be with a rational and honest regulatory body and suitable legal protection, the proper plan is for these scientists to meet with those of the regulatory bodies at the outset of toxicity testing; and to take independent advice. There are, as already indicated, clear advantages in having the definitive testing conducted by a contract organization, with its wealth of general background experience to add to the specific information possessed by the developers. Consultations with clinicians, engineers or others concerned with potential application of the candidate substance should also be feasible from the earliest possible stage if evaluation of safety in practice is to be attempted.

The organization of safety assessment should entail not only prospective but also retrospective studies. In the case of medicines or drugs, the interim and final results of clinical trials should be made available to the toxicologist, as should those from whatever form of postmarketing appraisal may be forthcoming. With non-therapeutic compounds there is a similar need for information at comparable stages, e.g. from field trials, residue studies, stability, the nature of degradation products, contamination, pollution and distribution following application or release into the environment. It is regrettable that concern for certain aspects of environmental safety should appear to have to rely upon the outbursts, demonstrations and sometimes alarmist publications of fringe groups, pressure groups and perhaps those who seek to gain politically or otherwise from "joining the bandwagon".

At the Royal Society meetings[11,15], Dr John Griffin and other then members of regulatory bodies who were present affirmed their wish to provide guidance on toxicity studies. This is an important step, to be consolidated or reinstituted in as many countries as possible; but only a first step. Toxicity studies need not only to be planned but also to be assessed during as well as after completion for them to take their rightful place in safety evaluation. This would be expected to result not only in more satisfactory and relevant test procedures but also in a shortening of the often inordinate amount of time taken from the emergence of a candidate substance and its eventual marketing[18].

ADDENDUM

Professor Dennis Parke has commented as follows:

It should be mentioned that pathological diagnoses should not be made only from examination of slides of histological sections. This is very important, and has caused a great deal of problems in a number of pharmaceutical companies within the last year or two.

Many pharmaceutical companies, in carrying out their chronic toxicity studies, keep the animals in one laboratory, kill them in another, have the tissues prepared commercially, and finally, have the sections examined by veterinarians and human pathologists working privately at home. In some cases the four aspects have been carried out in different countries! This practice has been shown to be quite unreliable and has been discouraged by the regulatory bodies.

The companies themselves have often come into grave difficulties when the histopathologists examining the final sections have made diagnoses, instead of merely recording their observations. Several companies have recently issued directives that diagnoses will be made only when all the pathology reports (postmortem, histopathology, clinical chemistry, haematology, etc.) are to hand, and can be considered collectively.

This matter is of considerable importance and should be mentioned in this chapter, as it is one that I continue to encounter frequently, as a member of various regulatory bodies, and one that can be very costly to any company involved.

REFERENCES

1. Worden AN (1986). The evidence supporting 6-month studies. In Walker SR and Dayan AD (eds) Long-term Animal Studies: their Predictive Value for Man. (Lancaster: MTP Press), pp. 83-86
2. Association of Food and Drug Officials of the United States (1955). Appraisal of the Safety of Chemicals in Foods, Drugs and Cosmetics. (Topeka, Kansas: Association of Food and Drug Officials of the United States, PO Box 1494)
3. Paget GE (ed) (1977). Quality Control in Toxicology. (Lancaster: MTP Press)
4. Medicines Act 1968, Chapter 67. ISBN 0-10-546768 5. (London: HMSO); see also Medicines Act Leaflets, (London: DHSS Medicines Division, Market Towers, 1 Nine Elms Lane, London SW8 5NQ)

5. Department of Health and Social Security (1986). Guidance on the Preparation of Data on Chemicals in Foods, Consumer Products and the Environment Submitted to the DHSS. Report on Health and Social Services, 30. (London: HMSO)
6. Data Requirements for Approval under the Control of Pesticides Regulations (1986). (London: MAFF) October.
7. Notification of New Substances Regulations 1982 (SI 1982 No 1496); (1981). See also Notification of new substances: Draft regulations and approved codes of practice, Health and Safety Commission Consultative Document. ISBN 0-11-883420 7. (London: HMSO)
8. Arrêté du 21 fevrier 1980 portant agrément d'experts analysts, pharmacologues-toxicologues et cliniciens pour les essais des spécialités pharmaceutiques (1980). Bulletin Officiel du Ministère de la Santé et de la Sécurité Sociale, Fasc. 80/10, Texts 18193-18228, 5 April.
9. See relevant Medicines Act Leaflets, cited in reference 4
10. Commission of the European Communities Council Directive 83/570/EEC (1985). See Notice to Applicants for Marketing Authorization for Proprietary Medicinal Products in the Member States of the European Community on the Use of the New Multistate Procedure. (Brussels: Directorate-General for Internal Marketing and Industrial Affairs, Communour of the European Committee, rue de la Loi 200, B-1049), July
11. Balls M, Riddell RJ and Worden AN (eds) (1983). Animals and Alternatives in Toxicity Testing. (London: Academic Press)
12. Griffin JP (1985). A comparison between guidelines on preclinical safety evaluation of medicinal products of the European Community, the Nordic countries, and Japan. ATLA, 13, 53-63
13. Cockburn A (1983). The need for flexibility. In Balls M et al. (eds). Animals and Alternatives in Toxicity Testing. (London: Academic Press), pp. 457-9
14. Conning DM (1983). Rapporteur on General Discussion on Regulations. In Balls M et al. (eds) Animals and Alternatives in Toxicity Testing. (London: Academic Press), pp. 467-9
15. Worden AN (1983). Consultation with the regulatory authorities. In Balls M et al. (eds) Animals and Alternatives in Toxicity Testing. (London: Academic Press), pp. 459-61 (ref. 11)
16. Parkes DVW (1983). Regulatory aspects. In Balls M et al. (eds) Animals and Alternatives in Toxicity Testing. (London: Academic Press), pp. 445-56
17. Chatfield DH and Green JN (1978). Disposition and metabolism of benoxaprofen in laboratory animals and man. Xenobiotica, 8, 133-44
18. Wardell WM (1978). The drug lag revisited: comparison by therapeutic area of patterns of drugs marketed in the United States and Great Britain from 1972 through 1976. Clin Pharmacol Ther, 24, 499-594

3

Animal Models of Responses Resulting from Short-term Exposures

V. K. BROWN

Predictive safety evaluation for all classes and all types of products is a recognized requirement on an international scale[1]. In devising predictive tests for short-term exposure investigations in toxicology, the problem of mimicking the infinite complexity of physiological systems has led to the simplistic acceptance that animal models can provide answers to questions that relate the interactive ability of chemical moieties to various physiological systems. The apparent success of this approach has led to the development of a very pragmatic attitude in relation to the needs of predictive tests for short-term exposure toxicology. Pragmatism is not wholly unacceptable as an approach to the problems of safety evaluation, but it is essential that responsible investigators have access to all available knowledge and experience in respect of the ways in which any product that is being tested will be used in practice, in order to avoid pseudo-respectable testing procedures that may be inappropriate[2].

It is convenient, and permissible, to consider short-term exposure in toxicology as being divisible into two categories. Firstly those situations in which the toxicant has a direct effect on one or more tissues, and secondly those in which the toxicant exhibits indirect (systemic) effects following absorption. The distinction between these two categories is not always rigorous and the two types of response may both occur with some toxicants.

Information derived from predictive short-term toxicity tests may be used to foretell the hazard rating of a product in situations of deliberate, adventitious or accidental exposure. Although the information from these tests may play a significant role in risk-benefit assessment it would be wrong to expect a simple relationship between actual risk and the experimental data because of the multiplicity of confounding factors that exist to affect the possible toxicology of any product. Too often those scientists responsible for generating data in predictive short-term exposure toxicology have been distanced from the application of their findings to real, as opposed to experimental, exposure situations. The need for the provision of predictive data in succinct form rather than in detailed discussive documentary format has often led to excessive reliance on numeric indices rather than more meaningful descriptive toxicological assessments.

There is a common misconception that predictive testing will somehow make a product safe. No amount of testing can protect against the follies of "human error" or even genuine accidents. The problems of relative risk are an integral part of life, and predictive toxicology testing can only contribute usefully to the relative risk assessment when the investigations are treated as being a serious scientific discipline and not relegated to the position of being "cheap and nasty" tests to be carried out by rote solely to achieve some numeric categorization.

Any consideration of the role of animal models in this area of predictive testing inevitably poses the ethical dilemma associated with health and safety in man, and occasionally other selected animals, versus the use of sentient species for investigative purposes. It is not the purpose of this paper to provide a discussion of the totality of the ethical and moral considerations that are involved in the use of living animals for experimental purposes. This contribution is presented from the viewpoint held by many toxicologists, and others, that tests that involve the use of sentient animals should be performed only when unequivocal justification can be demonstrated because no meaningful alternative is available. This contribution is addressing the real situation that products are, and will continue to be, developed, and does not seek to debate the issue of justification for all new products.

Just as there is a need for awareness of ethical factors in relation to the use of sentient sub-human species in predictive toxicology it is essential to be aware of the ethical and legal aspects of human exposure both in relation to deliberate investigative toxicology and also in relation to overall health and safety[3]. Although there are many guidelines and precedents for the testing of therapeutic agents in man (i.e. clinical trials) it is much more difficult to justify the deliberate exposure of people to other classes of chemicals for the intention of toxicological assessment. The problems associated with "informed consent" and "volunteer" are extremely inhibitory to experimental toxicologists, and some practices, such as encouraging members of the long-term prison population to volunteer (often with inducements), have largely disappeared. It must be made clear that some of these human exposure tests have always been prohibited in some countries. The principles underlying human experimentation of this type are clearly formulated in the Declaration of Helsinki.

Considering first the testing for direct toxic effects on tissues it is immediately apparent that it will be the skin, eyes and linings of the alimentary canal, respiratory tract and vagina that are most at risk. The corrosive and irritant properties of many products are well known, and it may be acceptable to avoid contact without the necessity for predictive in vivo testing to demonstrate the obvious. Corrosivity and irritancy may be markedly influenced by the nature of the exposure, and it may be necessary to carry out tests to investigate and establish what factors influence the rating. Clearly it would be much easier if products were either irritant or non-irritant, but it is the breadth of difference between the extremes that may be most important.

Taking the apparently most simple case of skin irritancy as an example: in order to provide a meaningful grading of the skin irritancy potential of any weakly or moderately irritant product in human volunteers it is necessary to use a large test population. Although it is correct to refer to the skin as an organ it is a remarkably variable entity; there is not only a major difference between the skins of different species but there can be major differences in sensitivity between individuals within a species, and very important differences in sensitivity between different anatomical locations within any individual. The value of skin irritancy testing that necessitates extrapolation of data from one species to another must be questioned.

Despite a very large amount of research into models of skin irritancy there has been little progress towards finding an acceptable alternative to the method initiated by Draize et al.[4] some 40 years ago. Perhaps the one factor in favour of the Draize test method is that it tends to over-emphasize the irritancy potential and hence errs on the side of safety. However, the method has been much criticized on numerous counts by experienced toxicologists and by dermatologists over the years[5].

Although there have been numerous other in vivo animal-based tests for skin irritancy none has proved more meaningful or useful, in general terms, than the test attributed to Draize. It may be argued that if the Draize test is restricted to screening for severe irritancy only, and is not used as though it is capable of providing data for ranking materials of low irritancy potential, then there may be some justification for the test being carried out, and the number of animals needed for a test may be minimized by performing the investigation sequentially (i.e. if the product is corrosive to the skin of one rabbit there is no justification for using more).

The Draize test[4] requires the exposure of the skin to the test product to be inside an occlusive dressing. With many products this use of an occluded site greatly enhances irritancy, and some products that might not be particularly irritant in normal use may appear to be very irritant indeed. If it is accepted that predictive testing for skin irritancy by the use of animals in vivo is justified then the test programme should be extended to include both occluded and non-occluded exposures.

It is unlikely that any chemical that exerts strongly irritant characteristics when applied to the skin will not be irritant to mucosa, but the converse is not the case. It has been accepted by some investigators and regulatory agencies that if a product is severely irritant to the skin it may be presumed to be irritant to the eyes, and no specific in vivo eye irritancy should be carried out. This is an excellent assumption on humane grounds but in reality the correlation between skin irritancy and eye irritancy is not very good.

Despite the obvious differences between the eyes of rabbits and human eyes the in vivo test method using groups of rabbits attributable to Draize[4] has remained the most commonly used predictive test. The Draize test[4] has been susceptible to various modifications, such as the use of ophthalmological instrumentation for assessing the effects of the product on the various parts of the eye, and the use of statistical refinement to the quantitative data obtained, but even so the test does not attract a lot of favourable comment[6].

Irritancy testing for the various mucosae may be carried out on any of a range of species. For some products the potential for irritancy to the mucosae is detected during investigations for other aspects of the short-term exposure (e.g. examination of the respiratory tract from animals used in inhalation experiments). With the development of pharmaceutical products that are intended for close contact with the various surfaces (e.g. vaginal pessaries) it is necessary to carry out specific irritancy tests, and many things are already known about the importance of pH values in this context.

There is no doubt that the total number of animals used for predictive short-term exposure toxicology can be reduced without serious loss of scientific integrity, but it is in the area of direct toxic effects on cells and tissues that the possiblity of achieving in vitro alternatives seems most plausible. In the current state of knowledge it is accepted that such important factors as inter-species and individual variabilities make in vivo predictive testing less than satisfactory, but so far, despite a large amount of re-search, the success rate in finding meaningful in vitro alternatives has been very limited. Although there has been an increased im-petus into research to develop alternative testing procedures for skin, eye and mucosa irritancy only partial alternatives are yet available.

Systemic effects resulting from absorption of chemicals follow-ing short-term exposure may be manifested in many different ways. Although the exposure is only acute or subacute the ensuing response may exhibit a rapid or a delayed onset and the effect may be transient, prolonged or even irreversible.

The magnitude of the exposure is generally critical to the toxicological importance of the sequalae. Sometimes replicated ex-posure to a product may be more harmful than a single exposure to a relatively larger amount of the same product, but this is not al-ways the case and the development of tolerance is also well known. These two possibilites are a major justification for predictive test-ing, including not only acute but subacute exposures.

In addition to the importance of the magnitude of any ex-posure the toxicological characteristics of any product are in-fluenced by the route by which the exposure occurs, and this may be greatly influenced by the physical presentation of the product to the target[2]. Ideally any model used to predict the response that will result from acute or subacute exposure to a product has to be capable of providing information on an infinite number of variables, and for this reason the in vivo animal model has enjoyed popularity with investigators; too often there is an over-simplistic assumption that physiological comparability is better than it really is.

For any short-term exposure investigation to be meaningful it is necessary to review the toxicokinetics and the toxicodynamics of the test product in the relevant species, and then to relate these findings to comparable data for humans. In this situation there is clearly a non-sequitur, for if the information on the toxicokinetics and the toxicodynamics in humans were available, the need for predictive testing in laboratory animals would disappear. Where information about the fate of a product in exposed humans exists the justification for additional laboratory animal investigation requires critical review.

Choice of animal species for use as in vivo models in predictive acute and subacute toxicology is more often governed by expediency than by scientific rationale. The majority of products are screened for their toxicological effects in rodents, particularly rats and mice, with scant effort being made to relate the fate and distribution of the test product in these species to the toxicokinetics and toxicodynamics in man. The ease with which rodents can be bred and maintained in laboratories has fuelled a preoccupation with quantification of toxic response[7]. Toxicometrics has developed at the expense of more detailed studies into the underlying biological significance of the toxicological interactions in the actual target species. This conflict of priorities is less apparent with pharmaceutical products because of the work of the clinical pharmacologists than it is with products that are not intended for deliberate human contact (e.g. many industrial chemicals); between these two extremes lie such products as pesticides and food additives, with the inevitability of human exposure.

It is apparent that acquiring a simple numeric index of acute toxicity and a derived index of subacute toxicity has become the prime objective for many investigators[8]. This objective has been encouraged by regulatory authorities, and it is necessary to establish the role of such indices as useful ancillary tools only. Too often it is assumed that indices, most often the LD_{50} values, are an adequate substitute for proper investigative toxicology[7,8]. This is not a condemnation of the concept of the LD_{50} value but a developing awareness that it is necessary to accept constraints on the desire for quantification; removal of the uncritical demand for LD_{50} values will lead to a reduction in the numbers of animals used in short-term exposure toxicology with no concomitant diminution in the usefulness of the information obtained, and hopefully, there may be an actual improvement in the meaningfulness of the data[7].

Any contemplation of the acute or subacute toxicology of a product must take into account peripheral influences, and this may profoundly influence predictive testing. For example many of the polymeric materials used in buildings, furniture, packaging, etc., are almost non-toxic unless they become hot, when pyrolysis can lead to highly toxic by-products. Conversely some highly toxic chemicals (e.g. some pesticides) can be formulated in such a way that the toxicity potential to non-target species is greatly diminished[9].

Many of the recent advances in therapeutics can be attributed to the techniques associated with getting the actual pharmacological molecule to the target within the patient. This awareness of pharmacokinetic manoeuvrability emphasizes the need for more attention to toxicokinetics in acute and subacute investigative toxicology. This point may be illustrated by reference to glyceryl trinitrate, a drug that has been in use for more than a century. Glyceryl trinitrate is broken down in the stomach, and is generally poorly absorbed if swallowed; hence in a conventional acute toxicity test in which the product is administered either by intragastric intubation or in encapsulated form, the acute toxicity rating would be very different from that experienced if the glyceryl trinitrate is absorbed in the buccal cavity (i.e. an absorption area not generally included in predictive acute toxicity tests). Now, to avoid the effects of gastric contents, there are therapeutic formulations of the compound that protect it from breakdown and allow efficient absorption from the gut[10]. Similarly controlled slow-release transdermal patches have been developed for glyceryl trinitrate for therapeutic application, whereas the acute percutaneous toxicity of the chemical administered in a conventional acute percutaneous toxicity test might have indicated that this route should be avoided[10].

Outside the reasonably well-defined needs for predictive acute and subacute toxicity testing for drugs and pesticides there are many other classes of chemicals for which predictive testing is required. Some of these products possess a high potential for acute toxic hazard, but in practice are associated with remarkably few incidents of acute intoxication. This apparent success is sometimes used as a justification for the pragmatic approach to predictive acute toxicology which justifies that importance shall be attributed to the use of indices based on data such as LD_{50} values, in isolation, for classification purposes; certainly this very basic approach to acute toxicology has the attractions of cheapness, ease and convenience but may be held to be lacking in scientific foundation and has been criticized on the basis of the ethics of living animal experimentation[8].

Few people would dispute that in the current state of knowledge the actual alternatives to the use of living animals for predictive acute toxicology are inadequate. This does not imply that the conventional test methods with the use of animals are always justified, and it is imperative that the objectives of the testing procedures that are in current use must be reviewed critically as an ongoing process and revised in the light of appropriate experience. The idea that any species can be used to mimic exactly the toxicological interactions that may occur in another species must be abandoned, and the pattern of events following short-term exposure to a product must be recognized as being functions of multi-compartmental processes which can vary considerably between species and even between individuals within a species. Sex-related differences in sensitivity to acute intoxication may not be common to all species for some products, and the differences in sensitivity that may be exhibited by different strains of the same species to particular classes of chemicals are further manifestations of the pitfalls that are associated with the extrapolation of toxicological findings[2].

The nature of acute intoxication may be profoundly influenced by the magnitude of the exposure. This is often most apparent with drugs where therapeutic dose levels produce a desired therapeutic effect but larger doses may produce quite different toxicological responses[11]. The same principle applies with other classes of chemicals where large exposures may affect receptor sites that are not apparently affected at lower exposure levels.

It must be emphasized that predictive acute toxicology investigations are not concerned solely with lethality, but rather with any adverse effects that may result from exposure to a product; sometimes it is found that subacute experiments are more revealing in terms of subtle toxic effects.

A major shortcoming of all predictive acute toxicity testing, whether carried out in vivo with laboratory animals or in vitro, is the inability to reveal symptoms of intoxication. The advantage of the in vivo methodology is the exhibition of signs of intoxication, whereas the in vitro techniques are not even able to reveal the most basic signs. Sometimes it is possible to speculate on the importance of in vitro changes in terms of the symptomatology; for example some in vitro experiments may indicate the ability of the toxicant to cause neuropathies and the investigator may, with limited confidence, anticipate that this is indicative of an ability to cause locomotor effects in the living target animal[12]. This level of speculation is not really satisfactory unless there are more supportive data[13].

Arguably the single most confounding factor in the whole of the imprecise science of predictive short-term exposure toxicology is the idiosyncratic response. However much may be known about the toxicology of any product there is always the possibility that a proportion of any exposed population will respond in an idiosyncratic way. Pharmacologically dramatic, sometimes fatal, responses occur among people exposed to remarkably small quantities of some chemicals, and this is generally associated with having been exposed to the same chemical on one or more previous occasions. This form of response is an immunological phenomenon, and occasionally cross-sensitization may occur between chemicals with certain molecular commonality in their structures. Apart from idiosyncratic systemic effects it is a common problem in dermatotoxicology that the skin may also become sensitized to many disparate chemical types. Although there is some recognition of the molecular characteristics most commonly associated with idiosyncratic effects it is still very difficult to assess the likelihood of a novel molecule creating clinical problems in predictive terms[14].

Quite apart from immuno-idiosyncratic influences it is essential to recognize that individual susceptibility to intoxication will be affected by other factors associated with the health status and pathophysiology of the individual. In the laboratory the essence of the investigative methodology depends on minimizing extraneous factors. For example the health status of laboratory animals may be controlled, to a considerable extent, by the use of appropriate husbandry. The use of specified pathogen-free (SPF) animals, the minimization of exposure to undefined secondary exposures by the use of carefully controlled diets and ambient atmospheres, put together with the use of controlled inbred or controlled outbred strains of laboratory animals help to refine the model and aid interpretation of findings. A move away from the simple alive or dead head-count approach to acute toxicology with more use of toxicokinetic measurements and selective detailed necropsies can refine the model even further.

No individual, including laboratory animals kept in near-optimal conditions, is ever exposed to only one type of chemical.

There is always the possibility of toxicological interaction, and it is common practice to ignore many of these effects until some obvious resultant difference renders the toxic effect apparent to the observer. Toxicologically important interactions sometimes occur as a result of the multiplicity of different drugs administered to some patients[15] and it is well known that toxicological interactions may occur between the therapeutic agent being used to treat a patient and some apparently innocuous component of the patient's food[15]. Outside the field of drugs, interactions are not uncommon, and there has to be an awareness of this within the chemical industry[1]. It is obvious that no investigative programme of predictive toxicology can take into account every possible permutation and combination of exposures, but it is practical to create useful matrices of combinations of molecules and to include these in the predictive testing. This combination matrix approach can be made flexible so that retrospective experience of interactions can be included to improve predictability.

Interactive effects may be sufficiently obvious to allow the investigator to draw conclusions on the basis of very limited testing. Often the interactions may be more subtle, and require the adoption of quantitative methods for detection and definition. The future development of acute and subacute predictive toxicity testing will have to come to terms with predicting interactive effects, and since many of these are associated with physiological function rather than either biochemical change or morphological effects it is difficult to foresee in vitro methods having much application.

The future of predictive toxicology in relation to acute and subacute exposure will depend largely on the refinement of in vivo methodology, but research into in vitro techniques will be increased by the current awareness of the need to minimize experiments that necessitate the use of living animals. Some reduction in the numbers of animals used for this purpose may result from the more efficient use of data banking, thus reducing replication of testing, but the problems associated with this type of data banking must not be underestimated (e.g. data verification and quality control, commercial security, legal problems, etc.), particularly on the international scale of operation.

Although it is essentially retrospective, the predictive value of data from exposed humans must not be underestimated or wasted. To this end there is need for an improved feedback of information from all relevant sources, and it may be suggested that the international poisons information centres should be provided with the resources necessary to function better as "brokers" for this information[16].

In a review of the future of predictive safety evaluation it may not be too provocative to recommend that an impartial review of the cost-effectiveness of predictive acute and subacute toxicology should be carried out, and as a concomitant of this review the risk-benefit of either partially or totally abandoning this aspect of predictive testing may be assessed.

REFERENCES

1. Martens, M, Mosselmans, G, Fumero, S, Jacobs, G and Lafontaine, A (1984). Some thoughts on a possible regulatory approach at EEC level on the classification and labelling of dangerous preparations. Reg Toxicol Pharmacol, 4, 145-56

2. Brown, VK (1980). Acute Toxicity in Theory and Practice. 1st edn. (Chichester: Wiley)

3. Fletcher, J (1977). Ethical considerations in biomedical research involving human beings. Bull WHO, 55 (Suppl. 2), 101-10

4. Draize, JH, Woodard, G and Calvery, HO (1944). Method for the study of irritation and toxicity of substances applied topically to the skin and mucous membranes. J Pharmacol Exp Ther, 82, 377-89

5. Weil, CS and Scala, RA (1971). Study of intra- and inter-laboratory variability in the results of rabbit eye and skin irritation tests. Toxicol Appl Pharmacol, 19, 276-360

6. Swanston, DW (1983). Eye irritancy testing. In Balls, M, Riddell, RJ and Worden, AN (eds) Animals and Alternatives in Toxicity Testing. (London: Academic Press) pp. 337-66

7. Brown, VK (1984). The LD50 value - a frequently misapplied concept. ATLA, 12, 75-9

8. Brown, VK (1983). Acute toxicity testing. In Balls, M, Riddell, RJ and Worden, AN (eds) Animals and Alternatives in Toxicity Testing. (London: Academic Press) pp. 1-29

9. Brown, VK (1975). Recommended classification of pesticides by hazard. WHO Chron, 29, 397-401

10. Abrams, J (1983). Nitrate delivery systems - a contemporary perspective. In Goldberg, AAJ and Parsons, DG (eds) Modern Concepts in Nitrate Delivery Systems. Royal Society of Medicine International Congress and Symposium Series No. 54. (London: Academic Press and Royal Society of Medicine)

11. Molinengo, L and Orsetti, M (1984). The principle of non-specificity and acute toxicity. Trends Pharmacol Sci, 5, 185-7

12. Dewar, AJ and Moffett, BJ (1979). Biochemical methods for detecting neurotoxicity - a short review. Pharmacol Ther, 5, 545-62

13. Dewar, AJ (1983). Neurotoxicity. In Balls, M, Riddell, RJ and Worden, AN (eds) Animals and Alternatives in Toxicity Testing. (London: Academic Press) pp. 229-95

14. Marzulli, F and Maguire, Jr, HC (1982). Usefulness and limitations of various guinea-pig test methods in detecting human skin sensitizers - validation of guinea-pig tests for skin hypersensitivity. Fd Chem Toxicol, 20, 67-74

15. Stockley, I (1977). Drug Interactions and their Mechanisms. (London: The Pharmaceutical Press)

16. Werner, B (1983). The use of acute toxicity data in poison information centres. Acta Pharmacol Toxicol, 52 (Suppl. ii), 263-8

4

Animal Models of Long Term Toxic Effects

A. N. WORDEN and S. R. WALKER

It might be seriously questioned whether or not there is a future for the long-term or chronic toxicity test as conventionally understood. Even before the first official or quasi-official pronouncement on the conduct and interpretation of this and other types of test was made - by the staff of the United States Food and Drug Administration (FDA)[1] in the publication entitled Appraisal of the Safety of Chemicals in Foods, Drugs and Cosmetics in 1955 - doubts had been expressed about its value. Alastair Frazer[2] in 1952 had suggested that a complete study of the physiology, biochemistry and pharmacology of the substance under test '....enables the chronic toxicity tests to be properly designed to cover any likely effect of the substance, directly or indirectly, on the bodily functions'. Barnes and Denz[3], in their critical review published in 1954, quoted Frazer's view and went on to say that: 'If such a complete study had already been made there would have been little need for a chronic toxicity test. A chronic toxicity test is always a make-shift affair to be replaced as soon as possible by a more permanent structure of knowledge built on the foundations of physiology, biochemistry and other fundamental sciences'. Barnes and Denz also emphasized the confusion that could arise in attempts to identify toxic lesions in ageing animals - a complication that has been lessened but not eliminated through the subsequent use of specific pathogen free (SPF) rodents.

Barnes[4] in 1963 went so far as to query whether official recommendations for the testing of drugs for toxicity were themselves dangerous: 'Testing procedures outlined by authorities whether national or international will either be so vague as to be not worth disseminating or become by necessity more precise. The recommended tests would then be carried out by scores of unthinking technicians who will supply a mass of data eventually to be pushed under official noses. The scientific study of toxicology will atrophy and the hazards from new drugs remain as much of a problem in the future as it is today'.

The intervening decades have seen much to suggest that the pattern of long-term testing procedures should be changed, but little to change it. The possible substitution of novel for what had become conventional procedures was, prior to the introduction of mutagenicity and other forms of genetic toxicity testing, approached with considerable caution, as is evident from the attempts to review the status of toxicological evaluation, or of some facet of it, during the past 25 years - see, e.g., Litchfield[5]; Bein[6]; Abrams, Zbinden and Bagdon[7]; Boyd[8]; Golberg[9,10]; Beyer[11]; Boyland and Goulding[12]; D'Aguanno[13,14]; Goldenthal[15]; Loomis[16]; Worden[17-20]; Frazer and Sharratt[21]; Benitz[22]; Hanley, Udall and Weatherall[23]; the Royal Society Study Group on Long Term Toxic Effects[24]; Page[25]; Wardell[26]; Lasagna[27]; Klaasen and Doull[28]; Weatherall[29]; Kesterson[30]; Zbinden[31]; Venning[32]; Homburger[33]; Suter[34]; and Rodricks and Tardiff[35].

The value of the conventional long-term test and its potential interrelationships with so-called alternative - mainly in vitro - procedures formed the subject of a 3-day meeting held at the Royal Society, London, from 1-3 November 1982 to discuss the report of the Frame Toxicity Committee (Balls, Riddell and Worden[36]). Here, Griffin stated that some toxicity studies were defective in protocol design, inappropriate or irrelevant, or conducted in a slovenly manner but concluded: 'Despite the many criticisms that can be made of long-term animal toxicity studies in terms of their design and conduct and, even when well conducted, of their predictability, they remain, in the current absence of any alternative, the best predictors of risk to man that we have'. He has since[37] stated that, while animal studies must not be regarded as infallible predictors, they '.....remain not only the best but, in the absence of any reasonable alternative comprehensive screening, the only predictors of potential hazard for man that we have. Animal studies do not have the potential to quantify risk'.

Laurence, McLean and Weatherall[38] obtained the collaboration of four pharmaceutical companies and were able to record the 'case histories' of bethanidine, bromocriptine, cimetidine, three beta-adrenoceptor blocking drugs (pronethanol, propanalol and practolol) and tamoxifen, based largely upon use of the detailed reports of work conducted within or for the companies concerned. The conclusions of the individual authors concerning the value of the relevant long-term studies - and of the toxicological profile in general - ranged from satisfaction with negative findings - and then subsequent repetition in man - through complaints of unnecessary time and expense to evidence of predictive failure in the case of practolol.

ANIMAL MODELS OF LONG-TERM TOXIC EFFECTS

Several attempts have been made to evaluate toxicological data with respect to the appropriate duration of chronic animal studies. In the sixties, Bein[6] collected data on 46 compounds which had been investigated at two independent research sites in order to assess any differences in the results obtained. He concluded from the toxicological assessment of 46 compounds studied at both centres, of which 19 were investigated with different durations and doses, that tests beyond 4 weeks did not disclose any new toxicologically salient effects. In addition, unwanted effects appeared more clearly in short-term tests employing high doses than with lower doses given for prolonged periods. Peck[39] studied the results of toxicological investigations with 11 compounds, 7 for both short (6 months or less) and long (greater than 6 months) periods. In only 1 case was there a new salient finding seen in the long-term tests and this may have been due to the absence of pathological examination between 1.5 months and 12 months.

More recently Lumley and Walker[40-42] obtained comprehensive toxicology data from repeated-dose animal studies from 13 pharmaceutical companies in the United Kingdom with the objective of determining what additional information is uncovered in studies of 12 or 18 months compared with those of 6 months duration. Having established a unique toxicology databank containing information on 74 compounds, with half of these having been investigated for 6 months or more, they carried out a retrospective analysis showing that there was little value in prolonging studies beyond 6 months apart from those designed to investigate carcinogenicity. Subsequently this databank was extended by pharmaceutical companies in Switzerland and Germany that also provided chronic animal toxicology studies. This European Databank now comprises information from 21 pharmaceutical companies on 124 compounds, the majority of which have been studied in more than 1 species, giving a total 214 case studies. Over half of the compounds have been studied for periods of longer than 6 months. From the results of this further analysis, Lumley and Walker[43] have concluded that there was no evidence to support animal toxicity studies of longer than 6 months duration. Unless the design of chronic animal toxicity studies is carefully examined when making these comparisons, e.g. the number of animals, choice and number of doses, recovery groups and the timing and types of interim and terminal tests, erroneous conclusions may be drawn regarding the value of long-term studies. Perhaps the shift in emphasis should be from the prolongation of investigations to identify toxicity in animals to post-marketing surveillance to determine safety in man.

A recent workshop at the CIBA Foundation addressed the issue of long-term animal studies and their predictive value for man[44]. The findings from this workshop were that, although there does not appear to be any possibility at the present time of replacing long-term animal studies, their predictive value is limited. However, with better design and more attention to mechanisms of toxicity their extrapolative value could be improved. It is widely, although not universally, accepted that with appropriate study design, except when carcinogenicity is being assessed, the majority of toxicological effects could be identified within 6 months and that there does not appear to be any justification for continuing studies to 12 or 18 months. The conclusion of the workshop was that more time and effort should be directed towards retrospective studies, both of animal toxicological data and clinical investigations, with comparative studies of the effects seen in animals and in man.

Heywood[45-47] emphasized the importance of the 'no-effect' level - a not-detectable effect level as defined by conventional toxicity studies (Zbinden[48]) - as a basis for assessing safety and establishing acceptable daily intakes. He stressed the influence of factors such as species and strain of animal used and suggested that in 60% of compounds the 'no-effect' level in rodents is higher, often by a 3-fold factor, than in non-rodent species.

Heywood also indicated the marked species variation in target organ toxicity. He studied the data for the dog and rat generated in studies on 39 drugs for pharmaceutical companies. In the rat, 79 target systems were identified, compared with 59 in the dog. Of the systems identified, 33% of those in the rat and 46% of those in the dog were predictable on the basis of known pharmacology. The best correlations of identified target systems between the rat and the dog were never greater than 20%, even including hepatotoxicity. This lack of predictability between species extends to experimental animals and man. Thus Fletcher[49] attempted to correlate toxicity in animals and adverse effects in man for 45 drugs and concluded that, for an individual drug, 25% of the toxic effects observed in animal studies may be expected to occur as adverse reactions in man. Vomiting and gastrointestinal disturbances had greater predictive capacity than had CNS signs such as ataxia, convulsions, sedation, salivation or tremor.

The vexed problem of the significance of adverse reactions as such in laboratory animals calls into question, as indicated at the commencement of this chapter, the value from this standpoint of long-term tests. Are they to be abandoned altogether, retained only to satisfy regulatory authorities and as some form of vaguely-worded insurance policy, or refined? Griffin[37] (discussion, p.106) suggested that '....toxicity testing was a crude business in which refinement seemed to have little place. What was being looked for was the potential of a substance to cause harm when it was let loose on an enormously variable human population, much of it sick or old or young or growing or pregnant. The best that could be hoped for was to gauge the extent to which the potential of a substance came up in toxicity studies'.

Certainly the long-term test has revealed many examples of an unexpected degree of toxicity. Worden[19] examined the records of the many results of long-term tests on compounds - over 705 of them from the pharmaceutical industry - handled over a decade by a large contract research laboratory. These were almost all substances upon which considerable amounts of time, expense and experimentation had been conducted prior to their being submitted for long-term investigation and were therefore considered good candidates, worthy of the relatively high cost and effort involved in a long-term study. In no fewer than 30% of the compounds studied, the contract research laboratory had advised that work should cease, since there was little chance that the side reactions that had been encountered would allow of the compound's acceptance. It is conceivable that some of these side reactions - or equally serious ones - would have been seen in man at therapeutic dose levels and that, equally, some potentially valuable therapeutic agents may have been lost.

It would seem on balance that, despite the limitations, pitfalls and interpretational pitfalls of the long-term tests and also advances made possible by molecular biology - as foreshadowed by Barnes and Denz[3] in 1954 and now being enunciated by Parkes[51] and his colleagues as described elsewhere in this book - there will remain a need for repeat-dose studies on intact whole animal models. Even taking into account the views of Griffin[52], however, considerable refinement of existing procedures must surely take place, primarily on scientific grounds but also to meet the need for savings in time and in the numbers of animals involved. It is not unreasonable to suggest that the following approach should become feasible within the near future:

(1)   Each study should be individually planned and its details discussed in advance - so far as confidentiality considerations allow - with experienced toxicologists, with expert pharmacologists and clinicians in the field or fields for which the compound is intended, and with regulatory authorities and their scientific advisers.

(2)   The study should not only be prefaced by detailed pharmacological, biochemical and kinetic observations on the test species but should also be accompanied by such observations during its course - and by related observations on the human subject.

(3)   Observations on the living animal should include, whenever feasible, the use of telemetry and nuclear magnetic resonance or other non-invasive procedures to seek patho-physiological and patho-pharmacological responses.

(4)   The chemistry of the test substance - with precise information on the dose form and on the role and physical state of any accompanying compounds - should be defined and a 'balance sheet' constructed of its fate following administration.

(5)   In all appropriate instances, probes, markers and other immunological techniques should be employed to elicit antibody response and any other effects, specific or general, that the test substance may exert upon the immune system.

(6)   Each animal should be in the care of sympathetic but proficient attendants and seen frequently by a veterinarian for careful observations for possible behavioural or clinical effects, including, e.g., ophthalmological changes, which were responsible for almost one-third of the severe reactions in the series summarised by Worden[19,50].

(7)   Each animal study would be complemented by appropriate in vitro procedures, not only initially but also during its course if circumstances so indicated[53].

(8)   Histochemical procedures would be employed, not only terminally but if so required during the course of the study.

(9)   Tissue samples would be obtained during the course of the study for identification or monitoring of morphological change at the cellular and subcellular levels.

(10)   Terminal morphological changes would be investigated more rapidly than at present, with sophisticated recording and analysis.

REFERENCES

1.   Association of Food and Drug Officials of the United States. Appraisal of the Safety of Chemicals in Foods, Drugs and Cosmetics. Topeka, Kansas: Association of Food and Drug Officials of the United States, P.O. Box 1494, 1955

2.   Frazer, AC (1952). The medical risks for the consumer and how they can best be minimized. Proc R Soc Med 45, 681-4

3.   Barnes, JM and Denz, FA (1954). Experimental methods used in determining chronic toxicity: a critical review. Pharmacol Rev, 6, 191-242

4.   Barnes, JM (1963). Are official recommendations for the testing of drugs for toxicity dangerous? Proc Eur Soc Study Drug Tox, 2, 57-66

5.   Litchfield, JT (1962). Evaluation of the safety of new drugs by means of tests in animals. Clin Pharmacol Ther, 3, 665-72

6.   Bein, HJ (1963). Rational and irrational numbers in toxicology. Proc Eur Soc Study Drug Tox, 2, 15-26

7.   Abrams, WB, Zbinden, G and Bagdon, R (1965). Investigative methods in clinical toxicology. J New Drugs, 5, 199-207

8.   Boyd, EM (1965). Toxicological studies. In Herrick, W and Cattell, McK (eds) Clinical Testing of New Drugs. pp. 13-22 (New York: Revere)

9.   Golberg, L (1965). The predictive value of animal toxicity studies carried out on new drugs. In Herrick, AD and Cattell, McK (eds) Clinical Testing of New Drugs. pp. 23-30 (New York: Revere)

10.   Golberg, L (1966). Liver enlargement produced by drugs: its significance. Proc Eur Soc Study Drug Tox, 7, 171-84

11.   Beyer, KH (1966). Perspectives in toxicology. Toxicol Appl Pharmacol, 8, 1-5

12.   Boyland, E and Goulding, R (eds) (1968). Modern Trends in Toxicology. (London: Butterworths)

13.   D'Aguanno, W (1968). Either low or high toxicity poses drug evaluation problems. Drug Res Rep, 11, 5-15 to 5-20

14.   D'Aguanno, W (1973). Drug toxicity evaluation - pre-clinical aspects. FDA Introduction to Total Drug Quality. DHEW Publication No. (FDA) 74-30006, 35-40

15.   Goldenthal, EI (1968). Current views on the safety evaluation of drugs. FDA Papers, 2, 13-18

16.   Loomis, TA (1968). Essentials of Toxicology. (Philadelphia: Lea and Febiger)

17.   Worden, AN (1968). Experimental and clinical evaluation of safety and effectiveness of new drugs. Jpn J Pharmacol, 10, 1177-84

18.   Worden, AN (1969). The Toxicity of Compounds of Veterinary and Agricultural Importance. Thesis, University of London

19.   Worden, AN (1974). Toxicological methods. Toxicology, 2, 359-70

20. Worden, AN (1984). Toxicology during René Truhaut's Life Time. In: Homage au Professeur Truhaut, 1220-1223. Paris, le 19 octobre 1984 (ISBN 2-9501065-0-1)

21. Frazer, AC and Sharratt, M (1969). The value and limitations of animal studies in the prediction of effects in man. In: Symposium on The Use of Animals in Toxicological Studies. London: UFAW, 22 January, 1969

22. Benitz, KF (1969). Measurements of chronic toxicity. In: Paget, GE (ed.) Methods in Toxicology. (New York: Academic Press)

23. Hanley, T, Udall, V and Weatherall, M (1970). An industrial view of current practice in predicting drug toxicity. Br Med Bull, 26, 203-7

24. Report. Long Term Toxic Effects: A Study Group Report. London: The Royal Society, 1978

25. Page, NP (1977). Chronic toxicity and carcinogenicity guidelines. J Environ Pathol Toxicol, 1, 161-82

26. Wardell, WM (1978). The drug lag revisited: comparison by therapeutic area of patterns of drugs marketed in the United States and Great Britain from 1972 through 1976. Clin Pharmacol Ther, 24, 499-594

27. Lasagna, L (1961). Toxicological barriers to providing better drugs. Arch Toxicol, 43, 27-33

28. Klaasen, CD and Doull, J (1980). Evaluation of safety: toxicological evaluation. In: Doull, J, Klaasen, CD and Amdur, MO (eds) Casarett and Doull's Toxicology: the Basic Science of Poisons. 2nd edn, pp. 11-27. (New York: Macmillan Publishing Co.)

29. Weatherall, M (1982). An end to the search for new drugs? Nature, London, 296, 387-90

30. Kesterson, JW (1982). Drug safety evaluation: animal toxicology studies and their interpretations. Drug Inf J, January/June, 22-34, 1982

31. Zbinden, G (1982). Current trends in safety testing and toxicological research. Naturwissenschaften, 69, 255-9

32. Venning, GR (1983). Identification of adverse reactions to new drugs. Br Med J, 286, 199-202, 289-92, 365-8, 458-60, 544-7

33. Homburger, F (1983). Introduction to method development session. In: Homburger, F (ed.) Safety Evaluation and Regulation of Chemicals. First International Conference, Boston, Massachusetts. pp. 191-192 (Basle: Karger)

34. Suter, KE (1983). Relevance of standard toxicological tests. Comparison of the experimental and clinical data of six pharmaceutical preparations. In: Zbinden, G et al. (eds) Current Problems in Drug Toxicology. Proceedings of an International Symposium 'Present Problems and Future Trends in Drug Toxicology', Paris. pp. 72-76 (London: John Libbey)

35. Rodricks, JV and Tardiff, RG (1983). Biological basis for risk assessment. In: Homburger, F (ed.) Safety Evaluation and Regulation of Chemicals. First International Conference, Boston, Massachusetts. pp. 77-84 (Basle: Karger)

36. Balls, M, Riddell, RJ and Worden, AN (eds) (1983). Animals and Alternatives in Toxicity Testing. (London: Academic

Press)

37. Griffin, JP (1983). Long-term toxicity - General Discussion. In: Balls, M, Riddell, RJ and Worden, AN (eds) Animals and Alternatives in Toxicity Testing. pp. 106 (London: Academic Press)

38. Laurence, DR, McLean, AEM and Weatherall, M (1984). Safety Testing of New Drugs: Laboratory Predictions and Clinical Performance. (London: Academic Press)

39. Peck, HM (1968). An appraisal of drug safety evaluation in animals and the extrapolation of the results to man. In: Tedeschi, DH and Tedeschi, RE (eds) Importance of Fundamental Principles in Drug Evaluation. pp. 449-71 (New York: Raven)

40. Lumley, CE and Walker, SR (1985). The establishment of a computer-based toxicology databank. Med Informatics, 10 (2), 173-4

41. Lumley, CE and Walker, SR (1985). What is the value of animal toxicology studies beyond 6 months? Br J Pharmacol, 84, 117P

42. Lumley, CE and Walker, SR (1985). A toxicology data-bank based on animal safety evaluation studies of pharmaceutical compounds. Human Toxicol, 4, 447-60

43. Lumley, CE and Walker, SR (1986). A critical appraisal of the duration of chronic animal toxicity studies. Regulatory Pharmacol Toxicol, 6(1), 66-72

44. Walker, SR and Dayan, AD (eds) (1986). Long-term Animal Studies: their Predictive Value for Man. Proceedings of the Centre for Medicines Research Workshop, CIBA Foundation, London, October 1984. (Lancaster: MTP Press)

45. Heywood, R (1981). Target organ toxicity. I. Toxicol Lett, 8, 349-58

46. Heywood, R (1983). Target organ toxicity. II. Toxicol Lett, 18, 83-8

47. Heywood, R (1983). Long-term toxicity. In: Balls, M, Riddell, RJ and Worden, AN (eds). Animals and Alternatives in Toxicity Testing. pp. 79-93. (London: Academic Press)

48. Zbinden, G (1979). The no-effect level, an old bone of contention in toxicology. Arch Toxicol, 43, 3-7

49. Fletcher, AP (1978). Drug safety tests and subsequent clinical experience. J R Soc Med, 71, 693-6

50. Worden, AN (1986). The evidence supporting 6 month animal studies. In: Long-term Animal Studies - their Predictive Value for Man. Proceedings of the Centre for Medicines Research Workshop, CIBA Foundation, London, October 1984. pp. 83-86. (Lancaster: MTP Press)

51. Parke, DV (1987). Molecular aspects of toxicology. In: This volume, pp. 3-38

52. Griffin, JP (1983). Repeat dose long-term toxicity studies. In: Balls, MR, Riddell, RJ and Worden, AN (eds) Animal and Alternatives in Toxicity Testing. pp. 98-104. (London: Academic Press)

53. Worden, AN (1986). Combined techniques. In: Animal Experimentation: Humane Uses and Alternatives. Dominguez (New York: John Wiley) (In press)

5

Inhalation Aspects of Toxicology Testing

D. G. CLARK

INTRODUCTION

Before discussing the future of inhalation toxicology it is worthwhile to restate just why the topic is, and will continue to be, so important: this is simply that breathing is mandatory. Of all the routes of entry of toxic chemicals into the body the inhalation route is the one least able to be controlled. We can refrain from drinking toxic chemicals and avoid splashes on the skin or in the eye. But we cannot stop breathing.

The potential for toxic insult via the respiratory tract is enormous. A man working 8 hours a day, 5 days a week for 45 years will inhale 30 million litres of his workplace air. Each and every one of us will inhale over 250 million litres of air as we pass through life from the cradle to the grave. This air can be contaminated with gases, vapours, fumes, aerosols, dusts, smogs, smokes or fibres. Exposure may be inadvertent, simply because the contaminated air is part of our workplace or general environment, or deliberate, as with cigarette smoking, glue sniffing or the inhalation of therapeutic drugs. All this contaminated air passes into the lungs, which contain delicate tissues designed to facilitate the passage of respiratory gases to and from the blood stream. Contaminated air thereby poses not only an indirect toxic threat to the body, but also a direct threat to the lungs themselves.

It is impossible to envisage any fundamental alterations in the nature of the toxic insult in the future. The respiratory system has been honed almost to perfection over several million years of trial and error, and the 15 years between now and the year 2000 are unlikely to see any further changes. The Utopian ideal of air free from contamination is also highly unlikely. Even a return to a pre-industrial society would pose toxic threats to the lungs, although of a different kind. Man will consequently still be breathing contaminated air - albeit a reduced amount - and inhalation toxicologists will still be attempting to predict or explain the effects in man using experimental models in the foreseeable future.

Unfortunately, many inhalation studies in the fairly recent

past have been inadequate for predictive purposes, and have merely paid lip service to science. The history of inhalation toxicology has been plagued by the rediscovery of the wheel, as new entrants to the subject have assumed it to be a blank sheet of paper on which they could write their own version of a new technology. Since the existing body of knowledge was not readily accessible in the open literature, and apparatus was not commercially available and had to be fabricated in-house, the temptation to take an independent route was almost irresistible. Inhalation studies seemed to be either animal or technical. The animal studies were generally conducted by biologists whose grasp of the complexities of atmosphere generation and analysis left something to be desired; the technical studies were conducted by chemists whose atmospheres were superb, but whose experimental animals were included almost as an afterthought. Recently, however, the publication of state-of-the-art textbooks and comprehensive reviews, the commercial availability of most apparatus, and the realization that inhalation toxicity is pre-eminently a team effort of biologists, chemists, physicists and engineers, has placed the subject on a firm scientific foundation[1-7].

At the time of writing, it was the year 1985. The point of this article is not how we got here, but where do we go?

The year 2000 is only five or six consecutive 2-year studies away. All the major factors that can influence inhalation toxicology in the future should already be clearly visible, and even some of the more speculative icebergs should have at least their tips visible. The future may therefore be regarded as a simple extrapolation of present trends, with political, social, commercial/economic and technical pressures accelerating or decelerating these trends.

The world of chemicals will be changing over the next 15 years. In the OECD the trend will be towards high value-added speciality chemicals and away from high tonnage commodity chemicals, and an increasing proportion of commodity chemicals will be manufactured in the newly industrializing countries. Traditional methods of manufacture may be complemented, and in some cases replaced, by biotechnological processes. The growing use of synthetic construction materials in buildings, coupled with the reduction in ventilation often resulting from the use of energy conservation measures, will serve to increase the amounts and range of chemicals to which we may be exposed in our daily lives. Nasal sprays will become more common in the administration of drugs to man, and novel methods of administering inhaled drugs via synthetic cigarettes may be developed. All will need sophisticated analysis by inhalation toxicologists. How will they be evaluated in the future, and what areas must be improved to allow better predictive evaluation?

EXPERIMENTAL FACILITIES

Chambers

The majority of exposure chambers have design defects that will have to be eradicated in the future.

A common problem is that it is difficult to detect toxic ef-fects during exposure. Animals must be visible at all times; not merely when they are fed and cleaned at the end of a day's ex-posure, in order that the time course of toxic effects can be determined. Whole-body chambers containing several layers of animals, often multiple-housed, make it virtually impossible to ob-serve the animals; whereas head-only chambers allow a clear view of all animals, but at the expense of restricting their movement so much that it is difficult to detect toxic signs.

Chambers are still not fully calibrated in terms of particulate distribution before being put to use. Calibration must be done using a range of chemical types and particle sizes, not merely with such a fine particulate atmosphere that it behaves almost as a vapour. The calibration must be done with the probes next to each animal, since the larger the chamber, the slower the air flow through the chamber and the more influence the animal's own ther-mals will have on the atmosphere distribution. Stirred chambers have much to commend them, and should be evaluated more thoroughly in the future.

The importance of temperature and humidity measurements within the chamber is well recognized, not only for the physiologi-cal well-being of the animals, but also for the condition of the at-mosphere, and is now a requirement of all inhalation toxicology guidelines. Practice, however, is not as easy as theory. It is no problem to measure temperature continuously, but humidity measurements are very difficult in a chemical-laden atmosphere. Ambient air devices presently used become contaminated with chemical; dewpoint apparatus gives excellent results until the sur-face film becomes contaminated. If humidity is to be measured ac-curately there is an urgent need for apparatus that automatically measures humidity after first separating out the chemical.

Larger chambers to accommodate larger numbers of animals leads to greater quantities of chemical to be disposed of. Chamber designs that rely solely on dilution into the outside atmosphere will be quite unacceptable in the future. A wide range of complex equipment will be needed to clean up the chamber exhausts, rang-ing from scrubbers to charcoal filters to incinerators, with even more specialized facilities for the disposal of chemicals such as chlorinated hydrocarbons.

Atmosphere generation

A wide variety of commercial apparatus is already available for use by inhalation toxicologists, and the range will undoubtedly increase in the future. But since the inhalation toxicology market is small, it is unrealistic to expect that commercial apparatus will be developed to cope with the wide variety of chemical types encoun-tered by an industrial laboratory in the future. Mixtures of plant streams containing volatiles, involatiles and thermally unstable chemicals, dusts of differing tackiness, and aerosols of liquid phase on a carrier will continue to pose such unique generation problems that they will only be solved by use of highly skilled in-house or consultancy engineering staff. Even an apparently simple problem, such as scaling up the generating apparatus from an acute study to a chronic study, will often tax the ingenuity of the engineers.

Atmosphere analysis

Current instrumentation for the automated analysis of chamber atmosphere is generally adequate, and any improvements can only be in terms of speed and efficiency. The advent of automated particle sizing apparatus has certainly transformed the monitoring of particulate atmospheres, although apparatus designed to cope with heavier atmospheres of larger particles would be a welcome improvement.

The use of precise automated equipment for the analysis of atmospheres, however, may be a mixed blessing. While it undoubtedly improves efficiency, there could be a danger that the inhalation toxicologist comes to rely so much on his "black boxes" that he loses the ability to evaluate critically the data he is being given. He may also neglect the importance of the equipment between the chamber and the analyser. What the analyser sees must be what is in the chamber. Pipe lengths, solenoid values, leaks, etc. will all influence the results in a variety of ways, and turn an apparently impressive experiment into an inadequate one. Validation of the whole system before an experimental animal is even thought of will thus become even more important in the future.

Animals

Rats and mice have been used for the vast majority of inhalation studies simply because they are convenient to handle in large numbers in cages in chambers. With such a large body of historic data there is often a reluctance to question the value of rats and mice, or the way in which they are used in inhalation studies. This should be done, however, if the maximum amount of relevant information is to be obtained from each chemical.

Rats and mice, in common with all the other species that are easy to handle, have respiratory anatomies markedly different from man - from their nasal passages to their mucus secretions. Dogs and monkeys are much closer to man in terms of anatomy and response, but their widespread use in the future will be restricted by non-scientific factors such as cost, ethics and public pressures. The domestic pig could be considered, in that it has some similarities to man in the development of the respiratory system, the distribution of mucus glands in the trachea, the thoracic, cardiac and coronary artery anatomy, and the general cardiorespiratory physiology. All that is against it is its size.

Despite their disadvantages the rat and mouse will continue to hold a pre-eminent position in inhalation toxicology, with other species confined to specialized studies if they are shown to be more appropriate for a particular chemical. The way that the rats and mice are used, however, could be subject to considerable change.

Rats and mice are nocturnal creatures. They are active at night and sleep during the day. A toxicologist is a daylight creature, and exposes his experimental animals between the hours of nine to five, whilst they are asleep. Not only are the animals not indulging in any behaviour that can be observed for chemical-induced changes, but they are also breathing at a minimum, and sleeping with their noses either buried in their own or another's fur. The pathway for the inspired air is lengthened, and an additional particulate filter is imposed between the experimental atmosphere and the lungs. Reverse-daylight chambers are the obvious solution so that the animals are exposed during their period of maximal activity. Unfortunately such exposure systems have not yet been evaluated, but will inevitably be tried in the future. Even if found to be of value, however, the use of reverse-daylight chambers as general experimental systems would involve a fine balance between improved, more scientific experimental conditions, and the undermining of the historic data base.

Nocturnal rhythms are only a small part of the cyclical changes in physiological function. There is a wide variety of changes related to season, sexual function, environment, noise, social contact, etc., that are known to occur in experimental animals. If, as seems likely, major organs such as the liver and kidneys are also subject to circadian rhythms, toxicity could be influenced by factors over which we do not yet have control. There is a considerable body of literature available, not readily accessible to toxicologists since it deals mostly with the biological phenomena of the rhythms themselves rather than their toxicological consequences. If the biologists do not extend their experiments to include toxicology, the toxicologists will have to consider more seriously the implications of these rhythms on the predictive value of their tests.

Automatic watering of experimental animals in their home cages and within exposure chambers is now almost universal, and automatic feeding will follow within the next few years. The advent of automatic feeding of precise quantities of food at predetermined times will sharpen the arguments about ad libitum versus restricted feeding in chronic rodent studies. The arguments have surfaced repeatedly over several years, but nothing positive has been done about "bored, sex-starved rodents eating themselves into premature old age". Although the arguments have generally been confined to long-term feeding studies, they apply equally well to long-term inhalation studies. The time for opinions and assertions based on prejudice and expediency has long passed, industry-wide ring tests are needed as soon as possible to provide the necessary base on which to make a final judgement.

Facilities for housing long-term rodent inhalation studies will have to improve. It has always been anomalous that chronic feeding studies are undertaken inside rigorously controlled, barriered animal houses to keep the animals free from the respiratory infection that would invalidate the experiment. And yet chronic inhalation studies have always been conducted with inhalation chambers inside ordinary laboratories. Since toxic insult to the lungs is likely to make experimental animals more susceptible to respiratory infection, it follows that chronic inhalation studies must be done inside a barrier-maintained specific-pathogen-free facility. Such a facility will be more expensive to build and run, and more inconvenient to operate, but must logically be the design for all future inhalation laboratories if standards are to improve.

MEASUREMENTS DURING EXPOSURE

The sheer effort and cost of mounting an adequate inhalation study with precisely regulated atmospheres will have to be reflected in the biological value of the results obtained. More biological measurements will have to be made during the course of the study so that the maximum of information is developed using the minimum number of animals.

Pharmacokinetics

Inhalation studies of industrial chemicals have all too often equated "chamber concentration" with "dose". Even in the simplest case of a chemical causing a direct toxic action on the lungs, the relationship between chamber concentration and dose is not linear, since although the experimenter may control the chamber concentration, the animal controls the dose by decreasing its respiration and activity. Once a chemical has passed the lungs and entered the body to be absorbed, metabolized and excreted, the relationship between atmospheric concentration and dose becomes even more tenuous, and simplistic views can lead to the generation of quite erroneous results. Future studies must take account of pharmacokinetic principles, particularly saturation kinetics. Although saturation kinetics may not be so important for high toxicity inhaled chemicals, where death intervenes before saturation is reached, they are vital for an understanding of many low toxicity chemicals. Vinyl chloride monomer and 1,1-dichloroethylene are only two examples of chemicals that serve to illustrate how important saturation kinetics are in understanding toxicity.

Functional measurements

Changes in function may be harbingers of more serious toxic injury that will eventually be detected by histopathological techniques, or they may be ends in themselves, detecting conditions such as asthma that are impossible to detect in other ways. They are often the only way to estimate the time course of a lesion and its reversibility, giving information on transient effects and adaptations, and the functional significance of histologically observed lesions.

Pulmonary function tests will become an essential feature of all subacute and chronic inhalation studies, with the inhalation toxicologist having a wide range of tests at his disposal, depending on the chemical under evaluation. The basic lung function measurement will be the plethysmographic determination of tidal volume and respiratory rate with computed minute volumes in marker animals throughout exposure. Indeed, an inhalation study without knowledge of the animals' minute volume will be regarded in the same way as a feeding study without food consumption measurements. Lung resistance, lung compliance and blood gases will be routinely measured in satellite groups of anaesthetized animals before, and at regular intervals during, exposure and diffusion and ventilation measurements will be made with selected chemicals. Following exposure, pressure/volume loops and cilia beat studies will be undertaken in vivo.

These techniques have already been developed for experimental animals, and most of the measurements can be made in small laboratory rodents as well as larger species such as dogs and monkeys. The spread of these techniques into general inhalation toxicology studies is presently inhibited because they are very labour intensive, with only a few animals able to be tested by a team of skilled technicians. Developments in automation and computer control with on-line data processing, however, are proceeding rapidly in laboratories such as Battelle, Geneva, and the whole battery of lung function tests will soon be possible on a simple routine basis in chronic studies.

As far as the effects on the rest of the body are concerned, the future needs of inhalation toxicology are no different from those of other areas of toxicology. But there is the additional complication that the animals are contained within a chamber where it is difficult to get the apparatus to them in order to measure the changes. Most of these other functional measurements can be loosely grouped as "mode-of-action" studies, which will be an essential feature of routine studies to explain how the chemical exerts its toxic effect. The range of possible studies is almost unlimited, but because of the close relationship between the cardiovascular system and the lungs, the study of functional changes in the cardiovascular system is worth particular attention.

The ECG can provide such a range of useful information that it will be an obvious addition to the range of functional measurements in inhalation toxicology in the future. It is relatively simple to measure with a rodent in a restraint tube during head-only inhalation exposure, but more difficult with the animal in a cage in a chamber. With the development of miniaturized ECG transmitters, radiotelemetry will allow continuous recording from small unrestrained animals throughout exposure, and in the home cage after exposure. Blood pressure measurements in small, conscious, freely moving rodents are extremely difficult to do, and so are rarely attempted on a routine basis. With the use of restraint, a wide variety of tail cuff methods can be used, but the fact that there is a wide variety of apparatus available indicates that none of it is truly satisfactory. The solution will lie in the development of miniaturized pressure transducers capable of being implanted in the aorta for radiotelemetric recording of the blood pressure when required.

One non-invasive technique that is potentially the most powerful tool at the disposal of the inhalation toxicologist is nuclear magnetic resonance (NMR). There are at least two types of spatially resolved NMR equipment that will have applications in toxicology. One takes spectra at selected points in the sample (topical NMR); the other maps out the density of resonant nuclear spin in one, two or three dimensions (imaging NMR).

Exposure to inhaled chemicals often gives rise to lung oedema because of irritation or cardiovascular failure, and often gives rise to density changes because of pulmonary fibrosis or emphysema. The recognition of such changes at present involves the destruction of the tissues at the end of exposure for lung weights and histopathology to be undertaken. NMR spin imaging, however, already shows promise in providing a non-destructive quantitative measurement of the development of lung oedema in experimental animals, and a means of quantifying regional differences in their lungs[8]. Topical NMR holds even greater promise, not only in inhalation toxicology but in all areas of toxicology, in that it will be capable of being used to measure chemical uptake and metabolism in specific organs without destruction or sampling, or interfering with the animal in any way. NMR is still a long way from becoming a workable technique for small animal toxicology, particularly in the provision of rodent-sized magnets, but development is proceeding at such a pace that it can be predicted with confidence that NMR will revolutionize experimental toxicology over the next 10 years.

SPECIAL TESTS

The majority of inhalation studies will continue to be conventional assessments of chemicals in animal models based on the assumption that all the human population exposed to the chemical are the same. But there are several areas where present-day conventional tests will not be sufficient to give adequate predictive safety evaluation, because it is known that the population at risk is not all the same.

One such area is the increased susceptibility to lung cancer of asbestos workers and uranium miners who also smoke cigarettes. Since it is unreasonable to expect that the half of the working population who smoke cigarettes will cease over the next 15 years, inhalation toxicology will have to pay some attention to the synergistic effects of cigarette smoking on other inhaled chemicals. The technology for exposing experimental animals to fresh cigarette smoke is already well validated; what is lacking is the recognition that there could be very real industrial or environmental problems.

A particularly potent synergism is known to result from exposure to mixtures of irritant gases and adsorptive environmental particulates such as soot. The role of such inert particulate matter in facilitating the penetration of gaseous environmental chemicals to the alveoli, and so enhancing their toxicity, will have to be given more serious consideration in the future.

A proportion of the cigarette-smoking working population also suffers from chronic obstructive bronchopulmonary diseases such as bronchitis and pulmonary oedema, as well as other temporary respiratory infections. The question will have to be asked if the results of inhalation studies in specific-pathogen-free rodents are really applicable to those whose respiratory defences are compromised by disease.

Not only is the working population not homogeneous with

regard to cigarette smoking or respiratory disease, but there are known to be subgroups with genetically determined differences in their responses to inhaled chemicals. The most obvious examples are α_1 antitrypsin deficiency predisposing to emphysema, and cystic fibrosis predisposing to acute and chronic respiratory infections. Undoubtedly, many other subgroups will be identified in the future, posing the dilemma of either developing appropriate animal models and testing for everything, or screening out susceptible workers.

One must hope that within the next 15 years the methodology for predicting respiratory sensitization to industrial chemicals will improve.

HUMAN EXPOSURES

Human exposures have always been undertaken in the development of new drugs, but only rarely in the development of new industrial or agricultural chemicals. The reason is obvious; drugs are intended to be taken by man, whereas industrial chemicals are, in general, intended not to be taken. However, since some exposure of workers or consumers is almost always possible, and since there is growing evidence of differences in susceptibility to toxic chemicals between individuals, the pressures for some form of biomedical monitoring will mount.

This could take two forms: development monitoring to identify the metabolic and pharmacokinetic differences between animals and man so that the most suitable experimental species could be used for extended toxicity tests, and biomedical screening to identify workers susceptible to the effects of particular chemicals. Both areas will be greatly influenced by the development of increasingly sensitive and selective analytical and immunological methods.

The use of man as an experimental species for the toxicological evaluation of industrial and agricultural chemicals will be influenced by the ethical and legal considerations pertaining in future years. It is difficult to predict how society will come to view these aspects, but if there is to be a move away from experimental animals, and the in vitro alternatives are inadequate, the only place to move to is man himself.

ALTERNATIVES TO ANIMALS

As with all areas of conventional toxicology there is a moral, practical and economic case to be made for the use of alternatives to live animals in inhalation toxicology. Indeed, because inhalation toxicology is the most technically complex, difficult and expensive area of all toxicology, the practical and financial pressures towards the use of alternatives are most pronounced. But there are important considerations in the search for alternatives. Since there is no alternative to breathing, and since the public demands greater safety with chemicals in the home, workplace and environment, there can be no compromise of reduced standards in the testing of chemicals for their inhalation toxicity. Any alternatives will have to give information at least as good as that provided by existing animal-based methods. The paradox is that, in validating the alternatives, more animals will be used in the short term in order to reduce the number of animals used in the long term. Validation will be the key to the acceptance of alternatives by professional, practising toxicologists and legislators. Many other methods have been developed, validated with a selected group of favourable chemicals and widely publicized as the panacea of the ills of animal toxicology. Unfortunately, general industrial chemicals do not conform to neat chemical types that are either water-soluble or oil-soluble, and the tests are often found to be of little use in the real world of industrial toxicology. A great deal of time and effort, and many animals, could be saved if there was an agreed list of typical industrial chemicals that could be used by those seeking to develop and validate alternatives.

Specific in vitro alternatives to animal inhalation studies are few and far between. Promising techniques that may be further developed over the next few years include the mouse peritoneal macrophage test for screening for lung fibrogenicity, and the use of cultured human fetal lung and tracheal explants[9]. Cell lines and short-term cell and organ cultures for use in lung toxicology have the limitations of all such techniques, in that the methodology for the isolation and maintenance of relatively pure populations of differentiated cells needs considerable further development.

The future for alternatives to whole-animal studies in inhalation toxicology does not seem too auspicious. The lungs are not only an organ of ventilation, but an organ of synthesis, release and degradation of many biological mediators, and an organ possessing a wide range of metabolic enzymes. The integration of these functions in ways not yet fully understood, and the paucity of knowledge of the underlying changes in many of the disease processes in the lungs, generally precludes the isolation of specific factors for an in vitro model development. Alternatives will probably be confined to empirical tests for screening large numbers of certain classes of chemicals causing certain types of specific lung diseases, rather than as complete substitutes for animal inhalation studies.

CONCLUSIONS

One thing that can be predicted with absolute certainty is that the cost of conducting inhalation studies will increase year by year. The increasing complexity and sophistication of the apparatus needed to generate and analyse atmospheres, and the increasing demands on the skills of the inhalation biologist in measuring toxic changes, will lead to greater specialization by the scientists in the inhalation team. The complexity and uniqueness of the apparatus, and the specialization of the scientists, will have important consequences for the future. To justify the massive outlay of capital to equip and run an inhalation laboratory to keep the experts expert and the standards high, will require a continuous throughput of chemicals for evaluation. Many laboratories will not have the throughput necessary to achieve the economy of scale, and decisions will have to be made as to whether they are wholeheartedly in the business of inhalation toxicology or not. There can be no half-way stage. Many companies will simply opt out of in-house inhalation toxicology completely, and will instead rely on specialist contract laboratories.

The inhalation laboratories that do survive to the year 2000 will be much more sophisticated than today. A wide range of screening tests will be used to select the chemicals to be assessed in the most appropriate experimental species. The traditional concept of a 2-year inhalation study in rats and mice will have been abandoned as a general-purpose model, to be replaced by a series of 3- to 6-month studies designed to elucidate the mode of action of the chemical using a battery of non-invasive functional studies. Selected species will be used to study particular facets of the chemical's toxicity.

The present purpose of the 2-year inhalation study - that of determining the carcinogenic potential of the chemical - will have been superseded by in vitro studies. Reliable short-term predictive tests using tissue culture to identify the neoplastic changes will have been developed following the characterization of the critical changes in chemical carcinogenesis at the gene/DNA level.

Over 30 years ago John Barnes[10] wrote:

The measurement of a toxic hazard can be properly based only on some knowledge of the fate and behaviour of a compound after its introduction into the body. A study of the absorption, distribution and elimination of a compound might take longer and prove more exacting than a routine feeding test. But such work could lead logically to biochemical and physiological studies. This approach would be scientific in contrast to the empirical method of chronic toxicity tests.

Is it too much to hope that the next 15 years will see the realization of this dream?

REFERENCES

1. Drew, RT (ed.) (1981). Proceedings of a workshop on inhalation chamber technology. Brookhaven National Laboratory, Formal Report No. 51318, Upton, New York
2. Leong, BKJ (ed.) (1981). Inhalation Toxicology and Technology. (Ann Arbor, MI: Ann Arbor Science Publishers)
3. MacFarland, HN (1983). Designs and operational characteristics of inhalation exposure equipment - a review. Fundam Appl Toxicol, 3, 603-13
4. Phalen, RF (1984). Inhalation Studies: Foundations and Techniques. (Boca Raton, FL: CRC Press)
5. Phalen, RF, Mannix, RC and Drew, RT (1984). Inhalation exposure methodology. Environ Health Perspect, 56, 23-34
6. Willeke, K (ed.) (1980). Generation of Aerosols and Facilities for Exposure Experiments. (Ann Arbor, MI: Ann Arbor

Science Publishers)

7. Witsch, H and Nettesheim, P (eds) (1982). Mechanisms in Respiratory Toxicology. Vols. I and II. (Boca Raton, FL: CRC Press)

8. Ailion, DC, Case, TA, Blatter, DD, Morris, AM, Cutillo, AG, Durney, CH and Johnson, SA (1984). Bull Magnetic Resonance, 6, 130-9

9. Brown, RC, Chamberlain, M, Davies, R and Gormley, IP (eds) (1980). The in vitro Effects of Mineral Dusts. (London: Academic Press)

10. Barnes, JM and Denz, FA (1954). Experimental methods used in determining chronic toxicity. A critical review. Pharmacol Rev, 6, 191-242

6

Testing For Reproductive Toxicity

A. B. G. LANSDOWN

INTRODUCTION

As the human diet changes, improved drugs are introduced and new methods are developed for agriculture, so thousands of new chemical compounds are introduced into the human environment. An element of hazard will accompany the use of many of these compounds, either through direct exposure or through complex food chains. In each case the nature of the hazard and its severity will depend upon the type and duration of the exposure. In the past few decades many new procedures have been adopted or advocated by legislative authorities and others in an attempt to identify potential hazards associated with environmental chemicals, thereby enabling appropriate precautions to be taken; these relate to reproductive as well as to other hazards.

In reproductive toxicology, as in other branches of the subject, the pattern of predictive safety evaluation adopted today has been precipitated by real-life problems. These have included the tragedies associated with the hypnotic drug thalidomide, and organic mercurial compounds (Minamata disease), in which deformed children were born to mothers who had inadvertently consumed the drug or ingested organic mercurials at critical stages in gestation.

The history of reproductive toxicology is coloured by many memorable observations dating from earliest times. Bizarre abnormalities involving human beings and domestic animals are depicted on the wall paintings of the ancient Babylonians and Egyptians, records have been seen from the Middle Ages and - until relatively recent times - their aetiology was attributed to the action of demons, curses or even acts of God. Man seems also to have been deeply concerned since the dawn of history with factors that could adversely affect - or correct - infertility and potency.

Although the thalidomide experience was undoubtedly the most significant event to influence present thoughts on reproductive toxicity evaluation, one may reflect upon the classical studies of Etienne Geoffrey de Saint-Hilaire[1] and his son in the early nineteenth century. The Saint-Hilaires induced anencephaly and spina bifida in chick embryos by shaking the eggs or by partly

77

coating the shells with an impervious material. Later they studied some human malformations and coined the term "teratology" to describe the study of monstrosities.

The application of embryological principles to teratology came at an even earlier stage. William Harvey[2] is reputed to have noticed that harelip, which occurs occasionally in malformed children, resembles a condition that is seen normally at an earlier stage in development. Thus, to Harvey, harelip represented a state of "arrested growth", a hypothesis that has been employed subsequently to explain the origin of such abnormalities as cleft palate, ectopia cordis and gastroschisis.

In the emergence of reproductive toxicology as a separate subject, much emphasis has been laid upon the incidence and severity of structural and functional defects in the offspring of mothers exposed to specific drugs or environmental agents during sensitive stages in gestation. However, evidence of infertility and reproductive failure in men following occupational exposure to lead, chronic alcoholism and possibly other environmental factors (kepone, methoxychlor, PCB, cadmium) emphasizes that, in predictive safety evaluation studies, experiments should not only embrace the period of intrauterine growth but should also take into account the influence of the test compound upon any aspect of reproduction. This should include a wide range of direct and indirect effects, since in mammals the whole organism becomes attuned physiologically, psychologically and structurally to the process of reproduction. Realistically, in such a broad safety evaluation, investigators should examine also the influence of test compounds upon the functional capacity of germ cells, motility and fertilizing potential (males), hormonal profiles and oestrus cycles (females) and the relevant behaviour of both sexes and of the offspring.

In recent years interest has increased in the study of nutritional factors, drugs and exposure to adverse environmental factors and their effects in late pregnancy. At these later stages most organogenetic events are in an advanced stage, but organs such as the heart, lung and brain are undergoing essential phases of "functional development". The fetal brain is particularly vulnerable to nutritional deprivation and to generalized fetal growth retardation during the stage known as the "brain growth spurt". Irreversible damage may result, which is appreciated post-natally as mental retardation etc.[3-5]. The prospect of catch-up growth occurring during post-natal development has been studied clinically and experimentally in many institutes. Behavioural teratology is a specialized study, and one which is becoming increasingly important.

An association between congenital abnormalities and neoplasms has been postulated, although there is no concurrence of malformations and tumours in man. Bolande[6] considered that teratogenesis and carcinogenesis were intimately related, and that teratogenesis was a more primitive response to chemically induced mutagenic injury. The two processes are almost certainly distinct[7], although such teratogenic agents as cadmium ion, X-irradiation, synthetic oestrogens and nitrosamines are also recognized carcinogens under appropriate conditions. Well known teratogens - including salicylates, thalidomide and some pesticides and food additives - are not presently known to be capable of inducing neoplastic changes. Prospectively, it is likely that tests will be developed to study the ability of exogenous chemicals to induce neoplastic changes in utero and the capacity of these changes to progress or regress postnatally.

The reproductive process in mammals is a complex process embracing a wide spectrum of events, each exhibiting its own peak of sensitivity to extrinsic factors. In a rational predictive safety evaluation programme it is essential to achieve a broad understanding of normal patterns of embryological and embryophysiological development and an appreciation of the fundamental mechanisms and pathogenesis of the common birth defects. In most regulatory-style experiments, authorities such as the Committee for the Safety of Medicines (UK), the Food and Drug Administration (US), ECETOC and the safety committees for many other countries tend to be concerned more about whether a particular test compound exhibits any positive evidence of toxicity in the reproductive process and under what conditions. Even so, a vast range of mechanistic studies has been conducted with well-known agents such as alcohol, rubella virus, X-irradiation, thalidomide, salicylates and trypan blue, all of which exhibit marked effects at one or more stages in the reproductive process in the human and/or sub-human species. These studies have proved beneficial in identifying sensitive stages during gestation and other information used in the design of methods currently adopted.

It is anticipated that, as the results of further basic research come to hand, so they will be incorporated in the design of sensitive tests which hopefully will provide the basis of future predictive studies.

It is perhaps inevitable, in view of the overwhelming significance of the thalidomide episodes in strengthening or developing legislation and codes of practice, that the official mind, the sponsor of the compound under test and even some investigators have concentrated their attention upon malformations or birth defects. Such concentration reflects public apprehension, and is largely emotive, although sponsors have to consider what tests are likely to be required or requested by the regulatory authorities - and are usually reluctant to go beyond this. It reflects the human tendency, already mentioned, to overestimate risks from rare or bizarre events.

It may reasonably be argued that emphasis upon birth defects has overshadowed the investigation of other adverse or potentially adverse effects of foreign compounds upon reproduction. In reality birth defects, although distressing, are among the least likely hazards to reproduction of a compound under test - but the proportion of effort put into assessing them is remarkably high - and has probably hindered lack of progress into the other aspects of reproductive toxicology.

Nevertheless there has to be acknowledgement of the public, political and commercial concern over the essentially teratological aspects of reproductive toxicity, to which much of this chapter is therefore devoted.

PRINCIPLES OF REPRODUCTIVE TOXICITY AND TERATOGENESIS

The entire mammalian organism is committed to the process of reproduction, which can therefore be affected indirectly as well as directly. Specifically, the reproductive process in mammals includes germ cell production and maturation in the parental generation, fertilization, conception and intrauterine growth of the offspring, and parturition and development after birth. In each case normal development depends upon the viability of the genotype and appropriate genetical instructions for morphogenic events. Constituent cells in the embryo/fetus will undergo a programmed sequence of cytodifferentiation, metabolic and functional changes, migration and even death in achieving normal organogenic events. Within a species these developmental patterns may show small variations, but for a particular strain or species these will fall within the "expected range". Small and subtle deviations in development are documented for most strains of laboratory animals commonly employed in reproductive studies.

Reproductive toxicology embodies several basic toxicological principles but also involves some specialized approaches and expertise. The period of intrauterine growth represents a highly vulnerable stage in development when the offspring are particularly sensitive to the toxic effects of exogenous agents, nutritional changes in the mother and adverse environmental physical factors. Maternal illness, inappropriate choice of drugs, hypoxia and hyperthermia have been implicated variously in reproductive failure, defective fetal development and reduced postnatal survival[8,9]. Epidemiological evidence suggests that up to 80% of human conceptions abort, and that at least 6% of live births are complicated by some structural or functional defect. Estimates of the frequency of these abnormalities vary greatly on account of the wide racial, socioeconomic and geographic variations in population studies. Statistics are also complicated by difficulties arising in the definition of "what constitutes an abnormality". The identification of minor deviations in human development is a further problem. In early fetal mortality and stillbirth it is quite likely that an undiagnosed deformity is present, possibly reflecting a mutagenic or functional defect.

Defects in reproductive performance may be due to genetic or environmentally induced damage in germ cell production, alteration in physiological factors, disease processes in male or female partner, or through immunological factors. In controlled laboratory experiments conducted under defined conditions most of these variables may be eliminated, such that the true influence of an environmental compound acting on a particular stage in the reproductive cycle can be assessed accurately.

In teratological studies, six general principles apply, each being supported by abundant clinical and experimental evidence[10] (Table 6.1). Some aspects of the scheme are discussed more fully below. As a generalization, the susceptibility of embryonic tissues to deformation or damage relates largely to the nature of the exogenous influence and its pharmacological influence on differentiating tissues at the time of exposure. In the embryo, each tissue system seems to possess a stage of critical sensitivity outside which it exhibits little or no response. In the case of the rat embryo exposed to trypan blue, dye accumulated in the lysosomes of the yolk sac endoderm leading to an impairment in fetal nutrition, and deformities. At later stages, when the function of the yolk sac placenta is superseded by the chorioallantoic placenta, trypan blue exerts minimal effect on fetal development[11]. Stockard[12] recognized these critical phases of development, which he indicated may occur at any stage from conception to birth and may involve functional or morphological parameters.

Table 6.1 General principles of teratogenicity

---

1. Susceptibility of a conceptus to a teratogenic agent depends upon its genotype and the manner in which this interacts with the environmental factor.

2. The susceptibility of a conceptus to a teratogenic agent relates closely to the developmental stage at the time of exposure.

3. Teratogenic influences act upon susceptible cells and tissues in the fetus by specific mechanisms to induce deviant development.

4. Manifestations of deviant development include growth retardation, structural deformities, functional disorders and mortality.

5. The influence of a teratogenic agent upon sensitive fetal tissues depends upon the nature of the agent and the route by which exposure occurs.

6. Manifestations of deviant development increase in degree as the dose levels of the teratogenic agent increase. They range from a no-effect threshold to a totally lethal effect.

Distinction should be made between the terms "embryo" and "fetus", with the corresponding adjectives. Although the distinction is not absolute, "embryonic" relates to period of differentiation of organ systems, and at this stage failure to differentiate results in malformation. At the fetal stage the main organs are formed, with differentiation at the cellular level, and failure leads to pathological changes or deformation. In humans, the embryonic stage lasts until day 58.

The genetic make-up of a conceptus is the setting in which teratogenesis occurs; genetic and extrinsic factors interact to varying degrees to initiate developmental abnormality. Responses range from embryolethality to no-effect, depending upon the teratogen and species of animal involved. Experience with such drugs as thalidomide, salicylate and anti-cancer agents has shown that the dose causing maternal toxicity is an unreliable guide to the level required to induce fetal deformity. Thalidomide exhibits a very low toxicity threshold in mothers but is highly teratogenic to the fetus at low concentrations. In contrast, the teratogenic dose of sodium salicylate in rats at least closely approaches that causing maternal toxicity[13]. Many examples exist to illustrate ways in which the mother exerts a protective effect against teratogenic influences. This is particularly true in the case of nutritional deficiencies. In the case of drugs, compounds are possible detoxified in the maternal liver. The placenta may act as a barrier for some toxic agents and infections (influenza virus). Occasionally, as in the case of cadmium and lead ions which are strongly teratogenic in rodents if they enter the circulation, substances ingested with the diet are poorly absorbed from the maternal gastrointestinal tract[14-16].

EPIDEMIOLOGICAL AND EXPERIMENTAL ASPECTS

The strongest evidence that a particular chemical or environmental condition is injurious to human reproduction is provided by large-scale population studies such as those conducted in Japan and Iraq in relation to accidental methyl mercury poisoning[17,18]. Chronic maternal alcoholism, rubella virus infection, ionizing radiation and exposure to drugs (thalidomide, warfarin) are further examples of teratogenicity and reproductive failure where irrefutable clinical evidence exists.

Occasionally, clinical studies suggesting that a particular agent or condition is responsible for increased numbers of stillbirths, congenital deformities and reproductive failures are equivocal. One such example concerned the potential teratogenic risks posed by trace levels of anaesthetic gases to pregnant nurses and other personnel working in hospital operating theatres[19,20]. These and other workers failed to identify a clear cause-effect relationship or to establish threshold levels of halothane, nitrous oxide or other gas necessary to cause toxic symptoms. Subsequent studies in which pregnant rats were exposed to high sub-anaesthetic levels of single or combinations of more than one gas failed to confirm teratogenicity[21-23]. Animals were exposed at periods of gestation, at which maximum teratogenicity occurs with other teratogens. Where embryofetal growth retardation was evident this was attributed to reduced food consumption through anaesthetic-induced drowsiness. It must be appreciated, however, that in such circumstances energy requirements are likely to be less. Although it would be unwise to extrapolate these observations in terms of a no-effect in humans without further wide-ranging trials, possibly employing other species, it is conceivable that the problems identified in the human cases resulted from a complex interaction of many factors, e.g. stress, tiredness.

Many examples exist of clinical evidence that a substance or environmental condition causes reproductive distress or teratogenicity where the results have be confirmed experimentally, e.g. thalidomide, salicylates, hypoxia, hyperthermia and various nutritional imbalances. Occasionally, however, reproductive or teratogenic risks identified through accurate clinical observations have not been reproduced under experimental conditions. Perhaps the best-known of these is the rubella syndrome, in relation to which studies have been conducted using a wide variety of laboratory animals, including sub-human primates. Although some congenital deformities have been produced resembling those produced by rubella infection in man, viraemia has not been recorded on many occasions and the true rubella syndrome of congenital heart disease, abortion, cataract and other changes has not been reproduced[8].

In the main, experiments currently designed to demonstrate teratogenicity or reproductive toxicity tend to be prospective rather than retrospective in outlook. It is hoped that, as a consequence of the experience gained in the past 35 years, the vast proportion of hazards presently in the environment or in permitted drug lists will be appreciated, and recommendations made accordingly. In the years ahead, through nationally and internationally controlled safety evaluation procedures, it is to be hoped that most hazards among new drugs, food additives, industrial processes and agricultural preparations would be identified before the human risk were encountered.

LEGISLATIVE REQUIREMENTS FOR REPRODUCTIVE TOXICITY TESTING

Reproductive toxicity is defined as that part of general toxicity dealing with the adverse effects produced by exogenous agents on the reproductive process[24]. Agents may act at any time during the reproductive cycle to impair fertility, prenatal or postnatal development. Teratogenicity represents a specific module within this framework and relates only to the effects of test chemicals on fetal growth and their ability to induce malformations recognizable at birth or at later stages, e.g. metabolic, cardiovascular, endocrine or central nervous system defects.

Early reproductive toxicity studies were conducted only on food additives, pesticides and agents for which exposure over several generations was expected. The test commonly used then was the two-litter test, where animals were dosed from before mating and through two complete cycles of mating, pregnancy and lactation. Studies would also be conducted on products which were likely to be administered to women of childbearing age. Toxicity was assessed on the basis of reduced levels of conception, litter size and postnatal viability. Although thalidomide was active in all three parameters, teratogenicity was not suspected.

The two-litter test failed to identify the teratogenicity of thalidomide, probably because repeated administration increased the effective "dosage" to such an extent that the embryos were killed rather than malformed[25]. The ability of thalidomide to induce limb and other deformities in babies following administration to pregnant mothers in the first 3 months of pregnancy was recognized by Lenz[26] in Hamburg and McBride[27] in Australia in the early 1960s. Since that time there has been a dramatic re-appraisal of reproductive safety evaluation requirements in the preclinical testing of new drugs, and various guidelines have been revised periodically as new information has come to hand.

The publication of "Guidelines for Reproductive Studies for

the Safety Evaluation of Drugs for Human Use", by the Food and Drug Administration (FDA) of the USA[28] is the basis of most of the predictive safety evaluation studies conducted presently. The recommendations are for single-generation studies for the evaluation of drugs and chemicals ingested by man over short periods or having short half-lives in the body. On the other hand, drugs used in long-term therapy, pesticides and food additives, which might be expected to concentrate in the body or which might be consumed over several generations, would be tested in multi-generation studies. These have often extended over three generations, but this is now generally regarded as unnecessary; two being sufficient.

Single-generation studies

The single-generation studies recommended under the FDA (1966) documents are more commonly known as the "three segment studies", on account of their provision for separate fertility studies with general reproductive performance (Segment 1), embryotoxicity and teratogenicity (Segment 2), and peri- and postnatal development (Segment 3) modules.

Experiments conducted under Segment 1 provide an overall insight of the potential risks involved with a test compound without identifying its target tissue or mechanism of action. Animals (rats or mice) are dosed for a sufficient time before mating to reveal effects on gametogenesis, through mating and gestation and to the end of lactation and weaning. Sacrifice of half of the females midway through gestation allows an investigator to assess effects on conception and fetal survival. Comparison of the number of corpora lutea in each ovary and conceptions in corresponding uterine horns allows pre-implantation loss to be assessed. It has sometimes been the case that, if non-pregnancy is diagnosed at this stage, a study will be terminated and repeated using lower dose levels. It would be more appropriate, however, to attempt to assess the results from sacrificed and reared litters and to design an experiment to find out why non-pregnancy occurred.

Segment 2 is sometimes termed the teratogenicity phase, since it seeks to examine the influence of a test compound upon post-implantation development, but it covers broader aspects such as embryolethality and altered growth. Rats, mice and rabbits are used, pregnant animals being dosed throughout the period of most active organogenesis. Experience with a wide variety of teratogens, drugs, viruses, X-irradiation and adverse environmental conditions has shown that highest rates of malformations occur when dosing is during this time. Dosing at earlier stages may lead to increased embryonic loss. Experiments are terminated shortly before delivery and parturition. This avoids the loss of deformed or dead offspring through maternal cannibalism. External examination of fetuses is made with the aid of a hand lens, and detailed examination for skeletal and soft tissue defects is mandatory.

Segment 3 of the single-generation studies for perinatal and postnatal effects is designed to evaluate the influence of a test compound upon later stages of fetal development, parturition and early postnatal development. Again the rat, mouse or rabbit are permissible species. Dosing is recommended during the latter third of gestation and through lactation and weaning. The main advantages of the perinatal and postnatal dosing study are that an investigator can determine the influence of a test compound upon the functional development of fetal organs such as the heart, lungs and brain. The scope of the recommended test may allow an appreciation of changes which would not be detected under Segment 1 or 2 recommendations. Behavioural and functional tests are conducted at the discretion of investigating scientists.

Where administration of a test compound to a pregnant animal leads to its excretion in the milk, the Segment 3 study will show this additional toxicity threshold. Progeny will be observed for:

1.   effects resulting from transplacental exposure,

2.   effects due to exposure through milk.

Segment 3 tests will also provide information concerning the ability of a test compound to impair the lactation and maternal behaviour of treated mothers. They will also indicate effects upon parturition, shown for example by all anti-inflammatory agents.

The basic three-module design for reproductive toxicity and teratogenicity has been criticized on the basis that it is inadequate in identifying the effects of test compounds upon fertility and reproductive performance[29]. Regulatory authorities in Great Britain and in the EEC recommend that there sometimes may be an advantage in conducting separate male and female fertility studies in Segment 1, with treated males being mated with untreated females and vice-versa. The modification allows a clearer appreciation of toxicity for a test substance than the FDA Guidelines permit. However, Palmer considered that the justification for this occurred with less than 1% of test compounds.

Multi-generation studies

Multi-generation studies are not always necessary, on account of the nature of a test compound and its anticipated usage. They are conducted where prolonged exposure in the human environment is envisaged[30]. They formerly often extended over three generations, which was time-consuming and costly, but today two generations are regarded as sufficient. In each case successive generations are examined for litter size, normality of the progeny and general reproductive capacity. For scientific and economic reasons, rats and mice are usually used. A proportion of offspring (50%) of each generation is sacrificed and examined macroscopically and histologically for abnormalities. The tests are modified by the different regulatory authorities, but these modifications generally apply to the number of animals in each test group and to specifications for sacrifice and evaluation of the toxicity.

Additional studies

Guidelines published by the various regulatory authorities for reproductive toxicity and teratogenicity are specific in their requirements, i.e. in the species to be used, the dosing period and the means of evaluation of toxicity. However, it is appreciated that the costs involved in conducting the entire spectrum of studies in intact animals can be prohibitively expensive. As a consequence, bodies such as ECETOC[24] encourage the development of short-term assays such as:

1.   male fertility and spermatozoal morphology tests,

2.   female fertility and toxic changes in oestrous cycles,

3.   in vitro tests for embryotoxicity,

4.   dominant lethal assay tests for mutagenicity.

Specific recommendations are not yet available for these tests. They are regarded as desirable on account of the reduced number of animals required, although this is not necessarily the case. Indeed, more animals may ultimately be required because of failure to recognize the integrated nature of the reproductive process, which may lead to lack of concordance between different aspects, human error and the need to do additional studies to tidy up loose ends. They also have the advantage in that they provide specific information in a shorter time than is possible with the more conventional approach described above.

The ECETOC[24] document considers that more emphasis should be placed upon developing and validating short-term assays for predicting toxicity in reproductive processes. It is anticipated also that, in due course, the tests will be harmonized by international authorities such as the Organisation of Economic Co-operation and Development (OECD).

MECHANISMS OF REPRODUCTIVE
TOXICITY AND TERATOGENICITY

Agents in the environment may adversely influence reproduction in the human and other species by their toxic action at any time from germ cell production and maturation in the parental generation to postnatal growth and development in the offspring. This toxicity may involve a specific stage in the reproductive cycle or be of a more general type. For simplicity, it is preferable to consider the action of the various agents according to whether they act directly or otherwise on germ cell production and reproductive performance in male or female parent, or alternatively are toxic in some way to postconceptional development of the progeny. It is recognized that normal development in the progeny either prenatally or postnatally depends upon the viability of the genotype and the way in which this interacts with its environment.

The role of detoxication and metabolic activation has been

reviewed by Parke[31].

Germ cell production and general reproductive performance

A wide range of exogenous agents including viral infections, metal ions, alcohol, anti-cancer and anti-viral drugs, pesticides and food additives may impair spermatogenesis leading to reduced reproductive capacity and perhaps to sterility in the long term. On occasions, defects in spermatozoal morphology have been linked with metabolic, functional and structural abnormalities in the surviving progeny, with perhaps doubtful validity. The action of the test compound in the male or female partner, leading to hormonal imbalances and to disturbances in reproductive cycles or in the movement of ova or spermatozoa, is a potential cause of reproductive failure. The changes may be recognized as a loss of libido in the male - difficult to evaluate in animals - and a depression of sexual activity in the female.

Reproductive activity may be depressed in event of ill-health. This frequently leads to altered physiological and endocrinological activity. It occurs with infections such as cytomegalovirus and several of the enteroviruses, conditions which are acknowledged causes of impaired development. Reproduction is inevitably linked with the overall physiological and psychological status of the adults, so that - as already indicated - reproduction may be affected indirectly.

Teratogenesis

Environmental agents may impair fetal development either by their toxic action in susceptible tissue or organ systems or through their detrimental action upon the health and nutritional state of the pregnant mother. By this latter mechanism, fetal growth is disturbed through imbalances in the intrauterine environment or through the non-availability of materials essential for optimal growth. The mother is unable to satisfy the physiological demands of her offspring.

In view of the extreme diversity of environmental agents capable of impairing fetal growth in one or more species, it is clearly impracticable to attempt to formulate a unifying hypothesis to explain the ways in which developmental abnormalities arise. For present purposes a simplified scheme is proposed where specific levels of toxic action are identified. In each case the text will be illustrated by research studies in specific chemical or genetically determined conditions. The scheme envisaged (Table 6.2) recognizes the cell as the main functional unit and identifies four principal routes of action[32]. This represents a considerable simplification of the mechanisms for abnormal development suggested by Wilson[33], who considered that it is possible to delineate up to ten possible ways in which sensitive tissues respond to toxic insults. In the present discussion it is recognized that cell sensitivity varies according to generative phase and to the gestational age of the individual.

Table 6.2 Levels of action of environmental agents in cells of the developing embryo/fetus

1.	INTRACELLULAR COMPARTMENT	
	(a) Nucleus	Mutagenesis Chromosomal damage Mitotic inhibition Impaired DNA synthesis
	(b) Cytoplasm	Defects in enzymic pathways and biomolecular syntheses
2.	CELL MEMBRANE	Defects in intercellular communication, recognition, induction, migration
3.	EXTRACELLULAR MATRICES	Deformities in structure and function
4.	CELLULAR ENVIRONMENT	Nutritional and physical defects

The four-level model for teratogenesis allows for the fact that certain teratogens including metal ions, hypervitaminosis A and some drugs influence tissues to different degrees according to their developmental state, functional condition and activity. It does offer a broad framework within which to discuss mechanisms of deviant development, avoiding many of the controversies that have arisen over the importance of primary and secondary routes.

The intracellular compartment

Genetic or chromosomal damage is an expression of changes resulting from exposure to toxic agents capable of altering DNA structure. On occasions this may be difficult to distinguish from responses due to such factors as ageing, irradiation or ultraviolet light, all of which are capable of mutagenicity[34]. Chromosomal damage is more frequently seen in patients with cancer or congenital defects but the reverse is not invariably true. The incidence of defects in the newborn attributable to chromosomal damage is an indication of clastogenicity minus the rate of intrauterine death[35].

In the human race the relative contribution of genetic factors to congenital defects is not known. Approximately 5% of malformations are attributed to somatic mutations, 10% to chromosomal damage and 5% to identifiable causes in the environment[36]. The so-called "inborn errors of metabolism" are included here. The mutation is often reflected in terms of an enzymic deficiency affecting a specific metabolic pathway.

The contribution of genetic damage to teratogenesis and chemically induced fetal growth impairment has been discussed[36], but often the data for a particular group of chemicals are incomplete and the interpretations questionable. Studies conducted with a range of well-known organochlorine and organophosphorus pesticides are an illustration[37] (Table 6.3). In summary, the mutagenic potential of these agents was a good indication of their carcinogenic potential in the tests used, but not of their teratogenic activity. DDT, for example, caused chromosomal damage in mice and in two cell-culture systems; it induced dominant lethal mutations in rats and mice but was not teratogenic in either species. Strangely, DDT actually prolonged reproductive life in rats by up to 5 months, and afforded protection against the teratogenic effects of salicylates, Benlate and chloridine. It has been concluded from multi-generation studies in rats that aldrin, carbaryl, dieldrin and malathion lead to infertility when tested over three generations[37], although the experimental evidence has not been altogether convincing in every case.

More consistent evidence of teratogenicity is seen with those agents which impair DNA synthesis and mitotic activity at periods of high organogenesis. Ionizing radiation is a well-known cause of mutation in human patients and an acknowledged cause of congenital abnormalities[38-40]. Whole-body radiation leads to the widespread production of free radicals and is also regarded as a cause of mutation[37]. Mitotic arrest, cell death and impaired cell proliferation occur with milder teratogenic influences such as rubella infection, folate antagonists, cortisone and agents which inhibit the mitotic spindle (the stathmokinetic agents). Impaired cell division in any tissue is a potential cause of asynchronous growth, hypoplasia and possibly agenesis depending upon the susceptibility of the tissue at the time of exposure. Neural crest cells are particularly sensitive to the effects of purine and pyrimidine antimetabolites. These agents will induce exencephaly, ancephalocoele and spina bifida if they are administered to the pregnant mother at the stage of neural fold formation in the embryo.

Defective regulatory mechanisms are a further teratogenic manifestation of intracellular toxicity. Anomalies in cell migration, proliferation and intercellular communication occur. Naeye and Blanc[41] concluded that hypoplastic development in the offspring of mothers infected with rubella early in pregnancy contained a subnormal number of cells, probably due to a virus inhibition of cell proliferation. The organs had in fact failed to achieve the "critical mass" for the particular gestational age and subsequent events were delayed or absent.

Vitamin A is an amphiphilic compound which readily penetrates the cell membrane to cause mitochondrial swelling, release of lysosomal enzymes and inhibition of DNA synthesis. Impaired cell division and migration occurring at critical stages in the development of the cephalic mesoderm leads to derangements in the overlying neuroectoderm and the formation of exencephaly, and spina bifida[42]. Cell death, mitotic arrest and defective migration patterns probably underlie the micromelias, cleft palate and cardiovascular deformities associated with cortisone, cadmium ion, salicylates and possibly thalidomide[43-45].

Table 6.3

Insecticide	Toxicity		
	Mutagenicity	Teratogenicity	Fertility
DDT	+(1,5),-(2,3)	-(a,b)	-(***)
Aldrin	-(3)	+(a,b)	
Dieldrin	-(1,3,5,6)	+(a,b)	+(**)
Endrin		+(a,b)	
Kepone		+(a,b)	+(***)
Chlordane	-(5)	-(a)	-(***)
Heptachlor	-(3)		
Mirex	-(5)	+(a,b)	+(**),+(***)
Lindane	-(3)	-(a,b)	-(**),-(***)
Dichlorvos	+(1,3,8),-(5)		
Malathion	-(3)	+(a,b)	
Parathion		+(a,b)	
Carbaryl	+(1,3)	+(a,b)	+(***)
Diazinon	-(3)		
Captan	+(1,4)		
Nitroso-carbaryl	+(1,4)		

Key:
1. Chromosomal damage in vivo or in vitro
2. Unscheduled DNA-synthesis
3. AMES TEST
4. DNA Base pair substitution test
5. Dominant lethal assay (rats or mice)
6. Heritable translocation test
7. Chromosomal damage in human peripheral blood culture
8. Chromosomal damage in Drosophila sp. salivary gland
a   Embryotoxicity
b   Teratogenicity
**   Oestrus changes in dogs, rats and rabbits with or without pregnancy failure
*** Reduced fertility
Data from ref. 37

The several genetical deformities operating at the cellular level seem to involve deficiencies in cytoplasmic enzyme systems. Phenylketonuria, lysosomal alpha-L-iduronidase deficiency (Hurler's syndrome) and diabetes mellitus are examples. As a consequence of the various enzyme deficiencies, some metabolites reach toxic levels, whereas others exhibit defective or alternative patterns of biodegradation. The defects are manifest as fetal mortality or as structural, functional or behavioural abnormalities which are appreciated in the neonatal period.

The cell membrane

Fetal development involves a complex pattern of cell aggregation, morphogenetic movements and cell migration, all of which depend to some degree on the characteristics of the cell membrane, and the intercellular passage of essential nutrients and inducer substances. Much of this subject is very unclear and speculative. However, some interesting genetic and non-genetic models exist to illustrate how damage induced in the cell surface can adversely affect morphogenesis and functional development.
 The vertebrate limb, for example, involves extensive cellular interaction in development. The early limb bud exists as a finger-like projection of mesenchyme ensheathed in ectodermal tissue. The apical ridge of this ectoderm exhibits a profound influence on the morphogenetic patterns of skeletal structures within the mesenchyme[46,47]. Extirpation, reversal or injury to this ridge of ectoderm has been shown to cause marked abnormalities in the limb bud[48]. Proper nerve connection with the limbs depends upon the mechanism of membrane marker production for limited cycles. (Although a large number of teratological agents do adversely affect the development of the limb bud, the mechanisms are probably not specific for that tissue but form part of a more complex condition.)
 Cell death is an important event in the morphogenesis of a number of structures including the limb bud, kidney and palate. This means that any teratogen selectively altering morphogenic patterns of cell death is a potential cause of structural abnormality in that tissue. Janus Green B for example has been shown to inhibit the degeneration of the interdigital tissues in the development of the limb bud, syndactyly being the resulting deformity[49]. Involutionary changes characterize the development of the thymus and thyroid from branchial pouch primordia, and also the derivation of the pituitary gland from Rathke's pouch of stomodeal origin. Defects in the degeneration of these primitive tissues result in a persistence of the embryonic tissues into postnatal life as "embryonic rests" or hamartomata. Such changes are occasionally seen as part of the normal background pathology in laboratory rodents, but occur rarely in other species[50,51].
 Morphogenetic cell death has an important implication in the normal development of the mammalian palate. Palatal primordia develop in the lateral mesenchyme of the buccal region and migrate towards the midline, where fusion occurs following the degeneration of the intervening epithelial tissues. Defects in this degeneration process underlie the formation of cleft palate commonly associated with cortisone treatment in fetal mice. This may, however, be a consequence of impaired maternal nutrition, resulting in physical effects, e.g. alterations of angle of the head. Cleft palate may also be attributable to defects in mucopolysaccharide synthesis and cell

division[52]. Although hypervitaminosis A is also a cause of cleft palate in various species, the mechanism is probably complex, involving changes in mesenchymal cells and their interaction with tissues of ectodermal origin[42,53].

The synthesis and composition of the extracellular matrix

Many fetal tissues are characterized by an intercellular matrix of specific chemical composition. Probably the best-known example is the ground substance of cartilage and bone, which is frequently deformed or absent in fetuses from mothers exposed to teratogenic agents in early or mid-gestation. Skeletal abnormalities are seen where exogenous agents or genetical determinants adversely influence the synthesis and degradation of mucopolysaccharides of cartilage matrix. Achondroplasia, chondrodystrophy and chondrodysplasia are all well-known conditions affecting bone development in humans, cattle and laboratory animals[54].

Teratogens impair the biosynthesis of chondroitin sulphate and lead to defective cartilage formation and ossification patterns. An example is seen with sodium salicylate, which has been shown to inhibit the sulphation of the polysaccharide moiety in early cartilage development[13]. Deviant cartilage formation with hypertrophy of chondrocytes was shown to impair subsequent ossification patterns. Damage in the skull and spinal regions led to manifestations of exencephaly and spina bifida in affected fetuses. Micromelias were also common observations.

Tetracycline, hypervitaminosis A and cortisone exhibit a pronounced effect on skeletal development in many species. The mechanism is complex. However, tetracycline shows a particular affinity for calcium ion in intact fetuses and in cultured tissues. Impaired skeletal development in this case is attributed to a state of "non-availability" of essential micronutrients[55].

Collagen and elastic tissue are other examples of intercellular tissues which may be abnormal in teratogen-exposed fetuses. Abnormal collagen formation is seen in cattle with the hereditary disease, dermatosparaxis. Affected individuals exhibit defects in procollagen synthesis[56]. Lathyrogenic agents such as beta-aminopropionitrile inhibit procollagen peptidase activity and abnormalities involving vascular and skeletal tissues are seen experimentally. Nutritional copper deficiency is a further well-known condition affecting collagen development. It is probably that copper acts in some way in the cross-linking of collagen fibres.

The cellular environment

In accordance with Wilson's[10] six principles of teratogenicity, embryonic or embryofetal development is determined by the close interaction between the fetal genotype and its environment. This environment relates not only to the intrauterine medium which is intimately linked to the state of health of the mother, but also the intrafetal conditions. This latter aspect reflects fetal nutrition, intercellular ionic balances and physiological conditions.

Maternal metabolic diseases, malnutrition and abnormal environmental conditions (hypoxia, hyperthermia, etc.) are well-known causes of distress in human pregnancies and they have been examined experimentally in several animal models. Often, conditions such as these are expressed at the fetal level in terms of nutritional insufficiency. This may arise through defects in uteroplacental circulation or through the inability of the mother to metabolize nutrients essential for normal fetal growth. The influence of maternal ill-health in pregnancy is well documented in the medical press.

A further aspect of maternal ill-health that has been well discussed is the role of viral infection in pregnancy, especially with influenza, rubella and herpes viruses. With influenza virus at least, where infection of the conceptus does not occur, fetal deformities and mortality are probably largely due to fever (hyperthermia) in the mother[57]. The work has been conducted in a number of experimental animal models; the structural defects seen closely resembled those seen in infected mothers. Metabolic imbalances attributable to disease processes are a further possible explanation.

Coxsackievirus infection in mice leads to a profound exocrine pancreatic atrophy within 2 days of infection and, as a consequence, mothers become incapable of digesting dietary protein[58]. Labile reserves of protein accumulated in the maternal liver become depleted, with the result that fetal development is retarded and mortality increased[59]. The level of fetal effect seen correlated well with the stage in pregnancy at which the infection occurred[60]. Subsequent studies demonstrated that this fetal distress could be prevented using immunological means or by feeding the animals with a diet containing protein in a digested form (i.e. casein hydrolysate). Fetal development, as determined by macroscopic examination and by analysis of serum alpha-fetoprotein and albumin levels, was within normal limits for the species[61].

Nutritional causes of congenital deformity are well documented with reference to the serious problems encountered in developing countries. Protein and/or deficiency in specific amino acids is associated with a range of defects involving the development of skeletal, vascular and nervous systems. However, these deformities probably form part of a more generalized pattern of growth retardation attributable to mitotic inhibition[62]. Deficiencies in essential vitamins, minerals, fats and amino acids occurring through starvation, metabolic deficiencies or through the chemical action of toxic compounds in the diet are discussed in more detail elsewhere[63].

EXPERIMENTAL CONSIDERATIONS

Species

Many strains and species of laboratory animal have been used in reproductive studies, but a majority of regulatory studies has been conducted in the popular strains of rat, mouse and rabbit. More rarely dogs, ferrets and pigs have been employed as non-rodent species. Species selection has usually been based on the convenience of the animals under laboratory conditions, a detailed knowledge of their reproductive biology, and their sensitivity to known human teratogens. Although monkey species are closer phylogenetically to human beings, they exhibit a number of metabolic and behavioural differences so that rarely have they been shown more suitable than rabbits and rats, which are less expensive to use and do not require the same level of expertise for their husbandry and management.

Test compounds are frequently administered in the diet or dosed intragastrically as in anticipated human exposure. Interspecies variations exist in gastrointestinal absorption of exogenous materials due to differences in gastric acidity, intestinal flora, metabolizing enzymes and in the characteristics of the mucosal surfaces. Preliminary studies are profitably conducted to examine this feature, since with many teratogens a close relationship has been stated between the level of agent in the maternal circulation and the fetal response. There may sometimes, however, be pronounced differences between plasma concentrations of the test substance levels in the conceptus according to the time of pregnancy. The rate at which a test compound is metabolized also has a marked bearing on levels of teratogenicity. Alcohol, for example, is metabolized more slowly in man than in the rat, and is appreciably more toxic. In contrast, imipramine is voided more slowly in rabbits and rodents than in man[64].

The reproductive biology and fetal development of rats and mice is well known, making them the choice species for many types of toxicity experiment[65]. Rats are the most commonly used, and were employed in the early two-litter test which preceded current predictive tests. Their use as the sole test species was limited on account of their lower sensitivity to thalidomide, and the rabbit is currently the main species for teratological studies, although even for these the rat and mouse are routinely adopted as second species. Rats - and mice infrequently - are regularly used in long-term and multi-generation studies[66].

The value of mice is limited in some teratological studies on account of their known susceptibility to "spontaneous" cleft palate[67]. This feature has, however, been used to advantage in demonstrating the interaction between environmental and genetical determinants of abnormality[68,69].

The sensitivity of the rabbit fetus to thalidomide-induced deformities is well known[70], but other features that make it a choice animal in teratogenicity studies include its spontaneous ovulation pattern and comparatively large size[71]. The rate of spontaneous malformations in the rabbit is slightly higher than in rodents but this is not deemed to be a serious disadvantage. In each study an increased number of abnormalities in test animals will be evidence of teratogenicity[72].

The ferret has been recommended as a non-rodent for teratological studies; it is a small carnivore and may offer advantages over other species[73]. At present its use is limited by the lack of background data and information on its sensitivity to known teratogens. In contrast, another rodent, the hamster, has been widely employed in a wide range of investigative experimental studies[74]. It is susceptible to many teratogens, is conveniently kept as a laboratory animal and has a comparatively short gestational period (16 days). It is difficult to dose intravenously.

The between-species difference in the case of the effect of corticosteroid drugs has not always been taken into account in routine teratological investigations. These steroids almost invariably produce teratogenic effects in rodents and lagomorphs, even in doses as low as those comparable with the human therapeutic regime. Although adverse effects in these species have been disregarded by some regulatory authorities, it would appear that companies assessing new corticosteroid preparations are still expected to conduct routine studies.

Dose of test compound and route of administration

The magnitude of the dose and the route of administration of a test compound to animals has a marked bearing on the outcome and pattern of embryofetal abnormality. Experiments conducted to examine the influence of dose level, time of administration and route of dosing have shown that these variables do not operate in isolation but interact in the production of abnormalities[75,76].

Experimental teratology differs from most pharmacological experiments in that test compounds are usually administered at doses calculated to produce an effect that is observable on the progeny. Occasionally the dose levels are artificially high and do not mimic the anticipated human exposures. In one such experiment[77], teratogenicity was demonstrated when sodium chloride was administered to mice at the massive dose of 1900-2500 mg/kg, a maximum dose which could be expected to lead to extensive ionic and osmotic imbalances in maternal and fetal tissues. Other experiments have sought to demonstrate the teratogenicity of caffeine in rats, but the doses administered were equivalent to that contained in 38-76 cups of coffee[78,79].

In regulatory studies, test compounds will normally be dosed to test animals by the route that is relevant to human exposures. Examples exist to show that whereas substances are without obvious risk under normal conditions of exposure, they may be toxic and teratogenic under unusual circumstances. Cadmium and lead ions are not teratogenic if dosed orally to hamsters or rats, but become so if they are injected subcutaneously or intravenously[80,81]. The relevance of this observation, in terms of human risk, is not clear. In the case of lead there is a reported ten-fold difference in the intestinal absorption in rats and in man[82]. Human beings have been reported to absorb 10% of an ingested dose of lead[83] but in its recent survey the Scandinavian Council for Environmental Information Workshop[87] concluded that lead is not a teratogen in human beings in the "classical" sense. It must be emphasized that biological properties cannot always be equated directly with risk. It is the circumstances that are of paramount importance, and exposure to the requisite dose at the requisite time is the more relevant factor.

Period of dosing

Environmental agents may impair the reproductive process in susceptible species at any stage from germ cell formation to postnatal
growth and maturation in the offspring. The sensitivity of fetal
tissues to deformation relates closely to the stage at which they
are exposed. For practical purposes, the reproductive cycle is
considered in three main phases: gamete formation; stage of
pregnancy; and postnatal growth and maturation. These factors are
taken into account by the various regulatory authorities in their
recommendations - and see also Johnson and Everett[84] and
Palmer[29].

Experimental studies have demonstrated that each fetal tissue
exhibits its own peak of sensitivity to deformation by exogenous or
genetic determinants, but for most species organ systems are most
likely to be subject to teratogenicity during early or mid-gestation
when organogenesis is optimal. In the mouse fetus, cleft palate was
regularly induced following administration of cortisone to mothers
at 11-13 days of pregnancy[69]. Exposure of rats to trypan blue,
sodium aurothiomalate or cadmium ion produced maximum
teratogenicity during the period 8-10 days of gestation when fetal
nutrition is largely by way of the yolk sac placenta. In the human,
maximum sensitivity to thalidomide is evident at about 37-50 days
of pregnancy[96]. Experimental evidence shows that in animals
treated with teratogens at different stages in the reproductive
cycle, the responses seen are specific for the stage of exposure
(Table 6.4).

Experimental observations

Identification of defects in reproductive performance or fetal
growth constitutes a vital part of any predictive safety evaluation
study. The quality of the results relates to the sensitivity of the
methods used and the experience of the investigator.

For comparative purposes the influence of environmental
agents administered to male and/or female animals before mating, or
to pregnant dams have usually been expressed under the following
headings: pregnancy index, conception index, fetal survival index,
malformation index, parturition index, and postnatal survival index. These indices are held to be useful in comparing the toxicity
of different agents (at comparable pharmacological doses) and in
examining the dose : effect relationship. They may nevertheless
have been something of a barrier to the increased understanding -
and therefore the development - of reproductive toxicology: they
fragment what is essentially a continuous integrated process.

Table 6.4 Range of reproductive effects and manifestations of teratogenicity as a function of the time of exposure to toxic agents during the reproductive cycle[*]

Stage of exposure	Response		
	Male	Female	Conceptus
Before mating	Reduced fertility Loss of libido abnormal sperm characteristics Spermatocyte mutation	Reproductive failure Abnormal oestrous cycles Hormonal changes Defects in ovum transport Mutation	—
During pregnancy	—	Generalized maternal illness Metabolic, hormonal and nutritional defects Circulatory and other functional changes Toxaemia	Preconception loss Stillbirth Intrauterine death Structural and functional abnormalities Biochemical changes Growth retardation Transplacental carcinogenesis Somatic mutations Postnatal distress
Perinatal and postnatal period	—	Failure in lactation Toxic metabolites in milk Prolonged gestation Deficiencies in maternal behaviour, weaning, etc.	Perinatal mortality Functional and developmental abnormality Mental and behavioural deformity Carcinogenic changes with mutations Postnatal toxicity through substances present in milk

[*]Excluding, e.g., the effects of compounds on the biogenesis of the sex steroids and prostaglandins

The pregnancy index is a measure of the effect of a compound upon germ cell production, reproductive behaviour and conception. Defects in the male animal may arise as a result of impaired spermatogenesis, sperm motility and fertilizing ability, hormonal changes or lowered reproductive behaviour. An analysis of sperm cell morphology (sperm head abnormality assay) and motility and fertilizing ability under in vitro conditions can provide useful information. Other tests that may be conducted include semen viscosity, pH and chemical composition. In the rabbit, sperm samples are readily obtained using the artificial uterus technique. In smaller animals, samples of sperm are obtained from the epididymis.

Reproductive activity in both male and female animals is sensitive to endocrine changes and disturbances in general health. Drug-induced oestrus changes are examined by vaginal smear and circulating hormone assays. In vitro fertilization is a further useful test.

A wide range of methods is available for determining the normality of fetal development in teratological development. Commonly, an investigator will count resorption sites, dead fetuses and stillbirths. Live progeny obtained by Caesarian section at near-term will be examined routinely by hand lens for evidence of gross abnormalities in the skull (especially in the facial aspects), limbs and general body proportions. The use of transverse sections or "steaks", as recommended by Wilson[10] can provide important information relating to visceral abnormalities. Skeletal abnormalities are commonly seen in teratological experiments where exogenous agents exert a direct influence on developing cartilage or bone, or where they lead to more generalized defects in fetal growth. The technique devised by Dawson[86] using alizarin red-S dye to stain the ossifying areas of fetuses macerated in potassium hydroxide, is still widely adopted in most laboratories. Counter-stains such as methyl green, methylene blue and methyl blue have been introduced on occasions to demonstrate cartilagenous abnormalities.

In perinatal and postnatal experiments, toxic changes are sought in the young animals. Methods available for this purpose are of two main types:

1. timing of specific developmental events, e.g. eyes opening, hair growth patterns, etc.;

2. behavioural teratology.

The second parameter is a specialized area and is employed to evaluate not only growth potential but also functional development in the brain. Different laboratories have acquired their own particular expertise and such methods as the righting reflex, open field exploration and movement, response to external stimuli, etc. are adopted[88]. In many respects the studies carried out closely resemble those used routinely in pharmacological studies.

EMBRYOS IN CULTURE

Fertilization and early development in the mammalian egg is not normally observable except through the use of tissue culture technology. However, by this means eggs of human and other species have been examined through fertilization and into the early stages of embryonic growth. Although much use has been made of this facility in overcoming reproductive problems in human patients, it offers opportunities for the toxicologist wishing to examine the influence of exogenous agents upon the early embryo in the absence of maternal influence.

Early studies used cartilage and bone explants from chick and fetal mouse limb to study the influence of various culture modifications and the influence of hypervitaminosis A[89]. Using a simple system where the explants were mounted on stainless-steel grids in a culture medium of serum-embryo extract, vitamin A induced a degeneration in the cartilage matrix probably due to an induced release of lysosomal proteases[90].

The technique for embryo culture has been modified on many occasions[91]. It ranges from the simple watch glass method employed by Fell[89] to more sophisticated apparatus using roller tube cultures and devices for circulating the culture medium. However, the chief limitation so far seems to be the duration for which embryos may be cultured and the normality of development. Several investigators have cultured rodent embryos from the late blastocyst through early post-implantation stages and the initial part of the organogenic phase, up to 13 days gestation. Mortality was probably due to an accumulation of waste materials or to changing nutritional or physiological requirements[92].

The value of culture techniques in teratogenicity evaluations depends upon the question "How normal is the developmental pattern?". One such appraisal demonstrated that fetal growth in culture proceeds at a slower rate than in utero, but the increases in somite number were within normal limits[93].

A range of known teratogens have been examined in whole embryo and fetal tissue explants. In many cases the observations have complemented those obtained using more conventional test systems. Thus trypan blue placed in culture medium was seen to concentrate in the yolk sac endoderm of rat fetuses as seen in intact animal experiments[94]. Resulting fetuses exhibited oedema and cardiac deformities. Rat fetuses cultured in the presence of vitamin A were retarded but displayed the characteristic pattern of neural tube defects attributable to an inhibition in neural crest cell proliferation and migration[85,95].

In summary, embryos cultured in the presence of exogenous agents can be used to provide useful supplementary information to that provided by the more conventional intact animal studies. They are likely to prove cost-effective and scientifically valid in evaluating mechanisms of teratogenic action of agents likely to have a direct effect on developing tissues. Clearly, in future years more expertise must be acquired in developing the technique to study older embryos. As the conference held at Reading concluded, these are other technological difficulties that make more reliance upon in vitro techniques some years ahead[7].

THE FUTURE OF PREDICTIVE SAFETY EVALUATION

SUMMARY

Reproduction and fetal development in humans and experimental animals may be adversely affected by a wide range of drugs and environmental agents. They may be toxic in the parental generation leading to impaired germ cell formation, loss of reproductive potential and infertility following chronic exposure. Deviant fetal development occurs as a consequence of cellular damage at sensitive stages in development. Changes seen range from intrauterine mortality and structural malformation to growth retardation with physiological and behavioural defects. Concepts on the mechanism of action of teratogens are discussed with reference to some better-known agents.

Presently, regulatory authorities prefer whole animal studies in predictive safety evaluation of substances to which a pregnant woman may be exposed. Tests are conducted over one or more generations and are designed to study the influence of test compounds upon general reproductive performance, fertility, fetal development and perinatal and postnatal behaviour. Experiments are designed to permit compounds to be tested under conditions resembling expected human exposure. Small rodents and rabbits are preferred species on account of their convenience as laboratory animals and the available knowledge regarding their reproductive behaviour, fetal development and known sensitivity to human teratogens.

Regulatory authorities express an interest in reproductive research and new methods for studying fetal growth patterns, especially the use of in vitro techniques. Future developments in the subject are unclear but it is anticipated that as useful information comes to hand, so regulatory requirements will be amended accordingly. Efforts will doubtless be made to develop more sensitive methods of investigation, but the cardinal principle remains that - as in other branches of toxicology and predictive safety evaluation - it is the circumstances in which adverse effects could occur that need understanding. Thalidomide is of low systemic toxicity when assessed by conventional means - and would almost certainly not be a teratogen in practice if it were to prove more harmful to either mother or embryo.

ACKNOWLEDGEMENTS

I am grateful to Professor A. Dayan for his constructive advice in preparing this review and to Professors Colin Berry[93,97] and H. T. G. Tuchmann-Duplessis[98] and to Mr. A. K. Palmer for their comments and suggestions.

ADDENDUM

Professor Parke has drawn attention to the importance of the ECETOC proposals for future short-term tests[24] and to the current research of Dr Diana Anderson and her colleagues at BIBRA on the teratogenic effects that have been observed from the action of

TESTING FOR REPRODUCTIVE TOXICITY

compounds on male germ cells. Reference has already been made to Parke's review of the development of detoxication of mechanisms in the neonate[31]. It has been shown that adverse effects in the fetus may arise simply by giving intraperitoneal injections as a bolus, with resultant very high blood concentrations that facilitate transplacental entry. Several cases of embryonic and fetal toxicity, including teratogenicity, have been traced to the use of bolus injections of the drug at weekends. It is now a requirement of most regulatory bodies to show that the pharmacokinetics of a drug in the pregnant animal do not differ widely from those in non-pregnant animals, and to ascertain information about the ability of the drug to cross the placental barrier. Attention should be drawn also to the publications of Snell[99] and Schardein[100].

REFERENCES

1.   Saint-Hilaire, IG (1832). Histoire Generale et Particuliere des Animales de l'Organisation chez l'Homme et les Animaux. (Paris: J. B. Balliere et fils)
2.   Harvey, W (1651). Exercitationes de Generatione Animalium Typis Du Gardianis; impensis Octaviani, Pulleyn, In: Coemetario Paulino, Amsterdam and London
3.   Dobbing, I and Sands, J (1971). Vulnerability of the developing brain. IX The effect of nutritional growth retardation on the timing of the brain growth spurt. Biol Neonate, 19, 363-78
4.   Dobbing, J (1974). The later growth of the brain and its vulnerability, Pediatrics, 53, 2-6
5.   Van Marthens, E, Harel, S and Lamenhof, S (1975). Experimental intrauterine growth retardation, Biol Neonate, 26, 221-31
6.   Bolande, RP (1984). Models and concepts derived from human teratogenesis and oncogenesis in early life. J Histochem Cytochem, 32, 878-84
7.   International Conference on Practical in Vivo Toxicology, University of Reading, 1985
8.   Lansdown, ABG (1978). Viral infection and diseases of the heart, Prog Med Virol, 24, 70-113
9.   Lansdown, ABG (1979). Clinical and experimental aspects of prenatal viral infection, In: Persaud, TVN (Ed). Advances in the Study of Birth Defects, Vol. 2, pp. 292-323. (Lancaster: MTP Press)
10. Wilson, JG (1959). Experimental studies on congenital malformations, J Chron Dis, 10, 111-30
11. Beck, F and Lloyd, JB (1963). The preparation and teratogenic properties of pure trypan blue and its common contaminants. J Embryol Exp Morphol, 11, 175-84
12. Stockard, CR (1921). Developmental rate and structural expression: an experimental study of twins, "double monsters" and single deformities, and the interaction among embryonic organs during their origin and development, Am J Anat, 28, 115-277

13. Lansdown, ABG (1970). Histological changes in the skeletal elements of developing rat foetuses following treatment with sodium salicylate. Fol Cosmet Toxicol, 8, 647-53
14. Gillette, JR (1977). Factors that affect drug concentration in maternal plasma. In: JG Wilson and FC Fraser (Eds). Handbook of Teratology, Vol. 3, pp. 35-78. (New York: Plenum)
15. Kennedy, LS and Persaud, TVN (1979). Acute alcohol intoxication in the pregnant rat. In: Persaud, TVN (Ed), Advances in the Study of Birth Defects, Vol. 2, pp. 223-38. (Lancaster: MTP Press)
16. Smith, RL and Caldwell, J (1977). Drug metabolism in non-human primates. In: Parke, DV and Smith, RL (Eds), Drug Metabolism from Microbe to Man, pp. 331-56. (London: Taylor & Francis)
17. Takeuchi, T and Matsumoto, H (1969). Minamata disease of human foetuses. In: Nishimura, H and Miller, JR (Eds), Methods for Teratological Studies in Experimental Animals and Man, p. 280. (Tokyo: Igaku Shoin)
18. Bakir, F, Damluji, SR, Amin-Zaki, L and Murtaiha, M (1973). Methylmercury poisoning in Iraq. Science, 181, 230
19. Knill-Jones, RP, Moir, DO and Rodrigues, LV (1972). Anaesthetic practice and pregnancy. A controlled survey of women anaesthetists in the United Kingdom. Lancet, 1, 1326-8
20. Corbett, TH, Cornell, RG, Endres, JL and Leiding, BS (1974). Birth defects among children of nurse anaesthetists. Anaesthesiology, 41, 341-4
21. Lansdown, ABG, Pope, WDB, Halsey, MJ and Bateman, PE (1976). Analysis of fetal development in rats following maternal exposure to sub-anaesthetic concentrations of halothane. Teratology, 13, 299-303
22. Pope, WDB, Halsey, MJ, Lansdown, ABG and Bateman, PE (1975). Lack of teratogenic hazards with halothane. Acta Anaesthesiol Belg, 26, 169-73
23. Pope, WDB, Halsey, MJ, Lansdown, ABG, Simmons, A and Bateman, PE (1978). Fetotoxicity in rats following chronic exposure to halothane, nitrous oxide or methoxyflurane. Anaesthesiology, 48, 11-16
24. ECETOC (1983). Identification and assessment of the effects of chemicals on reproduction and development. (Reproductive Toxicology). Monograph No 5, Brussels
25. Kreybig, Th. von (1965). Verschiedene Wirkmechanismen in teratologischen Experiment. Naunyn Schmiedeberg Arch Path, 251, 197-8
26. Lenz, W (1961). Diskussionsbemerkung Tagung der Rhein Westfah Kinderarzteverinigung. Dusseldorf, 11 November
27. McBride, WG (1961). Thalidomide and congenital abnormalities. Lancet, 2, 1358
28. Food and Drug Administration (1966). Guidelines for Reproductive Studies for Safety Evaluation of Drugs for Human Use
29. Palmer, AK (1981). Regulatory requirements for reproductive toxicology: theory and practice. In: Kimmel, CA and Beulke-Sam, J (Eds), Developmental Toxicology, pp. 259-87 (New York: Raven Press)

30. Department of Health and Social Security (1982). Guidelines for the Testing of Chemicals for Safety. Report No 27, 33-36

31. Parke, DV (1984). Development of detoxication mechanisms in the neonate. In: Kacew, S and Reasor, MJ (Eds), Toxicology and the Newborn, pp. 1-34. (Amsterdam: Elsevier)

32. Saxen, I (1976). Mechanisms of teratogenesis. J Embryol Exp Morphol, 36, 1-12

33. Wilson, JG (1972). Mechanisms of teratogenesis, Am J Anat, 136, 129-32

34. Kolata, GB (1980). Chromosomal damage: what it is, what it means. Science, 208, 1240

35. Carter, CO (1969). Genetics of common disorders. Br Med Bull, 25, 52-7

36. Wilson, JG (1977). Current status of teratology. In: Wilson, JG and Fraser, FC (Eds). Handbook of Teratology, Vol. 1, pp. 47-74. (New York: Plenum)

37. Sternberg, SS (1979). The carcinogenesis, mutagenesis and teratogenesis of insecticides: review of studies in animals and in man. Pharm Ther, 6, 147-66

38. Yamazaki, J, Wright, S and Wright, P (1954). Outcome of pregnancy in women exposed to the atomic bomb in Nagasaki. Am J Dis Child, 87, 448-63

39. Brent, RL (1972). Irradiation in pregnancy. Davis' Gynecology and Obstetrics, 2, 1-32

40. Wilson, JG (1964). Differentiation and reaction of rat embryos to radiation. J Cell Comp Physiol, 43, 11-37

41. Naeye, RL and Blanc, W (1965). Pathogenesis of congenital rubella. J Am Med Assoc, 194, 1277-83

42. Marin-Padilla, M (1966). Mesodermal alterations induced by hypervitaminosis A. J Embryol Exp Morphol, 15, 261-9

43. Saxen, L (1970). Defective regulatory mechanisms in teratogenesis. Int J Gynecol Obstet, 8, 784-804

44. Poswillo, D (1975). Causal mechanisms of craniofacial deformity. Br Med Bull, 31, 101-6

45. Andrew, FD and Zimmerman, EF (1971). Glucocorticoid induction of cleft palate in mice: no correlation with inhibition of mucopolysaccharide synthesis. Teratology, 4, 31-8

46. Cooke, J and Summerbell, D (1980). Cell cycle and experimental duplication in the chick wing during embryonic development. Nature, 287, 697-701

47. Saunders, JW and Fallon, JF (1966). Cell death in morphogenesis. In: Locke, M (Ed). Major Problems in Developmental Biology, pp. 289-314 (New York: Academic Press)

48. Wolpert, L (1976). Mechanisms of limb development and malformation. Br Med Bull, 32, 65-70

49. Menkes, B and Deleanu, M (1964). Leg differentiation and experimental syndactyly in the chick embryo. Revue Roum Embryol Cytol Serv Embryol, 1, 69-77

50. Lansdown, ABG and Grasso, P (1971). Histological observations on a Rathke's cleft abnormality in a laboratory rat. J Comp Pathol, 81, 141-4

51. Lansdown, ABG (1982). Multinodular splenic abnormality in a red patas monkey (Erythrocebus patas). Vet Rec, 110, 429-30

52. Ross, LM and Walker, BE (1967). Movement of palatine shelves in untreated and teratogen-treated mouse embryos. Am J Anat, 121, 509-22

53. Kochhar, DM (1968). Studies on vitamin A induced teratogenesis: effects on embryonic mesenchyme and epithelium and incorporation of H^3-thymidine. Teratology, 1, 299-310

54. Duffell, SJ, Lansdown, ABG and Richardson, C (1985). A clinical, radiological and pathological account of the occurrence of dwarf lambs. Vet Rec, 117, 571-6

55. Saxen, L and Kaitilia, I (1972). The effect and mode of action of tetracycline on bone development in vitro. Adv Exp Biol Med, 27, 205-18

56. Lenaers, A, Ansay, M, Nusgens, BV and La Piere, CM (1971). Collagen made of extended alpha-chains, procollagen in genetically defective dermatosparaxic calves. Eur J Biochem, 23, 533-43

57. Edwards, MJ (1972). Influenza, hyperthermia and congenital malformation. Lancet, 1, 320-1

58. Lansdown, ABG and Coid, CR (1974). Pathological changes in pregnant mice infected with Coxsackie virus B3 as a possible cause of retarded foetal development. Br J Exp Pathol, 55, 101-9

59. Lansdown, ABG (1976). Experimental studies in mice on the influence of Coxsackie virus B infections on foetal growth. Teratology, 13, 391

60. Lansdown, ABG (1975). Influence of time of infection during pregnancy with Coxsackie virus B3 on maternal pathology and foetal growth in mice. Br J Exp Pathol, 56, 119-23

61. Lansdown, ABG, Coid, LR and Ramsden, DB (1975). Mitigation of virus-induced foetal growth retardation in mice by dietary casein hydrolysate. Nature, 254, 599

62. Naeye, RL, Blanc, W and Paul, C (1973). Effects of maternal nutrition on the human foetus. Pediatrics, 52, 494-503

63. Hurley, LS (1977). Nutritional deficiencies and excesses In: Wilson, JG and Fraser, FC (Eds). Handbook of Teratology, Vol. 1, pp. 261-308. (New York: Plenum)

64. Harper, KH, Palmer, AK and Davies, RE (1965). The effect of imipramine upon the pregnancy of laboratory animals. Arzneim-Forsch, 15, 1218-21

65. Wilson, JG (1964). Teratogenic interaction of chemical agents in the rat. J Pharmacol Exp Ther, 144, 429-36

66. Manson, JM, Zenick, H and Costlow, RD (1982). Teratology test methods. In: Wallace Hayes, A (Ed). Principles and Methods of Toxicology, pp. 141-83

67. Loevy, H (1962). Developmental changes in the palate of normal cortisone treated strong a mice. Anat Rec, 142, 375-90

68. Pinsky, L and Di George, AM (1965). Cleft palate in the mouse: a teratogenic index of glucocorticoid potency. Science, 147, 402-3

69. Biddle, FG and Fraser, FC (1976). Genetics of cortisone-induced cleft palate in the mouse - embryonic and maternal effects. Genetics, 84, 743-54

70. Giroud, A, Tuchmann-Duplessis, M and Mercier-Parot, L (1962). Observations sur les repercussions teratogenes de la thalidomide chez la souris et le lapin. C R Soc Biol, 156, 765-8

71. Gibson, JP, Staples, RE and Newberne, JW (1966). Use of the rabbit in teratology studies. Toxicol Appl Pharmacol, 9, 398-408

72. Stadler, J, Kessidjan, M-J and Perraud, J (1983). Use of the New Zealand white rabbit in teratology: incidence of spontaneous and drug induced abnormalities. Fd Cosmet Toxicol, 21, 631

73. Beck, F (1975). The ferret as a teratological model. In: Neubert, D and Merker, HJ (Eds). New Approaches to the Evaluation of Abnormal Development, pp. 8-20. (Stuttgart: Thieme)

74. Ferm, VH (1965). The rapid detection of teratogenic activity. Lab Invest, 14, 1500-5

75. Fraser, FC (1964). Experimental teratogenesis in relation to congenital malformations in man. In: Fishbein, M (Ed), Proceedings of the Second International Conference on Congenital Malformations. International Medical Congress, New York, pp. 277-287

76. Mellin, GN (1964). Drugs in the first trimester of pregnancy and foetal life of Homo sapiens Am J Obstet, 90, 1169-80

77. Nishimura, H and Miyamoto, S (1969). Teratogenic effects of sodium chloride in the mouse. Acta Anat, 74, 121-3

78. Le Chat, MF, Borlee, I, Bouckaert and Mission, C (1980). Caffeine study. Science, 207, 1296-7

79. Palm, PE, Arnold, EP, Rachwell, PC et al (1978). Evaluation of the teratogenic effect of fresh-brewed coffee and caffeine in the rat. Toxicol Appl Pharmacol, 44, 1-16

80. Ferm, VH (1969). The synteratogenic effects of lead and cadmium. Experientia, 25, 56-7

81. McClain, RM and Becker, BA (1975). Teratogenicity, fetal toxicity and placental transfer of lead nitrate in rats. Toxicol Appl Pharmacol, 31, 72-82

82. Moore, MR, Hughes, MA and Goldberg, DJ (1979). Lead absorption in man from dietary sources. Int Arch Occup Env Health, 44, 81-90

83. Rabinowitz, MB, Wetherill, GW and Kopple, JD (1976). Kinetic analysis of lead metabolism in healthy humans J Clin Invest, 58, 260-70

84. Johnson,M and Everitt, B (1984). Essential Reproduction, 2nd edition. (Oxford: Blackwell Scientific Publications)

85. Morriss, GM and Steele, CE (1974). The effect of excess vitamin A on the development of rat embryos in culture. J Embryol Exp Morphol, 32, 505-14

86. Dawson, AB (1976). A note on the staining of the skeleton of cleared specimens with alizarin red S. Stain Technol, 1, 123-5

87. Scandinavian Council for Environmental Information (1977). Workshop on the utility of an evaluated data bank in teratology and its use for a state-of-the-art report on adverse ef-

fects of lead on reproduction and development. Nynashamn, Sweden

88. Barlow, S and Sullivan, FM (1975). Behavioural teratology. In: Berry, CL and Poswillo, DE (Eds). Teratology, Trends and Applications, pp. 103-20. (New York: Springer Verlag)

89. Fell, HB (1969). The effect of environment on skeletal tissue culture. Embryologia, 10, 181-205

90. Dingle, JT and Lucy, JA (1965). Vitamin A, carotenoids and cell function. Biol Rev, 40, 422-61

91. New, DAT (1978). Whole-embryo culture and the study of mammalian embryos during organogenesis. Biol Rev, 53, 81-122

92. New, DAT (1968). Growing embryos in the laboratory. Science J, 4, 50-5

93. Berry, CL (1968). Comparison of the in vivo and in vitro growth of the rat foetus. Nature, 219, 92-3

94. Turbow, MM (1966). Trypan blue induced teratogenesis of rat embryos cultivated in vitro. J Embryol Exp Morphol, 15, 387-95

95. Morriss, GM and Steele, C (1977). Comparison of the effects of retinol and retinoic acid on post-implantation rat embryos in vitro. Teratology, 15, 109-20

96. Lenz, W and Knapp, K (1962). Foetal malformations due to thalidomide. Deutsche Med Wochenschr, 7, 253-8

97. Berry, CL (1970). Coincidence of congenital malformation and embryonic tumours of childhood. Arch Dis Childh, 45, 229-31

98. Tuchmann-Duplessis, H (1984). Drugs and other xenobiotics as teratogens. Pharmacol Ther, 26, 273-344

99. Snell, K (ed) (1982). Developmental Toxicology. (London: Academic Press)

100. Schardein, JL (1985). Drugs as Teratogens. (Cleveland, Ohio: CRC Press)

7
Neurotoxicity

A. J. DEWAR

INTRODUCTION

Prediction of the adverse effects of a chemical on the nervous system poses many problems, and we are far from having a rational and comprehensive system of neurotoxicity screening. Furthermore, it is unlikely that such a system will have been fully developed and validated by the end of the century. Although some progress may be predicted with confidence the challenges in neurotoxicity testing are more likely to grow faster than our capacity to deal with them adequately.

THE PROBLEMS OF NEUROTOXICITY TESTING

The nervous system is by far the most complex organ in the body both functionally and structurally, and this complexity is reflected in the huge diversity of toxic actions that may be exerted upon it. Manifestations of neurotoxicity in humans include, amongst others, motor disorders, sensory disorders, disturbances of autonomic function, alterations in the state of excitability of the central nervous system, affective change and intellectual impairment; i.e. effects can be neurological, physiological, psychological or psychiatric. Similarly the term "neurotoxin" encompasses an ever-broadening spectrum of chemical types including industrial chemicals and solvents, metals, pesticides, psychoactive drugs, antimicrobials, chemotherapeutic agents, food additives and neurotoxins of biological origin.

Neurotoxic effects may be acute or chronic. Acute neurotoxicity generally follows a single large dose, and in most cases is caused by "pharmacological" actions on nerve cell membranes or synaptic transmission and is frequently reversible. In contrast, chronic neurotoxicity commonly requires repeated doses, involves degeneration of the cellular elements, is not readily reversible and may be caused by metabolic lesions in the neurons, their axons or the supporting cells (Schwann cells or glia), or interference with the vasculature. Some chronic effects, however, may result from a single dose (e.g. delayed peripheral neuropathy after a single exposure to certain organophosphates)[1] or be due to functional rather than degenerative changes (e.g. tardive dyskinesia after prolonged phenothiazine therapy)[2]. Many compounds may cause both acute and chronic neurotoxicity but at different doses and by independent mechanisms. N-hexane is a well known example - depending on the dose and duration of exposure it can cause either a reversible narcosis or a prolonged peripheral neuropathy[3].

Potential mechanisms of neurotoxicity are legion[4,5]. Toxins may selectively interfere with basic metabolic processes such as energy metabolism, lipid metabolism, protein and nucleic acid synthesis, with biochemical pathways responsible for myelin sheath maintenance, with axonal transport, with nerve membrane permeability or with synaptic transmission. As our knowledge of neurosciences grows so does the number of potential mechanisms that have to be considered. However, although a great deal is known of these potential mechanisms our knowledge of the precise modes of action of many neurotoxins is still relatively meagre - particularly of those that produce structural damage.

The effects of age are a further complicating factor. For example, the immature and developing nervous system has particular vulnerabilities to toxic insult, particularly during the period of cellular proliferation, myelination and synaptogenesis[6]. Many chemicals not overtly toxic to the mature system may have grave effects on the developing nervous system (e.g. inhibitors of DNA or cholesterol synthesis[6,7]). Some, such as lead, may affect both the mature and immature systems, but do so in different ways[8]. The ageing nervous system is also especially sensitive to some toxins (e.g. manganese)[9].

The above illustrates some of the inherent difficulties in devising a neurotoxicity testing strategy, and demonstrates why it is impossible to envisage a simple, rational, all-embracing "neurotoxicity test". Ideally, to make a reliable prediction of possible effects of a novel chemical on the nervous system acute and chronic exposures using aged, mature and neonatal animals are required. Since no one experimental technique would be capable of detecting all the potential neurotoxicological end-points a multidisciplinary approach is essential, i.e. full use should be made of clinical observation and appropriate behavioural, pharmacological, electrophysiological, biochemical and pathological methods. As in many other branches of toxicology, there exists the problem of the appropriateness of the animal model and the dangers of extrapolation of data to man. Moreover, there are some types of neurotoxicity that affect man (e.g. intellectual impairment) that are extremely difficult or impossible to detect by animal tests. A particular difficulty is that changes in neurological functions are on a continuum from normal to abnormal, and distinctions between exposed and control populations are relative rather than absolute. Moreover, the dose-response relationships for most neurotoxins are, as yet, unclear[9].

CURRENT TESTING AND ITS LIMITATIONS

For the reasons outlined above, neurotoxicity testing differs from other areas of toxicology where it has generally been possible to devise a relatively compact and economical testing strategy that can be applied across a wide spectrum of test compounds with a reasonable probability of detecting the type of toxicity in question. The detection of neurotoxicity requires a structured scientific investigation, the nature of which will differ considerably depending on the properties of the chemical under investigation. Consequently it is not readily amenable to the "Regulotox" approach and, so far, virtually no neurotoxicity tests per se have been specified in the various testing regulations[9-11]. It is tacitly assumed that many neurotoxic phenomena will be first detected during acute toxicity testing, or during chronic tests such as 13-week feeding studies or reproductive toxicity tests. However, as we have seen, it cannot be assumed that all types of neurotoxicity can be detected and characterized in the context of such routine procedures. There will always be a need for more specialized investigations.

In the space of a short chapter it is not possible to offer even a brief resumé of all the neurotoxicity tests that are at present available. There is a whole raft of techniques designed for a variety of very different purposes. Three broad categories of tests may be distinguished. At one extreme there are those appropriate for the primary detection of neurotoxicity of a novel compound of hitherto unknown properties. At the opposite extreme are tests for examining the neurotoxicity of a new member of a class of compounds whose neurotoxic properties and mode of action are known. In between these extremes are tests for particular types of neurotoxic effect (e.g. peripheral neuropathy) that are relatively specific but do not depend on a knowledge of the mechanisms involved. Also included under the broad umbrella of "neurotoxicity testing" are exploratory studies, i.e. investigations designed, after the primary detection of neurotoxicity, to identify the target system, describe the neurotoxic effect in more detail and if possible elucidate the mechanism.

The applicability of the various disciplines to each level of testing is shown in the form of a matrix in Table 7.1. It may be seen, for example, that behavioural tests are applicable at all levels of testing for acute and chronic neurotoxicity, and that there are behavioural tests suitable for the primary detection of neurotoxicity (e.g. the Irwin screen[12]), tests for identifying particular types of neurotoxicity (e.g. the discriminative Y maze test for testing for memory impairment[13]) and specific tests for detecting neurotoxic effects of known mechanisms (e.g. apomorphine-induced stereotyped behaviour for detecting extrapyramidal effects of neuroleptics[14]). In contrast, biochemical methods have limited applicability for the primary detection of neurotoxicity but provide useful second-order tests (e.g. the use of β-glucuronidase measurements for detecting and quantifying peripheral neuropathy[15]) and are particularly valuable for detecting neurotoxicity of known mechanisms (e.g. the neurotoxic esterase method for assessing the neurotoxic potential of organophosphates[16]).

Table 7.1 Summary of range and status of current neurotoxicity testing methods

		Clinical observation /behaviour		Neuropathology	
First-order tests (Primary detections of neurotoxicity) tests requiring no prior knowledge of the neurotoxic properties of the test compound	Acute	P/V	+++ (i)	N/A	
	Chronic	P/V	+++	P/V	++ (i)
Second-order tests Tests aimed at detecting the particular type of neurotoxicity but not requiring a knowledge of the mechanism involved	Acute	W	+++	N/A	
	Chronic	W	+++	W	+++
Third-order tests Tests for particular types of neurotoxicity based on a knowledge of the mechanism	Acute	W	+++	N/A	
	Chronic	W	+++	W	+++
Exploratory tests Studies carried out at elucidating the nature and mechanism of a neurotoxic effect once detected	Acute	W	+++	N/A	
	Chronic	W	+++	P/V	+++

Comments

(i) Behaviour is the outward expression of the net interaction between the sensory, motor, arousal and integrative components of the central and peripheral nervous systems. It is therefore one of the earliest expressions of neurotoxicity.

(i) Neuropathological examination is fundamental to the understanding of the effects of a structural neurotoxin on the nervous system. At present routine chronic toxicity testing commonly fails to use the most effective neuropathological techniques available.

Selected references   5,12-14,17-27   5,27-34

Key to ranking:
N/A = not applicable   - = methodology still under development
L = of limited usefulness   + = a few techniques available

NEUROTOXICITY

Electrophysiology		Biochemistry		Tissue culture	
L	+ (i)	L but could be W for pre-screening in vitro	-	L but could be W for pre-screening purposes	-
L	+ (i)	L	+	L but could be W for pre-screening purposes	+ (i)
L	++	L	+	L	-
W	++	W	++ (i)	L	+
W	++	P/V	++ (ii)	W	+
W	++	P/V	+ (iii)	W	+
P/V	+++ (ii)	P/V	+++	P/V	+
W	+++ (ii)	P/V	+++	P/V	++

Electrophysiology

(i) For most electrophysiological techniques to be chosen and applied effectively, some preliminary knowledge of the neurotoxic effect under consideration is required.

(ii) These techniques provide information not readily obtainable by any other method. Can be used in vitro

5,27,35-49

Biochemistry

(i) Neurochemical correlates of neuropathological change are of potential value for quantifying neuropathological damage and overcoming the sampling errors inherent in neuropathological methods. Techniques are available but are not widely used.

(ii) Many potential methods available, particularly for the assessment of effects on neurotransmission.

(iii) Very difficult to develop.

5,9,15,16,27,50-59

Tissue culture

(i) Potentially useful techniques have been developed but still require further validation

5,27,60-68

W	= of wide relevance	++ = techniques available
P/V	= of particular value	+++ = good techniques available and widely used

111

The table includes a subjective assessment of the relative degree of development and use of each type of technique. Thus it may be seen that neuropathological methods are relatively highly developed and widely used, whereas the potential of biochemical and tissue culture methods is relatively unrealized. Included in the table are a small number of references to relevant reviews and representative papers, and the interested reader should refer to these for more details (and bibliographies) regarding currently available methods.

In spite of the apparent multitude of tests reported in the literature it is possible to identify a number of major deficiencies in current neurotoxicity testing. These are:

1. The relative lack of rational testing procedures based on an understanding of the mechanism and a general underappreciation of the potential applications of the theoretical bases of modern neuroscience to neurotoxicology.
2. The relative lack of validated in vitro alternatives to animal tests.
3. A lack of integration of the many available tests and techniques into coherent, cost-effective and generally accepted (and validated) neurotoxicity evaluation strategies.

Before speculating on possible developments, some of the forces that could influence the future demands for neurotoxicology will be considered.

FACTORS INFLUENCING THE FUTURE OF NEUROTOXICOLOGY

General factors underlying all toxicological testing

The sociopolitical environment

This involves such factors as demographic change; health care expenditure; the global food situation and social attitudes to environmental issues and animal experimentation.

These general factors have already been considered in some detail in the introductory chapter (Volume 1) and require no extensive discussion here. The ageing of the population will be expected to result in a steep rise in the incidence of psychogeriatric disorders and this, in turn, will further exacerbate the problem of escalating health care expenditure (particularly hospitalization). Consequently one can envisage growing economic pressures to develop drugs for the management of chronic mental conditions.

The scientific and technological environment and the industrial environment

The principal features of these, i.e. the possibility of a new wave of chemically related innovations occurring by the end of the century, the consequences of the current restructuring of the chemical industry and the growing emphasis on high added-value performance chemicals, have also been reviewed in the introductory chapter and therefore do not need further consideration here.

Specific factors influencing neurotoxicology

Growing significance of mental health problems

It has been estimated by the US National Institute of Mental Health that nearly 19% of the US population suffer from at least one mental disorder over the course of any 6-month period[69]. Mental illnesses currently account for 52% of all US hospital beds. There are no reasons for believing that this incidence of mental health problems in the population will decrease. Many of the problems are believed to be associated with, or exacerbated by, the various stresses of modern lifestyles and, irrespective of economic scenario, the pressures are unlikely to diminish - whether it be the stresses of endemic unemployment or the stresses of the high pressure lifestyles associated with the emerging new industries[70].

Social attitudes to problems of neurotoxicity

Although in the public mind the risks of chemically induced cancer tend to be paramount (and this is reflected in the role of mutagenicity carcinogenicity as often the main criterion for regulating toxic substances), there have been many instances where neurotoxicity has been the central issue. Examples include such widely publicized incidents as the contaminated rape seed oil in Spain, methyl mercury poisoning in Japan and Iraq, Kepone in the USA, polyhalogenated biphenyls in Taiwan and the current controversies surrounding the more subtle neurotoxic effects of food additives and the lead in automobile emissions[9,72,73].

The new wave of innovation

The neurosciences are likely both to participate in, and benefit from, the new wave of innovation referred to above. The neurosciences have been developing particularly rapidly of late and the degree of intellectual excitement of this field is somewhat analogous to that in molecular biology in the 1950s and 1960s. Indeed, advances in molecular biology may be expected to make a massive impact on certain key problems in neurobiology[74]. Significant progress is now being made in understanding the mechanism of neuronal function at the molecular level and the underlying mechanisms of mental illness. It is highly probable that in the next two decades these advances will yield novel therapeutic strategies and be translated into pharmaceutical innovations[75]. Already the therapeutic implications of such recent discoveries as the existence of 30 small peptides in mammalian neurones are being investigated by drug companies[76]. Progress in microelectronics and biotechnology is contributing significantly to the speed of advance in the neurosciences. The increased data handling and information processing capability provided by the availability of powerful computers has been critical, and recombinant DNA techniques are being used to great advantage in neuropeptide research[77].

Implications for neurotoxicology

The trends identified above and in the introductory chapter have obvious neurotoxicological implications:

1.   There will be growing demand for therapeutic agents active in the nervous system, and the likelihood of radical advances in the neurosciences that could provide the basis for meeting this demand.   The adverse effects of such agents on the nervous system will have to be investigated.
2.   There is a strong probability of a new wave of chemical and pharmacological product innovation, due in part to the increased strategic emphasis being placed on product innovation by many chemical companies and the accumulating scientific and technological potential for such innovation.   Inevitably this will throw up novel neurotoxicological problems. What, for example, will be the neurotoxicology of such possible future developments as immunotropics, antivirals, biocompatible plastics, artificial blood, gene therapy, microbial pesticides and genetically engineered organisms in the environment?
3.   Even in the recent period of perceived low product innovation the number of new products manufactured each year far exceeded the capacity for complete animal toxicological evaluation.   The problem will worsen as the rate of innovation increases and societal demands for environmental conservation and safety increase.
4.   Neurotoxicological problems associated with the elderly will have to receive more attention than hitherto.
5.   Social and economic pressures towards the reduction of animal experimentation and the employment of in vitro testing methods will increase.

It may be concluded that neurotoxicology is likely to assume greater importance in the years to come, and regulatory agencies will be called upon to make an increasing number of regulatory decisions on the basis of neurotoxicological data.   At present (for the reasons previously outlined) the current state of the art of neurotoxicology is widely regarded as being inadequate for meeting these demands.   In the next section the prospects for remedying some of these deficiencies will be discussed.

FUTURE CHALLENGES AND DEVELOPMENTS

Tests based on an understanding of mechanism

Neurotoxins have played a considerable role in helping to elucidate underlying mechanisms of neurobiological function but, as yet, the theoretical base of modern neuroscience has been underexploited for assessing the neurotoxic potential of chemicals - certainly in comparison with the practical use made of advances in molecular biology and genetics in mutagenicity testing. Nevertheless, it has long been appreciated that testing methods based on an under-standing of mechanism could confer enormous benefits. A major challenge and opportunity for the future will be in successfully applying the discoveries of modern neuroscience in the service of applied neurotoxicology.

In view of the multiplicity of potential mechanisms for neurotoxicity there is no realistic prospect of a biochemical or electrophysiological predictive screening test (in vivo or in vitro) capable of detecting all types of neurotoxic phenomena. It is to be expected that many more potential mechanisms will be identified in the future - thus exacerbating an already virtually impossible task. Within the past 5 years, for example, the number of puta-tive neurotransmitters identified in the mammalian nervous system has jumped from 10 to over 40[76].

However, although it is not realistic to think in terms of a single comprehensive neurotoxicity test, there are many areas of neurotoxicology in which the biochemical or electrophysiological methods of assessment could be used to a far greater extent than at present. An area where one might realistically expect a growth in the use of biochemical methods is the assessment of acute neurotoxicity due to effects on neurotransmission. Chemical neurotransmission is a unique feature of the nervous system, and is therefore of considerable significance as a potential target for neurotoxins.

The neurochemical literature contains many elegant and sensi-tive methods for assessing neurotransmitter levels, synthesis, release, re-uptake and breakdown. Many techniques are also available for studying the dynamic aspects of transmitter metabo-lism and release in vitro using isolated nerve terminals[78] but, apart from a few examples, there has been little sign of these methods being used for neurotoxicity testing, although there is an extensive literature of the effects of toxicants on various aspects of neurotransmission[79,80]. Receptor theory of drug and neurotransmitter action provides a possible approach for predicting the action of novel compounds, and one that can often be corre-lated with the behaviour of the whole organism. Rapid systems for studying receptor function in vivo and in vitro have been developed, and have been advocated as a potential screening tech-nique in neurotoxicology[54]. However, the use of such methods is not yet widespread and further validation work is still required. It is to be expected that the number of such methods relevant to neurotoxicity assessment will grow - due to the growing importance of the CNS as a potential target for new drugs and to the economic forces that are driving pharmaceutical companies into developing more in vitro procedures for screening novel therapeutic agents[81,82].

The outlook for mechanism-based tests for assessing chronic neurotoxic effects is harder to predict. Biochemical methods have been used successfully for screening neuroleptic drugs for their capacity to induce extrapyramidal side-effects, but in this case the underlying cause involves effects on neurotransmitter-receptor interactions[53]. Methods for assessing the potential of chemicals for inducing structural damage to the nervous system are considerably more difficult to devise and, at present, only one test of this type exists. This, the exceptionally well validated neurotoxic esterase method for assessing the neurotoxic potential of organophosphates, was the outcome of over 40 years of basic research on the nature and causes of organophosphate neuropathy[1],[16]. It is based on the discovery that axonopathic organophosphates phosphorylate and inhibit a specific esterase known as "neurotoxic esterase" or NTE, and offers a particularly good illustration of the benefits and limitations of such methods. It is objective and, although commonly used in vivo/in vitro using hens, can be used wholly in vitro. It requires less test material and time than the conventional (and wrongly named) hen "demyelination" test, and is therefore considerably cheaper. Since it can also be carried out on post mortem human brain in vitro it has the capability of making realistic predictions of neurotoxicity to man[83]. Moreover it is now known that NTE is not exclusive to nervous tissue, being also present in more accessible tissues and cells such as placenta, lymphocytes and leukocytes[84]. This has opened up the possibility of using the inhibition of leukocyte NTE as a means of monitoring human exposure to axonopathic organophosphates.

The NTE method is therefore an extremely powerful one but, depending as it does on a specific mechanism, is inevitably of limited scope. The research effort required to generate methods of this type may be justified only in cases where many structurally related compounds are to be investigated in a search for "me-too" innovations. There is also the risk that because of the complexities involved in developing such sophisticated and powerful methods they would only become available after the greatest need for them had passed. To a certain extent this is true of the NTE method itself, because it appeared after the organophosphates had largely completed their development phase and the era of the next generation of insecticides, the pyrethroids, had begun.

There is no immediate prospect of comparable mechanistically based tests becoming available for other major classes of structural neurotoxins. There are, however, some grounds for considering that a biochemical test for assessing the potential of chemicals (as opposed to merely organophosphates) for producing distal axonopathy may be a possibility by the end of the century. This would be especially valuable since distal axonopathy is one of the most common toxic responses of the nervous system to exogenous chemicals. Considerable strides have been made in understanding the common metabolic basis of this type of lesion[85-89], but whether this will ultimately lead to a viable biochemical test for assessing the potential of chemicals for inducing distal axonopathy remains to be seen. Nevertheless the possibility has already been raised in the literature[90].

In spite of their many advantages, biochemical tests conducted totally in vitro do have some drawbacks. In vitro techniques in which the toxicant is added to the biochemical assay system allow direct interactions at the molecular level to be studied in a controlled environment. However, they eliminate such critical factors to in vivo toxicity as absorption, penetration of the blood/brain barrier, excretion, and secondary and indirect effects. Consequently it will always be necessary, at some stage, to perform tests in vivo/in vitro using tissue from dosed animals. Thus, even if a range of mechanism-based biochemical tests for neurotoxicity could be developed, the need for experimental animals would not be completely eliminated.

This discussion of neurotoxicity tests based on mechanisms has so far concentrated on tests physically carried out either in vivo or in vitro. However, in the future the use of computers to simulate chemical reactions and pharmacological interactions with receptors is expected to grow markedly, and one of its many potential applications will be in the study of structure-activity relationships of xenobiotics. Although with the present state of knowledge it is impossible to determine with any certainty the toxicological action of a drug or chemical solely from consideration of its chemical structure[91], structure-activity studies using computers will increasingly be capable of providing guidance which will enable toxicologists to focus on important structural aspects in selecting the optimum balance between therapeutic (or other bioactive) properties and neurotoxic properties of molecules. This may help to reduce significantly the need for in vivo screening. However, it must be remembered that with our present imperfect knowledge of structure-activity relationships of neurotoxins, there are many potential pitfalls. For example, chemicals with very different structures (e.g. triethyl-tin and hexachlorophene) are known to have very similar neurotoxicity, whereas some chemicals with very similar structures (e.g. triethyl-tin and triethyl-lead) can cause very different neurotoxic effects in vivo.

Neurotoxicity testing in vitro: tissue culture

In vitro toxicological testing methods may be based either on a detailed knowledge of the mechanism of the toxic effect under consideration (as discussed above) or on a structural model of the target system incorporating all the factors that could influence toxicity. It is, however, impossible to conceive of an in vitro system that could even approach the functional and structural complexity of the mammalian nervous system. Even if a model with all the requisite cell types, the ability to integrate sensory and motor output, the equivalent of a blood/brain barrier and a metabolic transformation system could be devised, problems such as the inability to detect behavioural disturbances would remain. An all-embracing primary neurotoxicity detecting testing system using a structural model is therefore not a realistic proposition.

This, of course, assumes that such a testing system should be capable of generating the toxic end-point as it occurs in vivo. However, if the primary purpose of a screening method is prediction with a relatively high level of confidence, it does not really matter how the prediction is made, provided that it is reliable. It has been argued that if many diverse neurotoxic substances killed carnations with 90% certainty, the death of carnations could justifiably be regarded as an acceptable end point for screening for neurotoxicity[92]. This is a perfectly valid pragmatic view, but unfortunately there is no such "carnation test" for neurotoxins at present, nor can one be predicted with any confidence.

The growing need for rapid inexpensive tools for toxicity testing and the experience of successful application of cell culture techniques to the prediction of mutagenicity and carcinogenicity have led to a growing appreciation of the potential usefulness of tissue culture in toxicological evaluation. However, despite the fact that nervous tissue was amongst the first to be successfully cultured, there remain many problems in the use of tissue culture in neurotoxicity testing.

Tests for carcinogenicity look for genetic mutations and disturbances in the control of cellular growth and proliferation. Abnormalities are clearly defined, and relatively simple cell cultures can be used. In contrast, for neurotoxicity assessment one is required to use differentiated cell systems whose principal component, the neurone, has lost the ability to divide. The problems involved in obtaining controllable and predictable nervous tissue cultures are legion, and techniques are time-consuming and expensive.

To date, most neurotoxicological studies in which tissue culture has been used have been concerned with the elucidation of mechanisms of pathogenesis - a task for which these techniques are particularly well suited. Toxicants can be administered to cultures in known pharmacological concentrations, and come into direct contact with the target tissue without the influence of complicating factors such as metabolic transformation or the blood/brain barrier. In addition, secondary effects on the nervous system due to the possible influence of the toxicant on other systems (e.g. vascular, renal, digestive, endocrine or immune) are eliminated. Since metabolic conversion and other indirect effects are absent these techniques can be used to determine whether a compound or one of its metabolites is responsible for its neurotoxic effects in vivo. By these means the metabolite 2,5-hexanedione was shown to be the primary neurotoxic agent in n-hexane and methyl n-butyl ketone neuropathies[93].

The very factors, however, that make tissue culture valuable for the study of mechanism limit its effectiveness as a predictor of in vivo toxicity and therefore the main usefulness of tissue culture in neurotoxicology is likely to remain (at least in the short and medium term) the study of mechanism. Nevertheless, in the longer term, tissue culture could come to have an important role in preliminary screening of chemicals to permit early rejection of some types of neurotoxic compound before effort is invested in in vivo studies or to generate information necessary for in vivo studies to be designed more effectively. For these purposes it will not be necessary to attempt to reproduce as much of the structural and functional complexity of the nervous system as possible in one culture system, but rather to develop a number of simplified systems for answering specific toxicological questions - e.g. systems for testing the relative sensitivity of cell types or organotypic cultures for detecting specific types of neuropathological damage.

Studies with a range of metal and organic compounds have,

on the whole, revealed a remarkable degree of conformity between the type and pattern of neuropathological change observed in organotypic cultures and that observed in vivo. For instance, phenomena such as the neurofibrillary tangles produced in sensory neurones by aluminium and the vacuolation of myelin produced by triethyl-tin have been reproduced in culture[94,95]. An organotypic system gaining acceptance in experimental neurobiology is that composed of structurally and functionally coupled fetal mouse spinal cord, dorsal root ganglia and striated muscle. When mature, this complex displays both morphological and electrophysiological features typical of mammalian neuromuscular tissues, and is capable of reproducing the principal features of aliphatic hexacarbon neuropathy[67,68].

It is probable that, in the future, simplified organotypic cultures may be used for screening for chemically induced peripheral neuropathy. However, before these and other systems can be used routinely, maintenance procedures must be simplified to reduce the costs and time involved, techniques of mass production of cultures to permit statistical analysis of data must be developed, nutrient media and culture conditions must be standardized to minimize interlaboratory and intralaboratory culture variations, and validation must be undertaken in a number of independent laboratories using a wide range of neurotoxins.

In response to intensifying social and economic pressures towards in vitro testing a number of schemes to develop in vitro toxicological screening programmes have been proposed[96]. These involve the use of a range of tests for assessing general cytotoxicity followed by a battery of tests for assessing adverse effects on the cellular functions of highly differentiated cells (hepatic, renal, myocardial, pulmonary, immune, reproductive and neurological). If such integrated approaches receive adequate research support progress in in vitro neurotoxicity pre-screening using tissue culture is likely to accelerate.

Future technological developments may help overcome some of the current technical limitations of tissue culture. The improvements in analytical techniques, biosensors and process control technology that will be necessary to meet the stringent demands of large-scale biotechnological processes involving genetically engineered organisms may well prove relevant to the parallel demands of maintaining the precise environmental conditions demanded by large-scale reproducible tissue culture. Continuing advances in cell biology, particularly the achievement of genetic engineering in eukaryotic cells, will also facilitate the more rapid development of in vitro cytotoxicology.

Validation will be the major rate-determining factor, and can only be undertaken once a consensus regarding culture types and conditions has been achieved. When one considers that validation of the (relatively) straightforward Ames test took over 10 years[97] one cannot be too sanguine concerning the rate of progress in the more contentious field of in vitro neurotoxicology.

Integration

As pressures grow on regulatory authorities to develop guidelines for neurotoxicity testing, the principal challenge will be how to consolidate the mass of disparate testing methods reported in the literature (and the many unpublished methods developed within industry) into a recommended multidisciplinary testing strategy for identifying all potential neurotoxins. Although the importance of an integrated approach to neurotoxicity testing is acknowledged[27], progress towards achieving this aim has not been encouraging. Attempts to reach agreement on a battery of neurobehavioural tests, for example, ran into severe difficulties[9]. The problem will undoubtedly grow as more tests (both in vivo and in vitro) are developed, and knowledge of nervous system vulnerabilities to toxic insult continues to expand. Even if a battery of tests could be agreed upon on scientific grounds, there is always the risk that it could prove prohibitively expensive to apply. This was one of the problems with devising a neurobehavioural test battery - many of the tests, even with advances in automation, were thought to be too expensive to apply across the board to all novel chemicals.

A more realistic aim might be to ensure that all those engaged in neurotoxicity testing are kept fully informed of validated tests that are available for specific purposes. Even now it is virtually impossible for working toxicologists to remain aware of all techniques available. At a time when the gathering, analysis and retrieval of toxicological information is being greatly facilitated by the growth of computerized information systems it is not unrealistic, technically speaking, to envisage the development of a comprehensive neurotoxicity testing data base available to (and contributed to by) those engaged in neurotoxicity testing[98]. Thinking further ahead, one could speculate that artificial intelligence and expert systems could prove an invaluable aid to the efficient detection and elucidation of neurotoxic phenomena. One could envisage an expert system that, on being given details of clinical signs observed during acute or chronic toxicity testing, could offer interpretations and recommendations for (and details of) further tests that would be appropriate for the next level of investigation. Similar systems are already being introduced in medical practice, and the approach is very similar in principle to that used for many years in chemical analysis. It is impossible to forecast when, or if, such systems could become a reality in neurotoxicity testing but there are no obvious technological barriers provided that the will to develop them was there. The first step would be the establishment of a credible interactive neurotoxicology data base to consolidate and structure the existing knowledge in the field. There are encouraging signs (e.g. the Neurotoxicology Information Repository[99]) that first attempts at setting up such systems are already being made.

Human studies

It is a salutary illustration of the inadequacies of past neurotoxicity testing that the properties of many well-known neurotoxins were not predicted on the basis of routine toxicological testing. Too often, effects were first identified as a result of accidental, occupational or therapeutic exposure in man, and were only subsequently reproduced in experimental models. Methyl n-butyl ketone is a good recent example[100]. It is to be hoped that with the increased awareness of the importance of neurotoxicity testing this situation will now improve. Nevertheless the importance and value of detailed studies of cases of accidental exposure in humans should not be underestimated.

Studies of neurotoxic poisoning have given infinitely more relevant information than even the most elegant of animal tests. For example, much of our knowledge of methyl mercury neurotoxicity was obtained from clinical, biochemical, electrophysiological and pathological studies on humans exposed during the notorious outbreaks of poisoning in Japan and Iraq. Similarly, it was study of post mortem human material that revealed the nature of the neurotoxic lesion produced by organic tin[71]. These epidemiological studies were "searching for causes"[101]. The other category of epidemiological study, "searching for effects", is considerably more problematic but the demand for such studies is likely to grow as the need to evaluate subtle effects of chemicals on human behaviour and intellectual performance (as in the case of food additives) increases.

Epidemiological investigations aimed at detecting neurotoxic effects in human populations labour under many difficulties[9,27]. These include:

1. Dose levels are usually too low to produce clearly defined symptoms and signs, and are frequently uncertain or unknown. Exposure may be to more than one toxic agent.

2. Signs and symptoms are frequently obscured by disease or other factors. Changes in neurological function are on a continuum from normal to abnormal; thus distinctions between exposed and control populations are more difficult to detect than, for example, the present or absence of tumours.

3. Neuroepidemiological data (particularly for psychiatric illness and those relating to intelligence) are unrefined in comparison with such clear conditions as cancer. In many cases criteria for diagnosis and classification differ markedly between practitioners.

4. The examination of human material before post mortem (e.g. nerve biopsies, cerebrospinal fluid) is rarely feasible. Post mortem tissue is frequently in a condition that precludes the use of optimal neuropathological techniques. It is difficult to see how these inherent disadvantages can be overcome in any radical way before the end of the century although some isolated advances may be expected. Biochemical measurements in peripherally available tissues (e.g. of neuropeptides) hold out some promise, particularly with the continuing refinements in analytical techniques such as radioimmunoassay. The possible use of leukocyte NTE measurements for monitoring exposure to axonopathic organophosphates has already been alluded to[84]. Perhaps the most significant advances are likely to occur through the dramatically increased

capability for collating and analysing epidemiological data afforded by the growing availability of powerful computerized information systems.

REFERENCES

1. Johnson, MK (1982). The target for initiation of delayed neurotoxicity by organophosphorus esters: biochemical studies and toxicological applications. Rev Biochem Toxicol, 4, 141-212
2. Burki, HR (1979). Extrapyramidal side-effects. Pharmacol Ther, 5, 525-34
3. Schaumburg, HH and Spencer, P (1976). Central and peripheral nervous system degeneration produced by pure n-hexane: an experimental study. Brain, 99, 183-92
4. Prasad, K and Vernadakis, A (eds) (1981). Mechanisms of Actions of Neurotoxic Substances. (New York: Raven Press)
5. Dewar, AJ (1983). Neurotoxicity. In: Balls, M, Riddell, RJ and Worden, AN (eds) Animals and Alternatives in Toxicity Testing. pp. 229-84. (London: Academic Press)
6. Suzuki, K (1980). Special vulnerabilities of the developing nervous system to toxic substances. In: Spencer, PS and Schaumburg, HH (eds) Experimental and Clinical Neurotoxicology. pp. 48-61. (Baltimore: Williams & Wilkins)
7. Suzuki, K and Zagoren, JC (1974). Degeneration of oligodendroglia in the central nervous system of rats treated with AY 9044 or triparanol. Lab Invest, 31, 503-9
8. Pentschew, A (1965). Morphology and morphogenesis of lead encephalopathy. Acta Neuropathol, 5, 133-60
9. Silbergeld, EK (1982). Current status of neurotoxicity, basic and applied. Trends Neurosci, 5, 291-4
10. Fisher, F (1980). Neurotoxicology and government regulation of chemicals in the United States. In: Spencer, PS and Shaumburg, HH (eds) Experimental and Clinical Neurotoxicology. pp. 874-82. (Baltimore: Williams & Wilkins)
11. Morton, DW (1981). Requirements for the toxicological testing of drugs in the USA, Canada and Japan. In: Garrod, JW (ed.) Testing for Toxicity. pp. 11-19. (London: Taylor & Francis)
12. Irwin, W (1964). Drug screening of new compounds in animals. In: Nodine, JH and Siegler, PE (eds) Animals and Clinical Techniques in Drug Evaluation. pp. 36-55. (Chicago: Year Book of Medical Publishers)
13. Vorhees, CV (1974). Some behavioural effects of maternal hypervitaminosis A in rats. Teratology, 10, 269-73
14. Worms, P and Lloyd, KG (1979). Predictability and specificity of behavioural screening tests for neuroleptics. Pharmacol Ther, 5, 445-50
15. Dewar, AJ (1980). Neurotoxicity testing - with particular reference to biochemical methods. In: Garrod, JW (ed.) Testing for Toxicity. pp. 199-217. (London: Taylor & Francis)
16. Johnson, MK and Richardson, RJ (1983). Biochemical endpoints: neurotoxic esterase assay. Neurotoxicity, 4, 317-26

17. Norton, S (1977). Observational techniques in behavioural toxicology. In: Zenick, H and Reiter, LW (eds) Behavioural Toxicology: an Emerging Discipline. pp. 63-72. (Research Triangle Park: US Environmental Protection Agency)

18. Tilson, HA and Mitchell, CL (1981). Models for neurotoxicity. Rev Biochem Toxicol, 2, 265-94

19. Tilson, HA and Cabe, PA (1978). Strategy for the assessment of neurobehavioural consequences of environmental factors. Environ Health Perspect, 26, 287-99

20. Fowler, JSL, Brown, JS and Bell, HA (1979). The rat toxicity screen. Pharmacol Ther, 5, 461-6

21. Brimblecombe, R (1979). Behavioural tests in acute and chronic toxicity studies. Pharmacol Ther, 5, 413-5

22. Perdue, VP, Eastman, WW, Burright, RG and Donovick, PJ (1984). Behavioural analysis of Kanamycin administration to mice. Neurotoxicology, 5, 101-12

23. Miller, MJ, Miller, MS, Burks, TF and Sipes, IG (1984). A simple sensitive method for detecting early peripheral nerve dysfunction in the rat following acrylamide treatment. Neurotoxicology, 5, 15-23

24. Comer, CP and Norton, S (1982). Effects of perinatal methimazole exposure on a developmental test battery for neurobehavioural toxicity in rats. Toxicol Appl Pharmacol, 63, 133-41

25. Roberts, NL, Fairley, C and Phillips, C (1983). Screening, acute delayed and subchronic neurotoxicity studies in the hen: measurements and evaluations of clinical signs following administration of TOCP. Neurotoxicology, 4, 263-70

26. Bogo, V, Hill, TA and Young, RW (1981). Comparison of accelerod and rotarod sensitivity in detecting ethanol- and acrylamide-induced performance decrement in rats: review of experimental considerations of rotating rod systems. Neurotoxicology, 2, 765-87

27. Hess, R, Krinke, G and Schaeppi, J (1983). The integrative approach. In: Balls, M, Riddell, RJ and Worden, AN (eds) Animals and Alternatives in Toxicity Testing. pp. 288-94. (London: Academic Press)

28. Cavanagh, JB (1973). Peripheral neuropathy caused by chemical agents. CRC Crit Rev Toxicol, 2, 365-417

29. Dayan, AD (1979). A morphologist's approach to detection and study of neurotoxicity. Pharmacol Ther, 5, 571-7

30. Sabatini, DD, Bensch, K and Barnett, RJ (1963). Cytochemistry and electron microscopy. The preservation of cellular structure and enzymatic activity by aldehyde fixation. J Cell Biol, 1, 19-25

31. Hayat, MA (1972). Basic Electron Microscopy Techniques. (New York: Von Nostrand Reinhold)

32. Spencer, PS, Bischoff, MC and Schaumburg, HH (1980). Neuropathological methods for the detection of neurotoxic disease. In: Spencer, PS and Schaumburg, HH (eds) Experimental and Clinical Neurotoxicology. pp. 743-57. (Baltimore: Williams & Wilkins)

33. Dyck, PJ and Lais, AC (1970). Electron microscopy of teased nerve fibres: method permitting examination of repeating

structures of same fibre. Brain Res, 23, 418-24

34. Spencer, PS and Bischoff, MC (1982). Contemporary neuropathological methods in toxicology. In: Clifford, L (ed.) Nervous System Toxicology. pp. 259-75. (New York: Raven Press)

35. Johnson, BL (1980). Electrophysiological methods in neurotoxicity testing. In: Spencer, PS and Schaumburg, HH (eds) Experimental and Clinical Neurotoxicology. pp. 726-42. (Baltimore: Williams & Wilkins)

36. Fullerton, PM and Barnes, J (1966). Peripheral neuropathy in rats produced by acrylamide. Br J Indust Med, 23, 210-22

37. Seppalainen, AM and Hernberg, S (1972). Sensitive technique for detecting subclinical lead neuropathy. Br J Indust Med, 29, 443-50

38. De Jesus, CPV, Pleasure, DE, Asbury, AK and Brown, MJ (1978). Effects of methyl butyl ketone on peripheral nerves and its mechanism of action. Final Report Contract CDG 99-766-16. Cincinnati: National Institute for Occupational Safety and Health

39. Mendell, JR, Saida, K, Ganansia, MF, Jackson, DB, Weiss, H, Gardier, RS, Chrisman, C, Allen, N, Couri, D, O'Neill, J, Meeks, B and Hetland, L (1974). Toxic polyneuropathy produced by methyl n-butyl ketone. Science, 185, 787-9

40. Takeuchi, Y and Hisanaga, N (1977). The neurotoxicity of toluene: EEG changes in rats exposed to various concentrations. Br J Indust Med, 34, 314-20

41. Liverani, SL and Schaeppi, U (1979). Electroretinography as an indication of toxic retinopathy in dogs. Pharmacol Ther, 5, 599-602

42. Niemeyer, G (1979). Electrophysiological testing of the function of the vertebrate retina. Pharmacol Ther, 5, 593-7

43. Glatt, AF, Talaat, HN and Koella, WP (1979). Testing of peripheral nerve function in chronic experiments in rats. Pharmacol Ther, 5, 539-43

44. Narahashi, T (1971). Mode of action of pyrethroids. Bull WHO, 44, 337-45

45. Narahashi, T (1980). Nerve membrane as a target of environmental toxicants. In: Spencer, PS and Schaumburg, HH (eds) Experimental and Clinical Neurotoxicology. pp. 225-38. (Baltimore: Williams & Wilkins)

46. Bercken, J van der, Akkermans, LMA and Zalm, JM van der (1973). DDT-like action of allethrin in the sensory nervous system of Xenopus laevis. Eur J Pharmacol, 21, 95-106

47. Wouters, W, Bercken, J van der and Van Ginneken, A (1977). Presynaptic action of the pyrethroid insecticide allethrin in the frog motor end-plate. Eur J Pharmacol, 43, 163-71

48. Bunney, BS (1984). Antipsychotic drug effects on the electrical activity of dopaminergic neurons. Trends Neurosci, 7, 212-5

49. Hasan, Z, Zimmer, L and Woolley, D (1984). Time course of the effects of trimethyltin on limbic evoked potentials and distribution of tin in blood and brain in the rat. Neurotoxicology, 5, 217-44

50. Rose, GP, Dewar, AJ and Stratford, IJ (1980). A biochemical method for assessing the neurotoxic effects of hypoxic cell radiosensitizers: experience with misonidazole. Br J Cancer, 40, 890-9

51. Clarke, C, Davison, KB and Sheldon, PW (1982). Quantitative cytochemical assessment of the neurotoxicity of misonidazole in the mouse. Br J Cancer, 45, 582-7

52. Dudley, AW, Chang, LW, Dudley, MA, Bowman, RE and Katz, J (1977). Review of effects of chronic exposure to low levels of halothane. In: Roizin, L, Shiraki, H and Grcevic, N (eds) Neurotoxicology. pp. 137-45. (New York: Raven Press)

53. Cattebini, F, Galli, CL, Groppetti, A and Racagni, G (1979). Significance of neurochemical parameters in the pre-clinical evaluation of neuroleptic drugs. Pharmacol Ther, 5, 563-70

54. Bondy, SC (1982). Neurotransmitter binding interactions as a screen for neurotoxicity. In: Prasad, KN and Vernadakis, A (eds) Mechanisms of Actions of Neurotoxic Substances. pp. 25-50. (New York: Raven Press)

55. Damstra, TE and Bondy, SC (1980). Neurochemical assay systems for assessing toxicity. In: Spencer, PS and Schaumberg, HH (eds) Experimental and Clinical Neurotoxicology. pp. 820-33. (Baltimore: Williams & Wilkins)

56. Sokoloff, L (1981). The deoxyglucose method for the measurement of local glucose utilisation and the mapping of local functional activity in the central nervous system. Internat Rev Neurobiol, 287-333

57. Johnson, MK (1977). Improved assay of neurotoxic esterase for screening organophosphates for delayed neurotoxicity potential. Arch Toxicol, 37, 113-5

58. Lotti, M and Johnson, MK (1978). Neurotoxicity of organophosphorus pesticides. Predictions can be based on in vitro studies with hen and human enzymes. Arch Toxicol, 41, 215-21

59. Rose, GP and Dewar, AJ (1983). Intoxication with four synthetic pyrethroids fails to show a correlation between neuromuscular dysfunction and neurobiochemical abnormalities in rats. Arch Toxicol, 53, 297-316

60. Richelson, E (1975). Tissue culture of the nervous system: applications in neurochemistry and psychopharmacology. In: Iversen, LL, Iversen, SD and Snyder, SH (eds) Handbook of Psychopharmacology, vol. I. pp. 101-36. (New York: Plenum Press)

61. Kasuya, M (1972). Effects of inorganic, aryl, alkyl and other mercury compounds on the outgrowth of cells and fibres from dorsal root ganglia in tissue culture. Toxicol Appl Pharmacol, 23, 136-46

62. Heilbronn, E and Walum, E (1979). Tissue cultured neuronal cell lines as test systems for toxic compounds. Abstr Int Cong Neurotoxicol, Varese, p. 79

63. Yonezawa, T, Burnstein, MB and Peterson, ER (1980). Organotypic cultures of nerve tissue as a model system for neurotoxicological investigation and screening. In: Spencer, PS and Schaumburg, HH (eds) Experimental and Clinical

Neurotoxicology. pp. 788-802. (Baltimore: Williams & Wilkins)

64. Heilbronn, E (1981). Cell cultures; an alternative in toxicology? - with special reference to the nervous system. Acta Pharmacol Toxicol, 49, 31

65. Trapp, BD and Richelson, E (1980). Usefulness for neurotoxicology of rotation-mediated aggregating cell cultures. In: Spencer, PS and Schaumburg, HH (eds) Experimental and Clinical Neurotoxicology. pp. 803-19. (Baltimore: Williams & Wilkins)

66. Honegger, P and Richelson, E (1976). Biochemical differentiation of mechanically disassociated mammalian brain in aggregating cell culture. Brain Res, 109, 335-54

67. Veronesi, B (1980). An organotypic model of hexacarbon dying back neuropathy, PhD thesis, New York: Albert Einstein College of Medicine

68. Veronesi, B, Lington, AW and Spencer, PS (1984). A tissue culture model of methyl ethyl ketone's potentiation of n-hexane neurotoxicity. Neurotoxicology, 5, 43-52

69. SRI International (1985). Patterns of change: mental health. Business Intelligence Programme Scan No. 2033, 7

70. Lahelma, E (1984). Does unemployment challenge public health? Scand J Soc Med, 12, 105-7

71. Le Quesne, PM (1981). Toxic substances and the nervous system: the role of clinical observation. J Neurol Neurosurg Psychiatry, 44, 1-8

72. Needleman, HL (1983). Lead at low dose and the behaviour of children. Neurotoxicology, 4, 121-33

73. Petit, TL, Alfano, DP and Le Bobtillier, JC (1983). Early lead exposure and the hippocampus: a review and recent advances. Neurotoxicology, 4, 79-94

74. Crick, F (1984). Memory and molecular turnover. Nature, 312, 101

75. Wells, G (1983). Pharmaceutical innovation: recent trends, future propects. London, Office of Health Economics.

76. Iversen, LL (1983). Neuropeptides - what next? Trends Neurosci, 6, 293-4

77. Milner, RJ (1982). Recombinant DNA strategies and techniques. Trends Neurosci, 5, 297-300

78. Bradford, HF (1975). Isolated nerve terminals as an in vitro preparation for the study of dynamic aspects of transmitter metabolism and release. In: Iversen, LL, Iversen, SD and Snyder, SH (eds) Handbook of Psychopharmacology, vol. I. pp. 191-252. (New York: Plenum Press)

79. Cooper, JR, Bloom, S and Roth, TRH (1978). The Biochemical Basis of Neuropharmacology. (Oxford: University Press)

80. Bondy, SC, Anderson, CL, Harrington, ME and Prasad, KN (1979). The effects of organic and inorganic lead and mercury on neurotransmitter high affinity transport and release mechanisms. Environ Res, 19, 102-11

81. Boeynaems, JM (1984). In vitro Methods for the Screening of Drug Activity. First Report: study contract EC1-1008-B-7210-83-B. Commission of the European Communities

82. Garattini, S and Spreafico, F (1984). Feasibility of Pharmacological Tests in Vitro. First Report: study contract EC1-

1007-B-7210-83-1. Commission of the European Communities

83. Lotti, M and Johnson, MK (1980). Neurotoxic esterase in human nervous tissue. J Neurochem, 34, 747-9

84. Richardson, RJ (1983). Neurotoxic esterase: research trends and prospects. Neurotoxicology, 4, 157-62

85. Schoental, R and Cavanagh, JB (1977). Mechanisms involved in the "dying-back" process; an hypothesis implicating co-enzymes. Neuropathol Exp Neurobiol, 3, 143-7

86. Spencer, PS, Sabri, MI, Schaumburg, HH and Moore, CL (1979). Does a defect in energy metabolism in the nerve fibre cause axonal degeneration in polyneuropathies? Ann Neurol, 5, 501-6

87. Sabri, MI and Spencer, PS (1980). Toxic distal axonopathy: biochemical studies and hypothetical mechanisms. In: Spencer, PS and Schaumburg, HH (eds) Experimental and Clinical Neurotoxicology. pp. 206-19. (Baltimore: Williams & Wilkins)

88. Graham, DG (1980). Hexane neuropathy: a proposal for the pathogenesis of a hazard of occupational exposure and inhalant abuse. Chem Biol Interactions, 32, 339-45

89. Cavanagh, JB (1979). The "dying-back" process. A common denomination in many naturally occurring and toxic neuropathies. Arch Pathol Lab Med, 103, 659-64

90. Sabri, MI and Spencer, PS (1979). Developing a test for axonal neurotoxins of environmental significance. Trans Am Soc Neurochem, 10, 63

91. Baumel, IP (1984). Design of safer chemicals: an EPA goal. Drug Metab Rev, 15(3), 415-24

92. Nardone, RM (1980). The interface of toxicology and tissue culture and reflections on the carnation test. Toxicology, 17, 105-11

93. Spencer, PS and Schaumburg, HH (1975). Experimental neuropathy induced by 2,5-hexanedione - a major metabolite of the neurotoxic industrial solvent methyl n-butyl ketone. J Neurol Neurosurg Psychiatry, 38, 771-5

94. Graham, DI, Kim, SU, Gonatas, NK and Gugotte, L (1975). The neurotoxic effects of triethyl tin sulphate on myelinating cultures of mouse spinal cord. J Neuropathol Exp Neurol, 34, 401-12

95. Seil, FJ and Lampert, PW (1969). Neurofibrillary spheroids reduced by aluminium phosphate in dorsal root ganglia neurons in vitro. J Neuropathol Exp Neurol, 28, 74-85

96. Roberfroid, M and Krack, G (1984). Feasibility of in vitro Toxicity Testing. Final report: study contract ECI-1009-B-7210-83-B. Commission of the European Communities

97. Balls, M (1984). In vitro toxicology. ATLA, 12, 108-10

98. Bawden, D and Brock, AM (1982). Chemical toxicological searching: a collaborative evaluation, comparing information resources and searching techniques. J Info Sci, 5, 3-18

99. Pellegrino, RG and Spencer, PS (1980). The establishment of a neurotoxicology information repository (N.I.R.). In: Spencer, PS and Schaumburg, HH (eds) Experimental and Chemical Neurotoxicology. pp. 899-901. (Baltimore: Williams & Wilkins)

100. Billmaier, D, Yee, HT, Allen, N, Craft, B, Williams, N,

Epstein, S and Fontaine, R (1974). Peripheral neuropathy in a coated fabrics plant. Occup Med, 16, 665-71

101. Friedlander, BR and Hearne, FT (1980). Epidemiological considerations in studying neurotoxic disorders. In: Spencer, PS and Schaumburg, HH (eds) Experimental and Chemical Neurotoxicology. pp. 650-62. (Baltimore: Williams & Wilkins)

8

Safety Evaluation – Carcinogenic Risks

J. H. WEISBURGER

INTRODUCTION

In our opinion three broad adverse health effects are most noticed by the public at large - mainly because they involve conditions that are irreversible. The first and probably most important of these is cancer, and the others, of increasing public awareness, are neurological impairment and birth defects.

Cancer, a set of chronic diseases, occurs in high incidence and mortality in many parts of the world. People throughout the world fear cancer more than most other diseases. Historic events have left in the mind of the public the view that chemicals are major causes of cancer. In many countries, therefore, the public demands of their political bodies protection from cancer risks by adequate control of suspected cancer-causing agents. An example expressing these fears and the consequent political action is the Delaney Clause of the Food and Drug Act in the United States. In other countries, similar concerns have been translated into legal regulations.

As these legislative activities were developed in the United States, the Congress in the past 40 years has voted increasingly generous sums designed to further the control of cancer through research. The American Cancer Society, a non-governmental organization privately funded, has found the public a willing contributor of personal funds in the expectation of solving the cancer question. In other parts of the world, likewise, cancer research has been supported by government action and by other agencies. At the same time, research efforts in the basic sciences and in medicine have led to important advances. Thus, in 1944 when Greenstein[1], in a major review dealt, with what was then known about nucleic acids, the field of molecular biology was not yet born. In contrast today, genetic research and engineering are being fruitfully applied to the development of new concepts in the area of cancer causation and detection.

MECHANISMS OF CARCINOGENESIS AND CLASSIFICATION OF CARCINOGENS

It now seems fairly well established that virtually all types of cancer represent a somatic mutation[2]. However, the specific genetic alteration is only a first step in a complex series of individual sequences eventually leading to an invasive neoplasm. The recognition that a series of steps is present in the overall carcinogenic process led to a classification of carcinogens into a number of subgroups. Some carcinogens are characterized by their reactivity towards DNA and the genetic material, and therefore since 1971 have been labelled "genotoxic" or DNA-reactive. The reaction of genotoxic carcinogens with DNA is followed by genetic alterations, including oncogenes, an area of research where knowledge is currently accruing rapidly, and promises a detailed insight into the important elements involved in carcinogenesis. Such understanding may also yield the tools for early diagnosis of neoplasia, and perhaps even its therapy.

Additional steps dealing with the growth and development of the altered cells with abnormal genomes have been discovered in the overall carcinogenic process. A controlling factor in the growth phase is the phenomenon of promotion. Early on, the concept distinguishing initiation and promotion stemmed from the pioneering studies of Berenblum and Shubik and of Shear. In contemporary terms, promotion, now an active subject of research, appears to relate to the effect of certain chemicals in modifying membranes and receptors, which, through mechanisms yet to be established, releases cells from growth control. These modes of action may involve epigenetic effects on intercellular communication, differentiation, and endocrine systems.

CAUSES OF HUMAN CANCER

In the past 30 years much has been learned also about the causes of important forms of human cancer[3]. First discovered, was the relationship between heavy exposure to certain chemicals at the workplace and the appearance of specific kinds of cancer, often decades later. The relationship between exposure to dye-stuff intermediates in chemical plants and cancer in the urinary bladder is one example, and more recently the incidence of hepatic angiosarcoma, seen in cleaners of reactor vessels for the polymerization of vinyl chloride, was related to exposure to the monomer.

More importantly, however, for the aim of eventual cancer prevention, was the finding that lifestyle accounts for the majority of the main human cancers[4]. Cigarette smokers or other users of tobacco products have a high risk of specific neoplasms, notably of the respiratory tract, pancreas, kidney, and bladder[5].

Snuff dippers or tobacco chewers are at high risk for cancer of the oral cavity and oesophagus[6]. Smoking also increases the risk of fatal heart attacks in the Western world. The customary use of salted, pickled, and smoked food is associated with cancer of the stomach, and in areas such as China it is associated with cancer of the oesophagus[7]. These same conditions are also connected with hypertension and stroke[8]. In the United States, and beginning also in other parts of the world, these diseases have dropped dramatically in the past 50 years with the advent of widespread home refrigeration, abolishing the need for salting, pickling, and smoking as a means of food preservation. Other kinds of prevalent human cancers in the Western world - specifically cancer in the colon, breast, prostate, ovary, endometrium, and in part, pancreas - are associated with the customary intake of a high level of total fat at about 40% of calories[9]. In contrast, these diseases formerly had a low incidence in equally developed and industrialized Japan, where the traditional fat intake used to amount to only about 15% of calories. A high level of dietary fat appears involved in the process of promotion for the development of these nutritionally linked cancers. This higher level of fat in the customary diets of the Western world, especially saturated fat from meats and dairy products, also represents a risk for atherosclerosis and heart disease[10-12].

As will be discussed below, in the context of safety evaluation, promotion is highly dose-dependent and in great part reversible. Thus current recommendations to lower the intake of fat in the diet in the Western world are designed to lower the risk of development of these prevalent forms of cancer. If governmental agencies, industrial management, and the public would agree to make greater efforts to alter nutritional traditions, and to decrease the use of tobacco products, risk for many major forms of cancer would be substantially reduced.

Clearly the main theme of this book, predictive safety evaluation, applied to carcinogenesis, will be absolutely useless unless people take advantage of what has been learned about the causes of cancer, heart disease, and stroke, and institute the appropriate preventive steps. Toxicology is useful only if its knowledge is translated meaningfully and realistically to public action. Actual or attempted bans of such environmental chemicals as food dye Red No. 2, nitrite, or saccharin will have no effect whatsoever on the incidence of many prevalent forms of cancer, because these products, under actual conditions of use, are clearly not human cancer risks.

Toxicologists, as well as lay people, must realize that actions intended to protect the public against real hazards require the carefully structured application of the results of research and testing, involving those elements that can be directly related to risk for neoplastic diseases, especially if the relevant mechanisms are understood. It is true that in the course of developing research approaches, situations occur where certain basic research efforts do not directly, or initially, bear on conditions actually representing human disease risk. Research of that kind is valuable, but the individuals performing it, and those interpreting it, should be aware that such basic research, while greatly adding to our broad base of knowledge, must not necessarily be applied to efforts for disease prevention or control if the investigational system is not appropriate to those ends.

CARCINOGENIC PROCESS

The current view of the carcinogenic process sees it as a multi-step series of events usually beginning with the conversion of an agent called a procarcinogen to an active form through metabolism[13,14]. This reaction, mainly carried out by the cytochrome P-450 metabolic system, is highly dependent on species, strain, and environmental conditions. In part, therefore, the ultimate incidence of cancer is determined by this early event. The reactive chemical produced interacts with the genetic material, specifically DNA, which upon cell duplication yields further gene alterations, including gene rearrangement and gene amplification. The cell with the abnormal genome so generated is conceived to be the latent tumour cell. This sequence of actions is part of the genotoxic pathway[15].

The growth and development of the abnormal cell requires the participation of host factors, as well as external agents operating as growth control elements, that may play a role in function and differentiation. These conditions bearing on growth and development are certainly quite different from those affecting genotoxicity. Environmentally important agents such as promoters may enhance this stage of the overall process. The conversion of a benign tumour, obtained in this sequence, to a malignant, invasive neoplasm or a highly differentiated cancer to an anaplastic, undifferentiated cancer has been labelled progression. The mechanisms whereby this process occurs are not known, although the operation of another alteration of the genetic apparatus seems likely.

Clearly, safety assessment means the capability to detect agents that are genotoxic, and other agents that act as promoters - or if future research indicates that progression is susceptible to external influences, to detect chemicals that affect that part of the process.

One direct means of safety assessment is the observation of cancer in humans exposed to specific chemicals. In the past this means of detecting carcinogens was concerned mainly with occupation-related cancer, while contemporary efforts aim to determine the nature of exogenous factors bearing on the aetiology of the common human cancers. Great progress has been made along these lines by establishing that, in the main, lifestyles related to smoking, excessive alcohol use, and nutrition, and in part, malnutrition are the major causes of most human cancers in most parts of the world.

The traditional approach to safety assessment involved the administration of test chemicals to animals (in recent years, mostly rodents). This scheme was based on the fact that known human carcinogens, when so tested, usually elicited neoplasms in such systems, and importantly, often did so in high incidence with a relatively short latent period. Thus any test compound with such properties, when administered to several strains or species of rodents, was construed to be a human cancer risk. Such chemicals were considered to be potent carcinogens.

With the development in many countries, especially the United States, of the use of large-scale animal bioassays, the data generated were interpreted as showing evidence of carcinogenicity by virtue of statistically significant, yet small, increases in the incidence of single types of neoplasms. Evidence of carcinogenicity often appeared in endocrine-sensitive tissues such as the adrenal or thyroid, and sometimes was seen in only one species. Because of the statistically significant increase in neoplasms, chemicals yielding such results were often labelled carcinogens. Based on legislation in some countries, and regulatory activities in others, action was often taken to control the use of chemicals displaying such limited effects. Yet it is questionable whether chemicals with such circumscribed ability to produce neoplasms are actually human carcinogenic hazards. In the absence of additional data with respect to genotoxicity or promoting properties, such a decision is most difficult and controversial. For that reason it is absolutely essential to generate additional information as to the broad toxicological properties of a given chemical.

SHORT-TERM TESTS

With the realization that the early events in carcinogenesis involved an alteration of the genome, efforts were made to develop rapid bioassays utilizing this property to detect carcinogens[16]. Based on the pioneering work of Rosenkranz, who developed indicators based on Escherichia coli, and of Ames who evolved systems utilizing Salmonella typhimurium mutants, large series of chemicals could be tested. In addition, a number of mammalian cell systems were introduced. In contrast, however, to recently explanted cells, many of these have been in culture for a number of generations, and they often have only low levels of the necessary metabolic activation systems. Thus most of the mammalian cell systems used also require an external supply of a metabolizing unit.

The procedures of Ames involved the use of a mitochondrial supernatant, including cytosol and microsomal fractions of rodent liver. This S9 fraction has found application also for the production of mutants, or to secure transformation of mammalian cells when these cells did not seem to have endogenous metabolic capability.

Of note is the fact that the S9 fraction of liver includes most of the required metabolic capability to convert procarcinogens to reactive products, but usually has quite low capabilities, in the absence of added co-factors, to produce type II conjugation reactions. Indeed, tests of chemicals under these conditions may yield false-positive responses because of the absence of type II conjugation systems that usually lead to detoxification. For example, a number of flavones, including quercetin, are positive in prokaryotic test organisms plus a liver S9 fraction, whereas in the presence of detoxication systems, and in vivo, such chemicals are negative[17].

Another important point is that the use of the S9 fraction, essential as it is, suffers from an inherent limitation. This limitation became apparent in several interlaboratory and international test series run on the same chemicals but utilizing different assays. A careful evaluation of the results obtained showed that in many instances the response with distinct prokaryotic or eukaryotic organisms was similar. The explanation may be that no matter which indicator DNA is used, any test is limited by the metabolic system utilized. If, in several different tests, the same kind of S9 fraction is utilized, it is the S9 fraction that is common to all tests and constitutes a limitation, based on metabolism, of these test systems. When a given indicator DNA in an organism can be shown to produce comparable sensitivity in the detection of altered DNA, use of such distinct tests involving an identical S9 fraction in a battery is redundant.

Yet it is quite clear that a carefully selected battery of tests is necessary to provide optimal information on possible genotoxicity of chemicals. It was noted above that any test system has several components. One is the biochemical activation and detoxication system used to mimic as closely as possible the situation prevailing in vivo in experimental animals and in man. The second is the indicator DNA and genetic material. The third is the transfer of any DNA-reactive metabolite from its site of production to the indicator DNA.

Because freshly explanted hepatocytes have a biochemical competence mimicking the in vivo situation better than the S9 fraction, this cell type is now widely utilized for in vitro studies. One problem with hepatocyte as an external means of biochemical change is that the metabolites produced need to pass across two membranes - first that of the hepatocyte, and second that of the indicator DNA cell system - which could be either mammalian or bacterial. With fairly stable ultimate reactive mutagens or carcinogens, this system may be adequate, but with metabolites with short half-life, this system may not be efficient.

One way of overcoming some of these limitations is to study the indicator DNA in the same cell that performs the metabolic conversion. In this instance the nuclear membrane only may be an obstacle to the efficient transfer of reactive metabolite. In fact in some instances, enzymes within the nucleus were found to convert a chemical to an active metabolite.

Thus the induction of DNA damage in freshly explanted hepatocytes, proposed by Williams[18] in 1976, and since validated by his laboratory and others, probably resembles most closely the overall biochemical and physiological features prevailing in vivo. Hepatocytes from several species, including human, have been used. Freshly explanted cells represent virtually the gamut of enzymic activities prevailing in vivo, and include activation as well as detoxication systems. The target DNA is in the same cell, alleviating the problem of transfer of metabolites through cellular membranes. This system has been exploited with two end-points, one of which is the development of DNA repair, a direct consequence of specific DNA damage. This test system has received fairly widespread support, and technically can be executed simply and reliably. There seem to be fewer discrepancies when this test is performed in different laboratories with the same chemical[19,20], in contrast to the variability sometimes encountered with the Ames Salmonella typhimurium system, as discussed above.

The second end-point is the development of mutants at the HGPRT locus, as revealed by sensitivity to antimetabolites such as thioguanine and azaguanine. Not only is this test system distinct from the bacterial mutagenicity assays, but it can also be readily and routinely performed. Thus this system should be considered an essential part of a battery of in vitro bioassay systems to detect genotoxic chemicals. Yet despite its clear theoretical and practical advantage this test system, now 10 years old, has not been adopted as widely as its promising sensitivity and specificity would indicate, although a trend towards its more general use has begun to appear.

A number of groups have utilized hepatocyte test systems in an in vivo-in vitro scheme[21]. The main reason for this variant is that under some conditions, such as nitroaryl compounds or conjugates with a glucosidic residue such as cycasin, such compounds are converted to reactive intermediates or proximate carcinogens by the action of bacterial enzymes from the intestinal tract. However, the Williams test can be adapted by adding specific enzymes such as glucosidases to the medium when the chemical to be tested is a suspected glucosidic or similar conjugate. Enzyme mixtures from bacteria can also be added in vitro to provide the necessary source of enzymes. The in vivo/in vitro scheme is much less economical because the test compound needs to be injected into a number of animals at several dose levels.

Other test systems involve cell transformation and sister chromatid exchange (SCE). Technically, cell transformation systems are much more demanding in staff skill and time. In many instances, especially if epithelial cells rather than mesenchymal cells are used, the end-points are difficult to visualize. More importantly, cell transformation has been obtained with chemicals that in other tests for genotoxicity were clearly negative. Thus cell transformation as an in vitro indicator needs to be construed as providing information on possible neoplasm-inducing properties in the broadest sense, rather than as a specific indicator of genotoxicity. The same position can be taken with SCE. The current status suggests that agents, not necessarily genotoxic, have yielded positive responses. Yet others that were clearly genotoxic did not. Nonetheless, because SCE can be detected not only in cells from tissues but also in formed elements from blood, SCE can be usefully extended to detect possible exposure to harmful chemicals in the workplace situation.

New approaches utilize the fact that specific immunoassays can be developed for specific carcinogen DNA or carcinogen protein adducts[22,23]. While such test systems are not useful to delineate the carcinogenic risks for unknown chemicals, they are accurate means of detecting individual exposure to specific known chemical carcinogens. No doubt these techniques will find broader and more general use in the future.

Human exposure to potential genotoxic agents can be visualized by examining urine for mutagenic metabolites. This technique, of course, requires current intake of the agent.

PROMOTION AND PROMOTERS

Mouse skin has been the classical model in which to investigate promotion in carcinogenesis[24]. In more recent years other organ systems - including colon, breast, liver, pancreas, and urinary bladder - have been shown to be susceptible to promotion[9,25]. Detailed laboratory studies and field observations have also demonstrated that human cancer causation at specific target organs is the result of initiation, cocarcinogenesis, and promotion. Thus complex tobacco smoke contains initiators, cocarcinogens, and promoters. Likewise, cancer at target sites, such as breast and colon, related to nutritionally linked carcinogenesis, depends to a considerable extent on the promoting phenomenon.

In addition, with experience in the evaluation of large-scale bioassays for carcinogens, it became clear that a number of environmentally important chemicals, pesticides such as DDT and solvents such as trichlorethylene or perchloroethylene, usually failed to induce significant cancer in rats or hamsters, but with great regularity led to neoplasms in the liver of the mouse strains used. These mouse strains normally display a certain incidence of spontaneous liver cancer. When these kinds of compounds or their metabolites were tested in in vitro tests for genotoxicity, little evidence appeared that they had the specific property of DNA reactivity[26].

Thus the conclusion could be formulated that such compounds induce liver cancer in specific mouse strains by the phenomenon of promotion. This distinction is important since, as will be discussed, agents that play a role as promoters in the overall carcinogenic process eventually need quite different public health consideration for cancer control purposes, compared with those agents that are definitely genotoxic.

It is important to develop test systems to delineate promoting potential. Such test systems should preferably be based on the specific properties of promoters. One fairly recent development in this area suggests that promoters may break gap junctions and lead to interruption of intercellular communication in cell culture. The groups of Trosko, Murray, Fitzgerald, and Williams, among others have utilized this specific property as a practical means of detecting promoters[27-30]. A number of chemicals such as certain halogenated hydrocarbons, the antioxidant butylated hydroxyanisole (BHA), or bile acids are all positive in such tests. Clearly, more research to reliably detect promoters, perhaps using additional end-points, in a battery of tests, as is available for genotoxic carcinogens, is desirable.

LIMITED IN VIVO BIOASSAYS

If the preceding test battery has provided qualitative evidence that a given chemical is either a genotoxic carcinogen or a promoter, validation of such properties and exploration of potency is necessary. A number of relatively rapid in vivo bioassays can be used since carcinogenesis is often organ-specific, usually as a result of the organ-related metabolic competence to form reactive metabolites, in contrast to detoxified products. Particular in vivo tests are selected based on comprehension of the probable mechanisms of action, whether genotoxic or promoting, of a given chemical.

The in vivo systems include the induction of abnormal foci in rodent liver, of skin tumours in mice, of mammary neoplasms in Sprague-Dawley female rats, and of pulmonary tumours in sensitive strains of mice[31]. Most of these tests can be conducted in less than 1 year. They should compare a series of test compounds with the action of a known positive control carcinogen. They should be conducted at a number of dose levels to indicate the slope of the dose-response curve of the test compound versus the known positive control.

Most of these systems can be designed to delineate potency and activity of genotoxic carcinogens as such. In other instances one or a few doses applied to target organs, or delivered systemically, followed by an appropriate promoter, can yield information of potency as an initiator. For mouse skin the usual promoter is the phorbol ester TPA; for rat or mouse liver, phenobarbital; and for mammary gland, a high-fat diet. In mice, however, phenobarbital itself yields liver neoplasms, and therefore the time of occurrence and slope of the dose-response curve are important criteria in evaluating the effect.

For agents suspected to act as promoters, a genotoxic carcinogen appropriate for the relevant target organ should be administered, followed by the test substance at four or five dose levels. Here again, the appropriate positive control promoter at several dose levels will indicate relative potency.

In all these studies utilizing in vivo bioassay systems, three end-points require consideration: (1) percentage of animals with histopathologically validated lesions, (2) the multiplicity and size of neoplasms, and (3) the time to occurrence of tumour.

An overall evaluation of results from the battery of in vitro tests and the limited in vivo bioassay tests often provides sufficient information for risk assessment and possible protection. As will be discussed under quantitative evaluation below, this set of in vitro and in vivo tests is especially revealing if the in vivo tests have been performed at a number of dose levels, four or six, so that a large enough data base exists to visualize the potency of a chemical based on the shape of the dose-response curve. Squire[32] and Wang[33] have reported on a semi-quantitative rating system, in which genotoxicity is taken into account.

Overall, the battery of data generated by in vitro tests for genotoxicity or promoting potential and properly designed limited in vivo bioassays most often will provide an adequate data base to protect the public. Thus chronic bioassays will be needed only infrequently.

BIOASSAYS FOR CHRONIC TOXICITY AND CARCINOGENICITY

Until recently, 2-year or even lifetime tests in rodents were the classic means of detecting carcinogenicity. With the advent of a better understanding of the mechanisms of cancer causation, the insight derived from the tests for genotoxicity, and the beginning development of rapid tests for possible promoting substances, the classic long-term bioassay may no longer be essential in order to protect the public against possible carcinogenic risks. Indeed, from the experience of the National Cancer Institute (NCI), now the

National Toxicity Program (NTP), large-scale bioassay programme, developed by Elizabeth Weisburger, Michael Shimkin, and John Weisburger beginning in 1962[34,35], it appears that the test results can be easily misinterpreted if the data obtained are not scrutinized with regard to the underlying mechanisms. In the early years, based on suspicion of carcinogenicity attached to certain chemicals because of insight into structure-activity correlations, series of chemicals such as monocyclic arylamines, halogenated hydrocarbons or specific types of pesticides, or drugs used in cancer chemotherapy, were selected for testing. As was expected, many of the chemicals so tested proved not only to be carcinogenic but also quite potent. That is, such chemicals were active in several species - mice and rats in particular - and led to the induction of cancer at one or more sites in substantial yield, often with a latent period of less than 18 months. Subsequently, with the development of short-term in vitro tests based on mutagenicity and genotoxicity, many of these compounds could be classified as genotoxic. An example is ethylene dibromide and the related dibromochloropropane that induce cancer reliably in high yield and actually in less than 9 months.

From this programme, test results for hundreds of chemicals are now available. Some chemicals were clearly negative, and some clearly positive. In a large number of cases, however, evidence of "carcinogenicity" was based on a relatively small, yet statistically significant, incidence, compared with simultaneous controls, of given neoplasms such as phaeochromocytomas, thyroid adenomas, or neoplastic nodules in the liver (without evidence of carcinomas). In such instances the chemical exhibiting this kind of result was tagged with the label "carcinogen". Furthermore, in vitro bioassays gave either no evidence of activity, or else activity was seen in perhaps one specific, often not widely used, test. In fact the evidence for genotoxicity might be based on the test of the chemical itself, without the simultaneous test of known positive controls, especially positive controls with structural features analogous to the chemical tested. A recent exchange of published letters[36] indicates that from 40% to 80% of chemicals tested were found "carcinogenic" in the US bioassay series. Do such numbers truly have meaning in relation to the actual risk of cancer for persons exposed to such a chemical? This question will be discussed later.

In any case, such far-reaching interpretations of bioassays, with possible regulatory implications, have led to questions not on the interpretation of results but rather on the procedures used in bioassays; especially singled out was the concept that one dose level should be high - the maximally tolerated dose, MTD. Nevertheless, there are good reasons for having such a dose level. Briefly, with known human carcinogens, testing at a high dose level has been necessary to demonstrate and reveal in the animal model the carcinogenicity obviously attached to such a chemical. For example, the classic human carcinogen 2-naphthylamine led to urinary bladder cancer in hamsters at 10,000 ppm but not at 1,000 ppm[31]. Another example stems from large-scale human studies involving cigarette smokers where the daily consumption of 40 cigarettes per day clearly represents a health risk, whereas the effect of four cigarettes per day is difficult to visualize.

Thus it is still necessary for in vivo bioassays to be conducted under conditions where at least one dose level is the MTD. With current knowledge, however, the decision to conduct a large-scale, expensive experiment will benefit from data on the presence or absence of genotoxicity. Based on such information, the definitive bioassay should employ four or more dose levels, including MTD. This scheme will provide information on the shape of the dose-response curve, and thus yield the essential data base for eventual health risk assessment. It is not proper, and as a matter of fact is scientifically unacceptable, to perform health risk assessments based on results available at only one or two dose levels. Every chemical has specific biological properties. For some, activity is apparent over a large range of dosages - as, for example, with dimethylnitrosamine or 2-acetylaminofluorene. For others, such as safrole, a sharp decrease in activity is seen as the dose is lowered. It is clear that the health risk formulation depends to a considerable extent on the quantitative data available.

Limited in vivo bioassays and standard chronic bioassays can be designed to reveal the effect not only of genotoxic carcinogens but also of promoters. In the latter instance, information is needed on the specific target organ where the promoter exerts its major effect. Pretreatment of the animals with an appropriate dose of a genotoxic carcinogen for that target organ, followed by a number of dose levels of the presumed promoter, provides quantitative information on the effect of the promoter. With a sufficient number of dose levels, taking into account possible human exposure, any no-effect level, presumed to exist with promoting substances, can be pinpointed. To facilitate statistical data management, a pyramidal increasing number of experimental animals with lower dose levels should be used. The untreated, and where indicated, vehicle-treated controls should involve the same larger number of animals as that used with the lowest dosage group.

DEFINITION OF A CARCINOGEN AS A POTENTIAL HUMAN CARCINOGENIC RISK

It is apparent from the preceding discussion of chronic bioassays that a chemical labelled "carcinogen" based on test results alone is not necessarily a human carcinogenic risk. How can we define and classify a human carcinogenic risk? In addition to strict statistical considerations it is important to involve sets of data bearing on mechanisms of action.

Most human carcinogens are also animal carcinogens. Not only is this a true statement, but it can be amplified as follows. Virtually all human carcinogens, when tested in the customary animal bioassays, usually induce cancer in several different species and do so in high yield, with 80-100% of animals affected, and with a latent period that is often relatively short, 12-18 months or less. Human carcinogens that are genotoxic, and most of them are, also reliably display activity in most of the in vitro short-term tests.

The reverse is likely to be true also. Thus a chemical (1) that is _reliably_ active in batteries of short-term tests (not just a single test) and that can thus be labelled genotoxic; (2) that is definitively active (high yield of tumours, latent period less than 18 months) in <u>several</u> in vivo bioassay systems; and (3) that exhibits activity over a range of dose levels, is likely to be a human cancer risk. Such a chemical requires appropriate worldwide controls to avoid cancer risk. For example, the recently discovered mutagenic heterocyclic amines formed during the frying of fish or meat fulfil these criteria. They display activity in most of the in vitro bioassays and carcinogenicity in every test so far performed in mice and rats (see ref.37).

When an unknown test chemical is active in only a few or only one of the in vitro bioassays, its classification as genotoxic requires careful analysis of the positive and negative experiments. For example, the plant flavone quercetin is active in the Ames test with metabolic activation but displays little activity in any other rapid bioassay test. It is negative in the Williams hepatocyte repair assay. Careful testing of quercetin in mice, rats, and hamsters has failed to demonstrate carcinogenicity[38]. One report indicates high-level feeding can induce liver tumours in low yield, consistent with a promoting rather than a carcinogenic effect[39]. Mechanistic analysis suggests that quercetin and related polyhydroxylated flavones may be positive in the Ames test because H_2O_2 or hydroxyl radicals might be generated under the conditions of the test. In mammalian systems, biochemical defence mechanisms protect against these reactive molecules or radicals; therefore tests in mammalian systems are usually negative. For these reasons a positive response in a single test alone requires careful analysis.

A limited response in a carcinogenicity bioassay also needs evaluation of the relevant mechanisms to reach sound conclusions appropriate for human risk assessment. For example, any lesions in endocrine-sensitive target organs such as the adrenal, thyroid, or pituitary gland may be due to the creation of hormonal imbalances, via mechanisms to be established. These, in turn, are usually highly dose-dependent and call for a multidose bioassay to determine the possible existence of no-effect levels.

Similar considerations apply for disturbances to other homeostatic systems where dose-response studies are absolutely essential to determine the linearity or non-linearity of an effect. These factors apply mainly to non-genotoxic agents, albeit even genotoxic agents under certain conditions could lead to possible disturbances in homeostatic balances.

Finally, ever more sensitive chemical analytical techniques can detect the existence of more chemicals in the environment. Do such small amounts have toxicologic significance, especially as regards cancer risks? Thus it is essential to acquire sound information on the quantitative aspects of an effect. Quantitation is especially indicated in the overall assessment of the causes of major types of human cancer that can involve complex interactions of genotoxic components present in relatively small amounts, and promoters that control the eventual development of cancer. For example, in nutritional carcinogenesis the genotoxic components may be generated during the cooking of food. The intake of dietary fat yields important promoting or enhancing elements at specific target organs such as breast or colon, but not in other organs such as the liver[4]. Understanding of this promoting phenomenon provides an accounting of why these newly discovered carcinogens formed during the cooking process do not seem to induce liver cancer in man, even though high-level intake in mice and rats suggests the liver as one of the target organs, in addition to colon and breast. In the absence of promoters, the liver is not affected.

Thus the data base required for risk assessment and the protection of man against cancer hazards involves systematic analysis of data as follows:

A.　Structure-activity relationships.

B.　Results of short-term in vitro tests yielding data

　　(1)　for genotoxicity
　　(2)　for non-genotoxicity
　　(3)　that are indeterminate (such as positive in one test and negative in another).

C.　In vivo bioassays yielding

　　(1)　high incidence of disease in mice, rats, and/or hamsters with a relatively short latent period
　　(2)　evidence of non-carcinogenicity
　　(3)　low but statistically significant incidence with a long latent period in:

　　　　(a)　endocrine-sensitive target organs, or
　　　　(b)　specific non-endocrine target organs.

Of these possibilities, the demonstration of genotoxicity and rapid powerful action in animal models on the one hand, or negative results in all bioassays, in vitro and in vivo, would be clear-cut eventualities and would require little discussion. In the first instance a carcinogen with such properties should be controlled or eliminated wherever possible. In the second instance there would be no risk. The third type of result needs detailed analysis and interpretation, as discussed above. In most instances it will be found that a chemical with such properties, displayed through systematic approaches in test series A, B, and C, is not likely to be a human cancer risk. No human carcinogen is known, after 60 years of carcinogenesis research, that has such properties.

QUANTITATIVE ASPECTS OF CARCINOGENESIS

DNA-reactive carcinogens

As is the case with other pharmacological agents, the response to chemical carcinogens is dose-dependent[40-42]. Nonetheless, carcinogens of the electrophilic DNA-reactive type are quite distinct from ordinary pharmacological agents in one way. Drugs, and toxic chemicals generally, exert their action rapidly. As the drug is metabolized and excreted the effect diminishes to the vanishing point, and in most instances no residual effect persists. Subsequent exposures act anew in the same manner, without any long-lasting effects. In contrast, while the onset of the interaction between a carcinogen and the cell is fundamentally similar, in that the chemical may undergo biotransformation, the key, biochemically activated, ultimate carcinogen reacts with tissue macromolecules, of which DNA is critical. During DNA synthesis and cell duplication, altered DNA can lead to gene or chromosomal mutations imprinting a permanent effect in the cell.

Therefore, with DNA-reactive, genotoxic carcinogens, a given dose can result in permanent abnormalities of cells. Subsequent dosages can add to such a change. After a sufficient number of such alterations have been produced, the multiplication of abnormal cells results in a detectable lesion, and eventually a neoplasm. Because the effects vary with the carcinogen and the tissue in which it exerts its action, the time required for a neoplasm to appear varies. Thus time as well as dose is a factor in assessing the properties of chemical carcinogens. It is primarily in this way that DNA-reactive carcinogens differ from ordinary toxic agents; a number of small doses may give no immediate evidence of their action, but in time they yield neoplasms within the lifespan of the host. Indeed, some carcinogens of the DNA-reactive type can induce cancer in animal models with a single dose. With toxins, comparably small dosages for acute effects would likely be completely innocuous.

DNA-reactive carcinogens are further distinct from other types of toxins, in so far as the same total dose, when administered as smaller doses over a longer period of time, may actually be more effective than when given as larger, yet fewer individual doses in a shorter period of time. In the extreme, several chemicals, such as 2-acetylaminofluorene, which are potent carcinogens when administered chronically, are not at all active when given as a single large dose. Administration of small single doses can also be disproportionately effective compared to larger doses, especially when accompanied by promotion[43].

In quantifying carcinogenic effects, the incidence of each kind of neoplasm in exposed groups compared with the control groups is essential information. More sensitivity is obtained if the parameters for evaluation include the latent period (time to tumour), often expressed as the time when the experimental group has reached a 50% incidence of neoplasms, or the total time required for all animals to manifest neoplasms. Another relevant parameter of effect is the multiplicity of specific neoplasms which, when considered in relationship to dosage, yields a more refined estimate of dose-response effects.

In numerous experiments using appropriate quantitative parameters, detailed dose-response relationships have been demonstrated. Two effects are usually observed with potent genotoxic carcinogens: with increasing dose (1) the percentage yield and multiplicity of neoplasms increases, and (2) the time required for neoplasm appearance decreases. In most cases the overall neoplasm yield in any specific organ is proportional to the total dose, but the speed or rate of neoplasm appearance is related to the amount in an individual dose or dose rate[41].

A controversial issue in dose-response relationships is

whether no-effect or threshold levels exist for chemical carcinogens. In a classic study by Bryan and Shimkin[44], 12 doses of
each of three polycyclic aromatic hydrocarbons were injected subcutaneously in mice. There were 40-80 animals in the lower dose
groups and 20 in the higher. The actual data show that two or
three of the lower exposure levels yielded no evidence of tumour.
Such observations, although clearly demonstrating thresholds
within the context of the experiment, have not been accepted as
evidence of thresholds for large numbers of subjects at risk because of statistical limitations.

To develop some information on the actual shape of the dose-
response curve at low levels of exposure, several relatively large-
scale studies have been conducted. In one study conducted at the
National Center for Toxicological Research in the USA, mice were
fed 2-acetylaminofluorene at seven doses ranging between 30 and
150 ppm, an overall range of only five-fold[45]. The data were interpreted as revealing a linear dose response for liver neoplasms,
but providing evidence for a no-effect level at 45 ppm for bladder
cancer. Another large-scale study performed at the British Industrial Biological Research Association[46] involved administration of
15 dose levels, from 16 to 0.033 ppm, of two nitrosamines to rats.
This study has also been interpreted to show a linear response for
liver neoplasms, but with a no-effect level for oesophageal cancer.
These studies thus suggest carcinogenic effects at low-level exposures in liver, but not in other tissues.

DNA-reactive carcinogens vary greatly in their potency. For
example, among liver carcinogens a greater than 50% incidence is
produced by lifetime administration of aflatoxin B_1 at 1 ppb, by
diethylnitrosamine at 5 ppm, by safrole at 1000-5000 ppm, and by
acetamide at 12,500 ppm. Relatively few studies have been done on
the effect of dose rate or even dose response with the weaker
DNA-reactive carcinogens. Shimkin and Stoner[47] examined the
potential of alkylating drugs of diverse structures to induce pulmonary tumours in mice. They found that the strong carcinogens
were active over a broad dose range, whereas the weaker ones
gave evidence of some carcinogenicity only at the highest, but not
at lower, dose levels. Long et al.[48] fed safrole in the diet to
groups of 50 rats at levels of 100, 500, 1000 and 5000 ppm. Malignant liver cancers were obtained only at the highest dose level,
and benign adenomas at the two highest, but not the lower doses.
Thus, available data show that a threshold or no-effect level can
be observed with some DNA-reactive carcinogens under standard
bioassay conditions. However, the question can always be raised
whether such thresholds would be seen if larger numbers of
animals were used, as in the two large-scale studies. Based upon
considerations of metabolism, the barriers to electrophiles in reaching critical targets in DNA, DNA repair processes, and the like, it
seems almost certain that for every carcinogen there must be a
threshold. It may be very low for powerful carcinogens, as suggested by the two studies on 2-acetylaminofluorene and the
nitrosamines, but seems to be correspondingly higher for weak
carcinogens.

These dose-response studies on DNA-reactive carcinogens
have provided the data for mathematical modelling. A number of

models have been proposed[49], and there is active debate as to which of these is most appropriate. One model, widely used by regulatory agencies because it is "conservative", consists of a linear no-threshold extrapolation. As noted, no proof has been found for any carcinogen that no threshold exists, and in fact thresholds have been observed in many studies, particularly with weak carcinogens. The assumption of linearity at low doses is also not well founded. Indeed, even for the less complicated process of chemical mutagenesis in vivo, a drop below linearity at low doses has been demonstrated[50]. Therefore, a "hockey stick"-shaped curve[51] probably best fits current data and concepts on carcinogenic effects at low levels of exposure.

Dose-dependent carcinogenic effects have also been observed in human exposure to carcinogens[52]. The most reliable quantitative data on human cancer resulting from exposure to specific carcinogens come from studies of occupational or therapeutic exposures. In these situations adequate data for several carcinogens show that human cancer incidence is proportional to dose, often measured by length of employment, since there are virtually no actual data on the prevailing levels of any chemical in the industrial environment, especially in the past. The cancer incidence in workmen exposed to benzidine, vinyl chloride, or bis(chlor-methyl) ether indicates a general relationship between exposure and disease occurrence. Workmen engaged in uranium or asbestos mining exhibited a risk of cancer broadly related to the length of time an individual was engaged in these particular occupations. Likewise, with the drug chlornaphazine, where intake was reasonably well established, the percentage of treated patients that subsequently developed bladder cancer was proportional to the amount of drug consumed. Many of the available dose-response relationships were observed in limited populations of people exposed iatrogenically[53].

As in experimental studies, the question of thresholds in human exposure to carcinogens is controversial. The issue has great contemporary importance in the light of the capability of analytic chemists to measure accurately, at the parts-per-billion and even the parts-per-trillion level, the presence of several types of carcinogens in the food chain and in the environment generally. Several chemicals such as nitrosopyrrolidine, found in bacon, can induce liver cancer in several species with appropriate higher dosages, of the order of parts-per-million to parts-per-thousand[54,55]. Primary liver cancer is rarely seen in populations that consume fried bacon. Is this evidence for a no-effect level? Similar questions can be raised for the trace amounts of powerfully carcinogenic mycotoxins such as aflatoxin B_1 currently permitted in food. Such considerations are controversial; opinions abound and facts are few[56]. It must be accepted that the issue is currently beyond the reach of exact science. Perhaps this is why decisions are based more on non-scientific considerations. The public are led to believe that they are being protected. Unfortunately, most of the time this is not so. Actions, mainly on essential lifestyle changes, that would lower cancer and other chronic disease risks, are rarely implemented, again for non-scientific reasons. Thus, real progress is slow because it depends chiefly on public education.

education.

Nevertheless, several lines of evidence suggest that in the human context thresholds do exist for DNA-reactive carcinogens. For example, hepatocellular carcinoma is relatively rare in much of the Western world even though unavoidable contamination of foods with the highly potent liver carcinogens aflatoxin and dimethyl-nitrosamine has occurred for decades, and continues to be found. Thus, there may be practical no-effect levels even for strong carcinogens, especially in the absence of promoting factors. Recently, additional documentation on this point comes from evaluating the effect of the powerful pulmonary carcinogen chloromethylmethylether. In one factory, evidence for a carcinogenic effect on workers was observed, but in another it was not[57]. Nonetheless, prudent policy dictates avoidance, wherever possible, of exposure to genotoxic carcinogens.

Epigenetic (non-genotoxic) carcinogens

For carcinogens that are not DNA-reactive and appear to operate by producing other biological effects, their carcinogenic effects might be expected to parallel dose-response relationships for their relevant biological effects. Unfortunately, relatively few dose-response studies have been done with carcinogens of the epigenetic type, and almost none with regard to underlying toxicological or pharmacological effects. Reasonable data exist for the chelating agent nitrilotriacetic acid, showing that kidney and bladder tumours are produced by exposures to about 75 mmol/kg diet and that this diminishes dramatically, in a non-linear fashion, when the exposure is reduced below 50 mmol/kg diet[58]. The mechanistic explanation is based on cytotoxicity of high levels of agent[59,60]. A recent dose-response study[61], in which saccharin was fed to large numbers of rats over two generations, shows that a 37% yield of bladder carcinoma plus papilloma was induced with 7.5% dietary saccharin, 20% with 6.25%, 15% with 5%, 12% with 4%, 8% with 3%, 5% with 1%, and 0.8% with 0%, the controls. Thus the data show a sizeable drop in incidence with less than a reduction of half of the dose; 3% and 1% saccharin appear to be no-effect levels.

For several types of epigenetic carcinogens, especially promoters, theoretical considerations, as well as available data from experimental studies, strongly support the existence of no-effect levels or thresholds. When such agents as DDT, phenobarbital, or butylated hydroxyanisole were tested by themselves for carcinogenicity in rats, an effect was evident only at the highest dose levels given in lifetime studies. These observations are supported by tests for promotion, where, after an appropriate genotoxic carcinogen is administered, neoplasms are induced in a shorter time with smaller numbers of animals. No-effect levels have been observed in promotion assays, after exposure to the appropriate tissue-specific genotoxic carcinogens, for saccharin in bladder cancer promotion[62], BHT or phenobarbital in liver cancer promotion[63,64], and BHA in gastric cancer promotion (Williams et al., unpublished).

145

These observations on dose response for non-genotoxic agents apply also to the human setting. Relatively few epigenetic agents have been carcinogenic to humans, but two examples are asbestos and diethylstilbestrol. There are no definitive, carefully collected dose-response data on their carcinogenic effects, although it is apparent that risk diminishes rapidly as exposure is reduced from the high levels associated with cancer causation[64].

Better data exist for the quantitative effects of promoting agents in humans. Bile acids are demonstrated promoters for colon cancer. In Western populations at high risk for colon cancer, the prevailing concentration of bile acids is 12 mg/g of faeces. In Japan, with a low-fat intake, or in Finland, with a high cereal fibre intake, the risk for colon cancer is low, and the concentration of faecal bile acids is about 4 mg/g, only one-third of the concentrations associated with high risk[9]. Complex tobacco smoke contains relatively small amounts of genotoxic polycyclic aromatic hydrocarbons, nicotine-derived nitrosamines, and certain heterocyclic amines. The major effect of tobacco stems from the promoting effect of the acidic fraction of the smoke[5]. It is established that an individual chronically smoking 40 cigarettes per day is at high risk, but with 10 cigarettes per day the risk is much lower, and with four cigarettes per day the risk is most difficult to evaluate accurately. This represents evidence that enhancing factors have steep dose-response curves in humans, as in experimental animals.

Human beings have been exposed to significant levels of a variety of epigenetic carcinogens such as certain of the organo-chlorine pesticides, phenobarbital, and natural estrogens without evidence of cancer causation[65,66]. Yet, carcinogens that are not DNA-reactive have produced human cancer, such as asbestos through occupational exposure and diethylstilbestrol (DES) at high pharmacological levels. Asbestos and DES are special cases. Inhaled asbestos fibres remain in the lung; thus there is lifelong continuing exposure of the tissue, even if the agent is no longer in the outside environment. Most lung cancers, however, are really caused by tobacco smoke, powerfully enhanced by asbestos. With high levels of transplacental DES there appears to be permanent imprinting of the endocrine system of the fetus, eventually expressed as a special type of endocrine-related neoplasm, clear cell carcinoma of the vagina, at puberty. The negative findings with other epigenetic agents therefore suggest that their exposure levels have been below the thresholds for cancer production and do not involve long residence in the body at sufficient levels or imprinting of a differentiating organ.

Thus carcinogens, both DNA-reactive and epigenetic, act in a dose-dependent fashion, although the dose-response relationship appears to be different. Thresholds have been observed for both types of carcinogens in experimental animals and humans. The thresholds for DNA-reactive carcinogens vary greatly and may be low. Those for non-genotoxic, epigenetic carcinogens, particularly of the promoter class, have been fairly high. These comments bear on design and interpretation of carcinogen tests to delineate human risk.

CONCLUSIONS

The overall aim of this volume is to assess future activities in safety evaluation. From the perspective of this chaper - namely, to define carcinogenic risks - many advances have been recorded through research in the past 20 years. Progressing from the historic means of assessing risk - namely, reports of cancer induced in man at the workplace or routine long-term bioassays in animals - it is now possible to provide this field with procedures and recommendations that can be carried out worldwide, economically and rapidly, to forecast possible carcinogenic hazards. These abbreviated procedures, based on current understanding of the mechanisms of carcinogenesis, are deemed no less efficient than the former cumbersome, time-consuming, and expensive bioassays. In fact, because the current and future procedures will entail critical components with yes or no answers related to mechanisms of action, the techniques actually provide enhanced quantitative decision-making potential.

At the present time, further advances in molecular biology may provide additional improvements in diagnosing potential cancer risks. Indeed certain oncogenic viruses and some chemical carcinogens have now been found to lead to specific gene rearrangements, especially the so-called onc genes. It is possible that this area might yield even more efficient means of determining, from a qualitative standpoint, whether or not a given product could eventually elicit cancer. Furthermore, improved knowledge in the area of the mechanisms of promotion may likewise contribute to the development of additional test systems that would facilitate the detection of materials with those properties.

As noted in the body of this chapter, toxicology and those who apply toxicological research results to public protection must be much more cognizant of the quantitative aspects and interactive events as regards carcinogenesis. The power of analytical chemistry is such that trace amounts of chemicals can be determined specifically and accurately. Claims have been made about the risk of disease associated with materials found in trace amounts in air and drinking water, that were "carcinogenic" based on the induction of liver neoplasms in mice. It seems reasonably certain that even powerful carcinogens at those low levels are toxicologically non-significant, and certainly agents that mainly induce mouse hepatomas are harmless under these conditions. In fact this writer is frustrated when, nationally or internationally, great efforts (incurred with large expense) are made to control such elements of dubious toxicological importance in relation to real protection of mankind. On the other hand, little official action is taken in many parts of the world on established health risks, whether this be the use of tobacco products, salted and pickled foods, too much total or saturated fat in the diet, or the relative absence of cereal fibre, and related lifestyle elements.

It was stated in this chapter, and is reiterated here, that safety evaluation covers only a single aspect of the overall comprehensive knowledge required, and in great part available, to reduce major diseases around the world. It is my hope that "safety evaluation" can be brought to where it really should be; namely, to be able to reduce major disease risks through research by the careful, deliberate application of sound research findings.

REFERENCES

1. Greenstein, JP (1944). Nucleoproteins. Adv Protein Chem, 1, 209-87
2. Searle, CE (Ed) (1984). Chemical Carcinogens, 2nd edn., ACS Monogr. 182. (Washington DC: American Chemical Society)
3. Hiatt, HH, Watson, JD and Winsten, JA (eds) (1977). Origins of Human Cancer. (Cold Spring Harbor, NY: Cold Spring Harbor Laboratories)
4. Wynder, EL, Leveille, GA, Weisburger, JH and Livingston, GE (eds) (1983). Environmental Aspects of Cancer: The Role of Macro and Micro Components of Foods. (Westport, CT: Food and Nutrition Press)
5. Surgeon General Report (1982). The Health Consequences of Smoking. Cancer, Chapter 5. US Govt. Pub. No. DHHS (PHS) 82-50179. (Washington DC: Superintendent of Documents, US Governmental Printing Office)
6. Hoffman, D and Adams, JD (1981). Carcinogenic tobacco-specific N-nitrosamines in snuff and in the saliva of snuff dippers. Cancer Res, 41, 4305-8
7. Weisburger, JH (1985). Nutrition and cancer prevention: gastrointestinal cancer. Gann Monog Cancer Res, 31, 275-283
8. Joossens, JV and Geboers, J (1983). Salt and hypertension. Prev Med, 12, 18-29
9. Reddy, BS, Cohen, LA, McCoy, GD, Hill, P, Weisburger, JH and Wynder, EL (1980). Nutrition and its relationship to cancer. Adv Cancer Res, 32, 237-345
10. Stamler, J and Cohen, JD (1985). Forum: The prevention of cardiovascular diseases. Prev Med, 14, 1-9
11. Truswell, AS (1985). Reducing the risk of coronary heart disease. Br Med J, 291, 34-7
12. Schaeffer, EJ and Levy, RI (1985). Pathogenesis and management of lipoprotein disorders. N Engl J Med, 312, 1300-10
13. Miller, EC and Miller, JA (1981). Mechanisms of chemical carcinogenesis. Cancer, 47, 1055-64
14. Conney, AH (1982). Induction of microsomal enzymes by foreign chemicals and carcinogenesis by polycyclic aromatic hydrocarbons. Cancer Res, 42, 4875-917
15. Williams, GM and Weisburger, JH (1986). Chemical carcinogenesis. In Doull, J, Klaassen, CD and Amdur, MO, (eds) Toxicology, The Basic Science of Poisons, 3rd edn. (New York: Macmillan)
16. Hollaender, A and deSerres, F (eds) (1971-83). Chemical Mutagens, Principles, and Methods for their Detection, vols. 1-8. (New York: Plenum Press)
17. Sugimura, T and Sato, S (1983). Mutagens-carcinogens in foods. Cancer Res, 43, 2415s-21s
18. Williams, GM (1976). Carcinogen-induced DNA repair in

primary rat liver cell cultures: a possible screen for chemical carcinogens. Cancer Lett, 1, 231-6

19. Upton, AC, Clayson, DB, Jansen, JD, Rosenkranz, HS and Williams, GM (1984). Report of ICPEMC Task Group No 5 on the differentiation between genotoxic and non-genotoxic carcinogens. Mutat Res, 133, 1-49

20. Brusick, D and Auletta, A (1985). Developmental status of bioassays in genetic toxicology. A report of Phase II of the U.S. Environmental Protection Agency Gene-tox Program. Mutat Res, 153, 1-10

21. Ashby, J, Lefevre, PA, Burlinson, B and Penman, MG (1985). An assessment of the in vivo rat hepatocyte DNA-repair assay. Mutat Res, 156, 1-18

22. Poirier, MC (1983). The use of antibodies to detect carcinogen-DNA adducts in vivo and in vitro. In Mirand, EA, Hutchinson, WB and Mihich, E (eds) 13th International Cancer Congress, Part B: Biology of Cancer (1), pp. 289-98. (New York: Alan R. Liss)

23. Weinstein, IB, Gattoni-Celli, S, Kirschmeier, P, Lambert, M, Hsiao, W, Backer, J and Jeffrey, A (1984). Multistage carcinogenesis involves multiple genes and multiple mechanisms. J Cell Physiol Suppl, 3, 127-37

24. Berenblum, I (1974). Carcinogenesis as a Biological Problem. Frontiers of Biology, vol. 34. (Amsterdam: North-Holland)

25. Wynder, EL, Weisburger, JH and Horn, CL (1983). On the importance and relevance of tumour promotion systems in the development of nutritionally-linked cancers. Cancer Surveys, 2, 557-76

26. Moriya, M, Ohta, T, Watanabe, K, Miyazawa, T, Kato, K and Shirasu, Y (1983). Further mutagenicity studies on pesticides in bacterial reversion assay systems. Mutat Res, 116, 185-216

27. Trosko, JE, Jone, C and Chang, CC (1984). The use of in-vitro assays to study and to detect tumour promoters. IARC Sci Publ, 56, 239-52

28. Murray, AW, Fitzgerald, DJ and Guy, GR (1982). Inhibition of intercellular communication by tumor promoters. In Hecker, E, Fusenig, NE, Kunz, W, Marks, F and Thielmann, HW (eds) Carcinogenesis. Vol. 7. (New York: Raven Press), pp. 587-92

29. Williams, GM (1983). Epigenetic effects of liver tumor promoters and implications for health effects. Environ Health Perspect, 50, 177-83

30. Newbold, RF and Amos, J (1981). Inhibition of metabolic cooperation between mammalian cells in culture by tumour promoters. Carcinogenesis, 2, 243-9

31. Weisburger, JH and Williams, GM (1984). Bioassay of carcinogens: in vitro and in vivo tests. In Searle, CE (ed.) Chemical Carcinogens, Vol. 2. (Washington DC: American Chemical Society), pp. 1323-73

32. Squire, RA (1981). Ranking animal carcinogens: a proposed regulatory approach. Science, 214, 877-80

33. Wang, GM (1984). Evaluation of pesticides which pose carcinogenicity potential in animal testing. 1. Developing a

tumor data evaluation system. Reg Toxicol Pharmacol, 4, 355-60

34. Weisburger, EK (1983). History of the bioassay program of the National Cancer Institute. Progr Exp Tumor Res, 26, 187-201

35. Cameron, TP, Hickman, RL, Kornreich, MR and Tarone, RE (1985). History, survival, and growth patterns of B6C3F1 mice and F344 rats in the National Cancer Institute Carcinogenesis Testing Program. Fund Appl Toxicol, 5, 526-38

36. Rosenkranz, HS, Klopman, G, Chankong, V, Pet-Edwards, J and Haimes, YY (1984). Prediction of environmental carcinogens: a strategy for the mid 1980s. Environ Mutagen, 6, 231-58

37. Tanaka, T, Barnes, WS, Weisburger, JH and Williams, GM (1985). Multipotential carcinogenicity of the fried food mutagen 2-amino-3-methylimidazo[4,5-f]quinoline in rats. Jap J Cancer Res (Gann), 76, 570-6

38. Stavric, B (ed) (1984). Symposium report. Mutagenic food flavonoids. Fed Proc, 43, 2454-8

39. Ertürk, E, Hatcher, JF, Nunoya, T, Pamukcu, AM and Bryan, GT (1984). Hepatic tumors in Sprague-Dawley (SD) and Fischer 344 (F) female rats chronically exposed to quercetin (Q) or its glycoside rutin (R). Proc Am Assoc Cancer Res, 25, 95

40. Clemmesen, J, Conning, DM, Henschler, D and Oesch, F (eds) (1980). Quantitative aspects of risk assessment in chemical carcinogenesis. Arch Toxicol, Suppl. 3, 1-330

41. Druckrey, H (1967). Quantitative aspects in chemical carcinogenesis. UICC Monogr, 7, 60-77

42. Eckardt, RK (1959). Industrial Carcinogens. (New York: Grune & Stratton)

43. Stenbäck, F, Peto, R and Shubik, P (1981). Initiation and promotion at different ages and doses in 2200 mice II. Decrease in promotion by TPA with ageing. Br J Cancer, 44, 15-23

44. Bryan, WR and Shimkin, MB (1943). Quantitative analysis of dose-response data obtained with three carcinogenic hydrocarbons in strain C3H male mice. J Natl Cancer Inst, 3, 503-31

45. Smith, J (1981). Re-examination of the ED_{01} Study. Overview. Fund Appl Toxicol, 1, 28-128

46. Peto, R, Gray, R, Brantom, P and Grasso, P (1984). Nitrosamine carcinogenesis in 5120 rodents: chronic administration of sixteen different concentrations of NDEA, NDMA, NPYR and NPIP in the water of 4440 inbred rats, with parallel studies on NDEA alone of the effect of the age of starting (3, 6, or 20 weeks) and of the species (rats, mice or hamsters). IARC Sci Publ. No. 57, 627-65

47. Shimkin, MB and Stoner, GD (1975). Lung tumors in mice: application to carcinogenesis bioassay. Adv Cancer Res, 21, 2-58

48. Long, EL, Nelson, AA, Fitzhugh, OG and Hansen, WH (1963). Liver tumors produced in rats by feeding safrole. Arch Pathol, 75, 595-604

49. Office of Technology Assessment (1982). Cancer Risk: Assessing and Reducing the Dangers in our Society. (Boulder, Co: Westview Press)

50. Russell, WL, Hunsicker, PR, Raymen, GD, Steele, MH, Stelzner, KF and Thompson, HM (1982). Dose response for ethylnitrosourea-induced specific-locus mutagens in mouse spermatogonia. Proc Natl Acad Sci, 73, 3589-91

51. Hoel, DG, Kaplan, NL and Anderson, MW (1983). Implication of nonlinear kinetics on risk estimation in carcinogenesis. Science, 219, 1032-7

52. Williams, GM, Reiss, B and Weisburger, JH (1985). A comparison of the animal and human carcinogenicity of environmental, occupational and therapeutic chemicals. In Flamm, WG and Lorentzen, RJ (eds) Advances in Modern Environmental Toxicology, Vol. XII: Mechanisms and Toxicity of Chemical Carcinogens and Mutagens (Princeton: Princeton Scientific Publishers Inc.), pp. 207-48

53. Schmähl, D, Thomas, C and Auer, R (1977). Iatrogenic Carcinogenesis. (Berlin, Heidelberg: Springer-Verlag)

54. Preussmann, R and Stewart, BW (1984). N-nitroso carcinogens. In Searle, CE, (ed.) Chemical Carcinogens, 2nd edn, Vol. 2, ACS Monogr. 182. (Washington, DC: American Chemical Society), pp. 643-828

55. O'Neill, IK, Von Borstel, RC, Miller, CT, Long, J and Bartsch, H (1984). N-Nitroso Compounds: Occurrence, Biological Effects and Relevance to Human Cancer. IARC Sci Publ No. 57 (Lyon: International Agency for Research on Cancer)

56. Symposium on safety assessment: the interface between science, law and regulation (1984). Fund Appl Toxicol, 4, S255-S434

57. McCallum, RI, Woolley, V and Petrie, A (1983). Lung cancer associated with chloromethyl methyl ether manufacture: an investigation at two factories in the United Kingdom. Br J Indust Med, 40, 384-9

58. National Cancer Institute (1977). Bioassays of nitrilotriacetic acid (NTA) and nitrilotriacetic acid trisodium salt monohydrate ($Na_3NTA.H_2O$) for possible carcinogenicity (NCI-CG-TR-6). DHEW Publ. No. (NIH) 77-806

59. Kanerva, RL, Francis, WR, Lefever, FR, Dorr, T, Alden, CL and Anderson, RL (1984). Renal pelvic and ureteral dilation in male rats ingesting trisodium nitrilotriacetate. Food Chem Toxicol, 22, 749-53

60. Ved Brat, S and Williams, GM (1984). Nitrilotriacetic acid does not induce sister chromatid exchanges in hamster or human cells. Food Chem Toxicol, 22, 211-15

61. Schoenig, GP, Goldenthal, EI, Geil, RG, Frith, CH, Richter, WR and Carlborg, FW (1985). Evaluation of the dose response and in utero exposure to saccharin in the rat. Food Chem Toxicol, 23, 475-90

62. Nakanishi, K, Hagiwara, A, Shibata, M, Imaida, K, Tatematsu, M and Ito, N (1980). Dose response of saccharin in induction of urinary bladder hyperplasias in Fischer 344 rats pretreated with N-butyl-n-(4-hydroxybutyl)nitrosamine.

J Natl Cancer Inst, 65, 1005-10
63. Maeura, Y and Williams, GM (1984). Enhancing effect of butylated hydroxytoluene on the development of liver altered foci and neoplasms induced by N-2-fluorenylacetamide in rats. Food Chem Toxicol, 22, 211-15
64. Goldsworthy, T, Campbell, HA and Pitot, HC (1984). The natural history and dose-response characteristics of enzyme-altered foci in rat liver following phenobarbital and diethyl-nitrosamine administration. Carcinogenesis, 5, 67-71
65. Clemmesen, J and Hjalgrim-Jensen, S (1981). Does phenobarbital cause intracranial tumors. A follow-up through 35 years. Ecotoxicol Environ Safety, 5, 255-60
66. IARC Monographs Suppl. 4 (1982). Evaluation of the Carcinogenic Risk of Chemicals to Humans. (Lyon: Internatl. Agency for Research on Cancer, WHO)

PART 3
Nutrition and Toxicological Prediction

9

Diet and the Future of Drug Safety Evaluation

D. L. FRAPE

9.1 INTRODUCTION – LABORATORY DIETS

It has been assumed frequently that diet is a passive entity in so far as both the testing of drugs and their use in practice are concerned. There has been insufficient recognition that diet forms part of the model when laboratory animals are used in the development of drugs. Scant attention has been paid to diet in texts on laboratory animals. Even as recently as 1984, a standard text on animal models simply recommends for rats "a standard commercial rodent diet, usually in the form of firm dry blocks or pellets, without any type of supplemental feeding". The same diet is recommended for gerbils, which may be supplemented with limited amounts of green food such as lettuce, spinach, or carrots. The author commented simply that sunflower seeds are not satisfactory as a total diet because they are low in calcium and high in fat content. There is thus an enduring assumption that diet has no impact on the modelling process. That diet may act as a vehicle of disease; that many forms are unscientific by not being reproducible; and that diet is frequently far removed from that consumed by the species being mimicked, are facts too often ignored. An objective of this review is to demonstrate that diet is able to play an active role both in the development of drugs and in their clinical application. In so doing, diet can make a substantial contribution to the model if it complies with certain basic criteria of scientific significance. Compliance with such criteria will not only further the development of medicine, but incidentally could expand more rapidly the general fund of knowledge concerning the interaction between xenobiotes and nutrition.

Many diets that have been used do not lend themselves to any worthwhile scientific description in that it is impossible to avoid unwitting, or known, variation in chemical, or other, composition from batch to batch, and from the description given it is impossible to reformulate the diet faithfully. Variable diets not only induce variable reactions to test substances, but as breeding diets they can lead to variable reserves in offspring. Rader et al.[1] commented that successive batches of the standard diet NIH-31 not only differed in their elemental composition but that this dif-

155

ference led to variable tissue concentrations in weanling rats.

NUTRIENT REQUIREMENTS

The minimum dietary requirement for a particular nutrient has been misleadingly interpreted as a much more precise and definitive concept than can be justified. At the very most, the minimum quantity of a nutrient required per day, or per unit weight of diet, is a gross approximation of that necessary to support normal growth of weanlings of a given species. The quantity of any one nutrient required is valid only when all other nutrients are present at their required minimum levels. Furthermore, both the array of nutrients and the quantities required are different where response criteria other than growth are used. Alternative criteria include reproductive characteristics, maximum lifespan, various measures of metabolic health, resistance to transmissible disease, or cancer. Added to this the requirements for entire males and females compared to castrated and ovarectomized individuals differ. The presence in the diet of many hazardous or benign non-nutrient substances may influence the absolute or quantitative need for a particular dietary nutrient. For example, the addition of cellulose to a biotin-free diet brought about a growth response in weanling rats possibly due to a stimulation of intestinal biotin synthesis[2]. A response to a particular nutrient can be induced in a species that normally is capable of adequate tissue synthesis of the nutrient in question. For example, the toxicity of several metals is modified by supplementation of ascorbic acid. Furthermore the toxic effect of certain elements may depend on interaction with the nutrient status of the host, or it may be dependent upon the simultaneous intake of a modifying nutrient[3].

TYPES OF DIET

Three types of diet have been recognized:

1. natural ingredient diets,
2. semi-purified diets, and
3. chemically defined diets.

Their facility for scientific definition, and generally their cost, are least for the first of these and greatest for the last. The cost of feeding studies with laboratory animals for the achievement of a given objective is, however, unlikely to show the same progression where the possibilities of dietary manipulation in the modelling process are fully exploited. A purpose of this review is to facilitate that manipulation by describing the role of diet in certain metabolic diseases that are prime targets of drug development.

DIET PROCESSING

Complete raw diets for laboratory animals are traditionally

processed in a number of ways with the principal objectives of increasing their appeal to many animal species, reducing dustiness and compacting, destroying micro-organisms, arthropods, parasite eggs and other unwanted potentially infectious, or destructive, living organisms. Where heat processing is adopted, a number of natural heat-labile potentially hazardous substances, mainly of plant origin, are inactivated, destroyed or substantially reduced. Vigorous cooking procedures such as expansion achieve these effects comprehensively, reducing moisture activity of feedstuffs and destroying intracellular catabolic enzymes that can otherwise accelerate deterioration of disrupted cellular matter. These effects lower the rate of deterioration and extend shelf-life of products. Spencer[4] demonstrated that the shelf-life of irradiated diet is at least 12 months, although changes in vitamin A potency occurred that could influence certain metabolic processes even though minimum requirements may be met. Cooking has an immediate destructive impact on heat-labile nutrients. This is not of great importance as allowance for the loss can be made in formulation, and account is taken of it in the post-manufacture analysis. Other cooking or processing techniques - such as steam pelleting, irradiation, or particularly autoclaving - achieve the objective in varying degrees and with differing destructive effects. Gassing, as for example with ethylene oxide, can leave unwanted residues of the gas in the diet, or can itself react with the diet. More subtle effects can be incurred by treatment. For example, thermally oxidized corn oil causes an increase in colonic activity of benzo(a)pyrene hydroxylase in rats[5]. Thus the colon is a possible specific site for alteration of mixed-function oxidase activity by the products of thermally oxidized oils.

NUTRIENTS AVAILABLE TO THE ANIMAL

An essential characteristic of a laboratory diet is an adequate description, entailing appropriate physical, chemical, biological and microbiological characteristics. The particular attributes assessed must depend partly upon the objectives of the study, in order that excessive costs are not incurred. However, chemical analysis is frequently not adequate without some biological assessment of nutrient availability, where a chemical method for availability is non-existent. Measurements of availability are necessary across the entire spectrum of nutrients from carbohydrates, amino acids, vitamins to minerals. Differences in the availability of various phosphorus sources are widely appreciated, and in turn the effect of this nutrient - and those of calcium, copper and fibre - on the availability of zinc is widely accepted. For some elements there is an enormous range of availability - for example that of iron may differ from diet to diet by as much as a hundred-fold[3].

The scientific description of diets normally relates to the time immediately after manufacture, or the time of sale, although some estimate of shelf-life, or expiry date, is also given. This information is demanded but can be misleading. For many characteristics and nutrients no detectable change occurs during storage so long as the conditions of storage are satisfactory. In the case of labile nutrients the product is subject to a continuous change. The disruption of plant cells during manufacture accelerates the rate of autocatalysis. This rate may be further accelerated by elevated dietary moisture activity and elevated storage temperatures in the presence of active micro-organisms, insects and the like. Several of these accelerating conditions are present in the animal room itself, a sometimes neglected factor, as the only relevant diet is that which is actually consumed.

The animal is capable of compensatory reactions to a declining potency of nutrients and to other metabolically active compounds so that there can be a range of individual potencies over which the animal's reaction changes little. Nevertheless it is not possible to assume that this is the case; nor is it possible to assume that the interaction between diet and test substance does not also change in important ways. The shelf-life of a diet is intended simply to indicate the limiting time at which the most labile nutrient still just meets the minimum dietary requirement.

Laboratory animal responses to diet

The concept of minimum dietary requirement for a nutrient is a useful baseline for diet formulation, but it ignores the widely accepted evidence that incremental doses of individual nutrients above the minimum requirement concentration can have metabolic effects and lead to animal responses.

There is a continuum of interactive effects with other nutrients, non-nutrients, drugs and other test substances over the whole range of possible dietary concentrations of nutrients.

The way in which diet is offered has an impact on its utilization and the metabolic pathways of energy metabolism that predominate. Increasing amounts of information and interest have been shown in the effects of level and pattern of feeding on the response to diet both of laboratory animals and man. Restricted intake of feed obviously causes a lower rate of fat deposition, but it also introduces change in the preponderance of different pathways of the metabolism of energy-yielding nutrients. Thus the interaction of diet with any particular test substance can be altered by changing both the pattern and rate of daily feeding.

HEAVY METAL CONTAMINATION OF DIET

Lead

Many raw materials that are feed ingredients or that are used as foods contain low and variable amounts of lead and other heavy metals. The amount present can be estimated readily by chemical analysis. However, the biopotency, or toxicity of these metals depends not only upon their chemical form, but also upon the amounts present of a number of other dietary constituents.

A dietary deficiency of vitamin E has been demonstrated to increase the toxicity of lead in the diet of rats. The addition of vitamin E to the diet decreased lead toxicity more effectively than did the addition of selenium, although excessive dietary seleniur had some ameliorating effects[6]. The addition of 400 mg iron pe kg diet has similarly been shown to decrease the toxicity of dietar lead[7]. Dietary inadequacies of calcium, zinc and copper exacerbat the toxicity of lead and inadequacies of calcium, iron and coppe increase the toxicity of cadmium[8]. A deficiency of dietary protei increases the toxicity of both lead and cadmium[9]. Selenium i protective in the toxicity of dietary mercury and methy mercury[10]. It seems to decrease the toxicity of methylmercury b liberating it from sulphydryl bonds in body tissue proteins[11] Very high levels of a number of dietary nutrients seem to enhanc the protective effect against heavy metal toxicity. These includ excessive levels of calcium, zinc, iron and selenium[6,8]. Truelov et al.[12] concluded that dietary phytates depress the absorption o dietary lead, and probably also that of mercury.

Several dietary factors may stimulate lead absorption, an the observation that dietary fat stimulated the uptake of lead in duced Quarterman et al.[13] to conclude that the stimulation to bil secretion by dietary fat in turn led to an improved absorption o dietary lead. Dietary lactose also seems to stimulate lead absorp tion, but it may also reduce retention of lead in bone an kidney[14].

Natural toxicants in feedstuffs

A major difference between purified diets and natural diets is th presence in natural raw feedstuffs of organic compounds that inter fere with nutrient utilization, or that possess other toxi properties.

A number of proteins have been isolated from the seeds of large number of leguminous species that have anti-protease or anti amylase properties, or that are known as lectins (haemagglutinins) These substances are protein in nature and can be inactivated i many cases by heating. The degree of heating required to inac tivate some lectins is very substantial. A number of compound found particularly in cruciferous species possess goitrogeni properties that are also destroyed by heating. A wide range c plant species contain cyanogenic glycosides that have the potenti for releasing HCN. Species include linseeds, lima beans, sorghum cassava roots and many legumes.

Several species of the pea family contain substances calle lathyrogens, that cause lathyrism, induced as a consequence c persistent consumption of members of these species. Cooking ha apparently little effect on the potency of these toxins. Certai members of the bean family can cause haemolytic anaemia and othe characteristics of favism.

Other toxic compounds widely distributed in the plar kingdom include oxalic acid, saponins, polyphenolic compound (tannins) and gossypol, found in cotton seeds. A further ex tremely large group of compounds of variable toxicity from ex tremely high to slight potency are the alkaloids found in a wid range of plant species.

Protease inhibitors, lectins, saponins and polyphenolic com

pounds exert their effects by depressing digestion, or by influencing the metabolic utilization of proteins. By contrast, phytic acid, oxalic acid, glucosinolates and gossypol express their effects by reducing the solubility of, or interfering with the utilization of, mineral elements.

A number of toxins are introduced into feedstuffs by the growth of bacteria, e.g. Clostridium botulinum, and moulds. Carson and Smith[15] demonstrated that the lignin component of alfalfa was effective in overcoming the toxicity of the T-2 toxin produced by Fusarium, Myrothecium, Trichoderma, Cephalosporium, Verticimonosporium and Stachybotrys. Alfalfa lignin increased the faecal excretion of the T-2 toxin. The effect was similar to that observed by Frape et al.[16], who demonstrated that lignin increased the faecal excretion of aflatoxin B1.

The use of chemically defined diets or semi-purified diets considerably reduces the risks attendant upon the use of natural-ingredient diets. Threshold levels of toxicity may exist for most toxins, but below these dietary concentrations it is likely that many have enzyme induction properties which influence the metabolism of test chemicals.

Purified diets

The incidence of metabolic disorders is greater, generally speaking, when purified diets, rather than natural-ingredient diets free from toxins are used in longer-term studies. It has been asserted that the differences are accounted for by differences in dietary fibre content and Wise[17], and Sherrill et al.[18,19] have demonstrated differences in xenobiote and toxin metabolism by caecal micro-organisms when fermentable fibre sources are added to purified diets. However, Medinsky and colleagues[20] observed that Fischer 344 rats given diet AIN 76A, a purified diet containing 5% cellulose, developed a much higher incidence of periportal lipidosis and possessed livers with a higher liver to body weight ratio, some developing severe haemorrhagic lesions, than was found in rats receiving a cereal-based diet. The inclusion of abnormally high concentrations of sucrose in many purified diets is recognized as a cause of certain metabolic upsets. It should also be noted that the inclusion of large amounts of purified fat in rodent diets may be necessary in the modelling of human diets, even though such amounts may accelerate the onset of atherosclerosis and related disorders. On the other hand it is apparent from some evidence that extended lifespan of rodents may be achieved by a reduction in the daily intake of metabolizable, or net, energy. This of course could be achieved, despite the use of high-fat diets, by restricted access to food.

Adult DNA may be more sensitive than juvenile DNA to chemical lesions, so that the adult rodent may be a more suitable model for measuring the disruptive, or protective, influence of diet on DNA integrity in the assay, xenobiote x diet oncogenic effects. However, the adult may be a less variable and more reliable experimental animal for this purpose only if its previous dietary history is known, and has been constant. Where these prerequisites are met, a previous dietary history represented by purified diet is likely to provide a more satisfactory adult test animal in the study of oncogenesis.

What is the correct test diet?

In order to give some partial answer to this question it is helpful, but not essential, to understand the mechanisms of action of test substances and the mode of any interaction with the diet. Information on this should enable one to formulate diets that increase, or decrease, the potency of the test substance, or that promote or suppress metabolic disorders which the test substance is designed to combat.

Test diets should be as far as possible completely controlled variables. An adequate scientific definition of a diet should be available, and this same definition should apply to successive batches of the same diet. The definition should enable other research workers to reproduce an identical diet. A sufficient exploration of dietary interactions should have been undertaken so that the product has as wide an application as is necessary to the likely range of clinical and dietary environments that may be encountered by those using it. An objective of this review is to assist those wishing to attain these objectives.

An awareness of recent research into the interaction of drugs and dietary constituents, and into the role diet plays in the major metabolic diseases that afflict mankind, is essential to objective formulation of diets for drug development and safety evaluation. As there has been no recent review of the whole subject it has been considered necessary to do so before conclusions may be drawn on the future role of diet in that evaluation.

REFERENCES

1. Radar, JI, Wolnik, KA, Gaston, CM, Celesk, EM, Peeler, JT, Fox, MRS and Fricke, FL (1984). Trace element studies in weanling rats: maternal diets and baseline tissue mineral values. J Nutr, 114, 1946-54
2. Radar, JI, Gaston, CM, Wolnik, KA, Fricke, FL and Fox, MRS (1985). Growth and tissue minerals in weanling rats fed purified biotin-free or fiber free diets. Ann NY Acad Sci, 447, 417-9
3. Fox, MRS (1978). Nutritional consideration in designing animal models of metal toxicity in man. Environ Hlth Perspect, 25, 137-40
4. Spencer, KEV (1985). Long term storage of irradiated rodent diet. 8th ICLAS/CALAS Symposium Vancouver, 1983. (Stuttgart/New York: Gustav Fischer)
5. Perciballi, M and Pintauro, SJ (1985). The effects of fractionated thermally oxidized corn oil on drug-metabolizing enzyme systems in the rat. Food Chem Toxicol, 23, 737-40
6. Levander, OA, Morris, VC and Ferretti, RJ (1977). Com-

parative effects of selenium and vitamin E in lead-poisoned rats. J Nutr, 107, 378-82

7. Suzuki, T and Yoshida, A (1979). Effect of dietary supplementation of iron and ascorbic acid on lead toxicity in rats. J Nutr, 109, 982-8

8. Levander, OA (1977). Nutritional factors in relation to heavy metal toxicants. Fed Proc, 36, 1683-7

9. Suzuki, S, Taguchi, T and Yokohashi, G (1969). Indust Hlth, 7, 155

10. Ganther, HE, Goudie, C, Sunde, ML, Kopecky, MJ, Wagner, P, Oh, SH and Hoekstra, WG (1972). Science, 175, 1122

11. Sumino, K, Yamamoto, R and Kitamura, S (1977). A role of selenium against methylmercury toxicity. Nature, 268, 73-4

12. Truelove, JF, Gilbert, SG and Rice, DC (1985). Effect of diet on blood lead concentration in the Cynomolgus monkey. Fund Appl Toxicol, 5, 588-96

13. Quarterman, J, Morrison, JN and Humphries, WR (1977). The role of phospholids and bile in lead absorption. Proc Nutr Soc, 36, 104

14. Bushnell, PJ and De Luca, HF (1983). The effects of lactose on the absorption and retention of dietary lead. J Nutr, 113, 365-78

15. Carson, MS and Smith, TK (1983). Effect of feeding alfalfa and refined plant fibers on the toxicity and metabolism of T-2 toxin in rats. J Nutr, 113, 304-13

16. Frape, DL, Wayman, BJ, Tuck, MG and Jones, E (1982). The effect of gum arabic, wheat offal and various of its fractions on the metabolism of ^{14}C-labelled aflatoxin B_1 in the male weanling rat. Br J Nutr, 48, 97-110

17. Wise, A (1985). Caecal microbial metabolism. Workshop W8 - Laboratory Diets and Response to Drugs. XIII International Congress of Nutrition, 18-23 August, Brighton

18. Sherrill, JM, Debethizy, JD and Hamm, TE Jr (1983). Influence of diet on gastrointestinal microfloral composition and metabolism in the rat. Proc Am Soc Microbiol, New Orleans

19. Sherrill, JM, Debethizy, JD and Hamm, TE Jr (1984). Dietary effects on the gastrointestinal microflora in the Fischer-344 rat. Proc Am Soc Microbiol, St Louis

20. Medinsky, MA, Popp, JA, Hamm, TE and Dent, JG (1982). Development of hepatic lesions in male Fischer-344 rats fed AIN-76A purified diet. Toxicol Appl Pharmacol, 62, 111-20

9.2 INTERACTION OF DRUGS AND NUTRIENTS

D. L. FRAPE

APPETITE AND INDUCED NUTRIENT DEFICIENCIES

Apart from the anorectic agents such as diethylpropion, fenfluramine and dexamphetamine there are many other drugs that can reduce appetite. In some metabolic states this can be advantageous, as for example with most Type II diabetics who are overweight. Drugs in the digitalis group used in cases of cardiac cachexia are a major contributor to the anorexia that may develop. Many other drugs, including glucagon, indomethacin, morphine, mustine, and cyclophosphamide, are amongst those likely to reduce appetite. Some drugs stimulate appetite. These include sulphonylureas, oral contraceptives, the androgens and anabolic agents, the corticosteroids and insulin.

Many pharmacological agents can produce a nutrient deficiency by (1) inhibiting the absorption of the nutrient, (2) increasing the rate of turnover of the nutrient and (3) competing with the nutrient at the site of action.

NUTRIENT SYNTHESIS AND ABSORPTION

A number of drugs influence the intestinal synthesis of vitamins. Many antibiotics, especially those which are poorly absorbed, decrease the intestinal synthesis of folic acid. Neomycin and other poorly absorbed broad-spectrum antibiotics may reduce intestinal bacterial synthesis of vitamin K, and neomycin and other antimitotic agents interfere with absorption of nutrients from the gut. Neomycin, and to a lesser extent kanamycin, can induce steatorrhoea and other characteristics of malabsorption in man but not in animals[1] and flattening of the jejunal mucosa has been detected[2]. Colchicine, phenindione, sodium aminosalicylate (PAS) and indomethacin can have similar effects. Neomycin, bacitracin[3], PAS[4] and several other antibiotics cause the malabsorption of vitamin B_{12} and folic acid. The prolonged use of drugs that inhibit bacterial growth is likely to be of significance in terms of vitamin K status.

As a lipid-soluble substance vitamin K is subject to the same drug-induced disturbances of absorption as vitamins A and D. Its absorption is reduced in the absence of bile, and hepatotoxic drugs causing biliary obstruction may indirectly cause vitamin K deficiency. Excessive and continued use of purgatives can sometimes result in vitamin K deficiency by minimizing the effectiveness of synthesis by colonic bacteria. Regular use of purgatives can also produce potassium depletion.

Coronato and Glass[5] produced evidence to suggest that cholestyramine inhibits absorption of vitamin B_{12} by impairing the formation of the intrinsic factor-vitamin B_{12} complex, essential for the absorption of the vitamin. Cholestyramine is an anion-exchange resin that binds bile acids in the intestine, increases their excretion in the faeces and thus reduces fat, and fat-soluble vitamin absorption and plasma cholesterol concentration. Cholestyramine contains chloride ions that increase bone resorption, and its subsequent urinary excretion is associated with increased calcium excretion.

Long-term treatment with slow-release potassium chloride has led to vitamin B_{12} deficiency with associated megaloblastic anaemia, possibly through acidification of ileal contents[6].

Chlortetracycline inhibits pancreatic lipase[7]. Tetracycline compounds can chelate minerals such as calcium, magnesium and iron. Co-administration of tetracycline and substances such as antacids, milk and iron preparations, that contain these metals, can reduce the absorption of both the tetracycline and the mineral with a loss of potency of both.

Women taking oral contraceptives tend to have lower serum red cell folate concentrations, and occasional cases of megaloblastic anaemia have been documented[8]. Although the absorption of folate monoglutamate is apparently not disturbed, the impaired absorption of polyglutamic folate may result from interference with jejunal folate conjugase[8]. Methotrexate can reduce folate activity, and vitamin B_{12} deficiency may occur during methotrexate therapy possibly due to impaired vitamin B_{12} absorption[10]. Vitamin B_{12} malabsorption can be produced also by the hypoglycaemic drug phenformin[3]. The sulphonylureas, the most common oral hypoglycaemic agents, are chemically analogous to sulphonamides, which are antifolic acid agents, but nutritional effects may be only slight.

Isoniazid, an antagonist of nicotinic acid, binds pyridoxine and can produce pellagra symptoms that are responsive to niacin[3]. The antagonism of this drug with pyridoxine leads to the formation of pyridoxal hydrazone, which is excreted in the urine and can deplete body stores of the vitamin[11].

BINDING AND TRANSPORT IN THE BLOOD PLASMA

The use of oral contraceptives is associated with an increased urinary excretion of folate metabolites and an increase in a serum folate binding factor[12,13]. The binding factor is thought to be a hormone-induced protein analogous to corticosteroid-binding globulin, which is also elevated during pregnancy and during use of synthetic oestrogen. Oral contraceptive treatment reduces circulating vitamin B_{12} levels in European and African women, for what is probably a similar reason to that affecting folate[14].

Aspirin has been shown to reduce vitamin C binding to serum albumin, but the clinical relevance of this is uncertain[15].

METABOLISM OF NUTRIENTS

Isonicotinic acid hydrazide and cycloserine, widely used drugs in the treatment of tuberculosis, impair the actions of vitamin B_6. The drugs may react directly with pyridoxal phosphate. Methotrexate, sulphamethoxazole and the combination of trimethoprim and sulphamethoxazole are folic acid antagonists[16]. These drugs interrupt folic acid metabolism. Methotrexate is a structural analogue of folate, and it owes its cytotoxic action to competitive inhibition of folate reductase. The side-effects include anaemia and diarrhoea. It is used in the chemotherapy of malignant disease, for immunosuppression and in psoriasis. The closely related compounds aminopterin; pyrimethamine, an antimalarial drug; pentamidine isothionate, an antiprotozoal drug; trimethoprim; and triamterene, a diuretic are folic acid antagonists as a consequence of similarity in chemical structure with the vitamin[17]. Co-trimoxazole and methotrexate interfere with phenylalanine metabolism[18].

All contraceptives may promote a more efficient utilization of absorbed folate, as oestrogen has been shown to facilitate the conversion of the vitamin to the co-enzyme form. Oral contraceptives may also accelerate the rate of ascorbic acid degradation in tissues[19]. Oestrone sulphate inhibits tryptophan metabolism in rats, resulting in a considerable reduction in the synthesis of nicotinamide nucleotide coenzymes[20]. This effect has been put forward as an explanation of the higher incidence of pellagra in women receiving marginal tryptophan diets, and the administration of oral contraceptives may be a precipitating factor in pellagra.

Oestrogens are frequently used to treat postmenopausal osteoporosis as they inhibit parathyroid hormone-induced bone resorption. Similarly oestrogen-containing oral contraceptives increase the incorporation of these minerals into bone, and reduce their circulating levels and their urinary excretion[21].

Doses of aspirin used in the treatment of rheumatoid arthritis may uncouple oxidative phosphorylation, deranging glucose metabolism, depleting glycogen stores, decreasing plasma free fatty acids and increasing the oxidation of ketones[22].

Anticonvulsant drugs pheneturide, phenytoin and phenobarbitone, together with the hypnotic glutethimide, apparently not only inhibit the conversion of vitamin D to its 25-hydroxy form in the liver, but they may also enhance the conversion of vitamin D to inactive metabolites[23]. Corticosteroids increase the rate of vitamin D metabolism in the same way as do anticonvulsant drugs. Hypocalcaemia rickets, or osteomalacia, may be precipitated. These effects have been diagnosed in epileptics receiving anticonvulsants[24]. Anticonvulsants and sedatives also accelerate vitamin K metabolism[25].

DRUG POTENCY

Drugs and other foreign compounds are metabolized in the body by a group of non-specific mixed-function oxidases (MFO) that are found predominantly in the liver. The activity of these enzymes falls with increasing age, and so does the extent to which they may be induced by the administration of drugs. These enzymes require folic acid as a co-factor, and the folic acid status of the individual or animal can influence the potency of many drugs. Moreover many other nutrients influence MFO activity.

EFFECTS OF DRUGS ON NUTRIENT REQUIREMENTS

Phenytoin has been shown[26] to inhibit DNA synthesis in vitro in human bone marrow. This could increase the requirement for folate, yet the administration of folic acid to epileptics tends to lower blood phenytoin levels and can precipitate fits[27]. The most likely explanation is that anticonvulsant drugs induce hepatic MFO enzymes, which are known to require folate as a co-factor[28].

Dopa and methyldopa require vitamin B_{12} and folic acid for metabolism, suggesting increased vitamin B_{12} and folic acid requirements for individuals receiving large amounts of these drugs[29].

Diuretics increase the excretion of sodium and water, and can lead to sodium depletion in some patients if severe sodium restriction is simultaneously imposed. Some patients receiving chronic thiazide diuretic therapy have serum potassium levels below the normal range[30]. The action of digitalis and other cardiac glycosides is modified by potassium and magnesium status. Digitalis has a much greater toxicity in the magnesium-depleted subject[31].

GASTRIC EMPTYING

The presence of food in the stomach postpones the time at which drugs reach the general circulation. This effect may not matter when drugs are given repeatedly, because the rate of absorption may have no influence on the steady state concentration. For a few drugs (griseofulvin, lithium, nitrofurantoin, diazepam and riboflavin)[32] the gastrointestinal absorption increases after meals, owing possibly to delayed gastric emptying and gastrointestinal transit, allowing more complete dissolution, or prolonged residence at sites of optimal intestinal absorption. Compared to liquid meals, solid meals almost double the emptying time of the stomach[33].

The biopotency of drugs is influenced by their solubility and stability in gastric juices, as well as by the lipophilic character of the dissolved drug molecules, e.g. whether the drug is ionized and thus relatively resistant to absorption, or not ionized and hence readily traverses lipid membranes, at gastric pH. A few drugs are destroyed in the acid environment of the stomach, or are metabolized by the gastric mucosa (levodopa). In these instances food may reduce both the rate and extent of absorption. The role of pH in drug absorption is illustrated by the effect of antacids in altering rate but not extent of diazepam absorption[34]. In general relatively little drug absorption occurs in the stomach compared to that in the small intestine; therefore by retarding stomach emptying food delays drug absorption. Weak basicity or transportation by active carrier mechanisms, renders some drugs more likely than others to be absorbed in the small intestine[32]. Prolonged residence in the acidic environment of the stomach is likely to delay dissolution of acidic compounds and to accelerate dissolution of basic molecules. Although some acidic and neutral compounds are absorbed directly from the stomach, the optimal site for absorption is the small intestine.

The extent of absorption and toxicity of a large number of organic acids and bases and also of inorganic ions is increased with increasing compound dilution also stimulating stomach emptying; whereas concentrated drug solutions may be sufficiently hypertonic to delay stomach emptying and rate of absorption from the small intestine.

The absorption of erythromycin stearate by healthy volunteers was shown to be reduced by the presence of food and by a reduced fluid volume, but the absorption of erythromycin estolate was increased by food[35]. The estolate is relatively acid-stable and it is reasonable to suspect that delayed stomach emptying may delay absorption but may also increase overall absorption efficiency owing to increased dissolution in the stomach[36]. Similarly, the absorption of diftaline was shown to be increased 2.6-fold, with a 2.8-fold increase in overall bioavailability, by administration after a meal compared to fasting conditions, possibly for similar reasons[37]. In vitro studies, rather than the further use of laboratory animals, are likely to facilitate and accelerate the acquisition of data of this kind.

INTESTINAL BLOOD FLOW

Meal-induced increases in splanchnic blood flow should accelerate drug absorption from the gut lumen to the capillary bed. Blood flow can be doubled by a high-protein liquid meal and slightly reduced by a liquid glucose meal[38]. Food stimulates intestinal motility, not only accelerating dissolution of solid particles but accelerating their motion through the intestine with indeterminate effects on absorption.

Ingestion of food increases gastric secretion of hydrochloric acid, and also of enzymes that may affect drug dissolution and degradation. Increased secretion of bile after food, especially fatty food intake, may accelerate the dissolution of poorly soluble compounds. On the other hand drug absorption may be impeded by accelerated bile flow due to bile salt-drug complexation[39].

Loss of a variety of nutrients may result from prolonged use, or overuse, of laxatives because of drug-induced hyperperistalsis, or the trapping of fat-soluble nutrients in the laxative itself (mineral oil).

Cations in foodstuff, principally calcium, will chelate with most tetracyclines to reduce their intestinal absorption. Some other drugs have been shown to complex with proteins[40].

EFFECT OF DIET ON DRUG METABOLISM

Meals seem to elevate the plasma concentrations of drugs subject to an extensive first-pass effect. These drugs include propranolol, metoprolol and lidocaine[32]. After high-protein meals the increase in oral bioavailability of drugs subject to a large first-pass effect has been attributed to enhanced hepatic blood flow associated with such meals. Enhanced blood flow presumably serves to allow such high-extraction drugs to pass rapidly through the liver, thereby escaping hepatic removal, and causing higher drug concentrations in systemic circulation. However, Svensson et al.[41] observed that the meal-induced increase in hepatic blood flow was of too short a duration to explain the extent to which the bioavailability of an oral dose of propranolol rose. The hepatic metabolism of orally administered labetalol is diminished in the presence of food[42]. Possible explanations include an increased rate of drug absorption and altered blood flow through the liver. Alternatively, blood and the drug might be shunted either within the liver or around it. Both laboratory animals and in vitro tissue studies can advance knowledge in these areas.

DIET AND DRUG EXCRETION

A number of food items can contribute to acidification, or alkalinization, of urine. Balanced protein diets usually produce an alkaline urine. Citrus fruits, vegetables and milk products are likely to contribute to acid urine. Tricyclic antidepressants are generally excreted as a weak base. Their excretion is enhanced in an acid urine[43]. Lithium, a highly water-soluble cation, substitutes for other body fluid cations. Lithium is excreted unchanged almost entirely through the kidney, and sodium balance is an important factor in regulating this excretion. Any appreciable decrease in dietary sodium for hypertension, for example, can lead to lithium retention and possible lithium toxicity[44]. An excessive intake of alkaline ash beverages (citrus juices) can influence quinidine excretion. The beverages increase urinary pH and may be responsible for increasing the proportion of un-ionized quinidine, thus enhancing renal reabsorption of the drug[45].

BINDING OF DRUGS IN PLASMA AND OTHER TISSUES

Malnutrition has been demonstrated to reduce the plasma phenylbutazone half-time $t_{\frac{1}{2}}$, and to cause larger clearance than in controls[46]. Under-nutrition may reduce the binding of phenylbutazone to albumin with a corresponding increase in drug availability for metabolism and elimination[32]. Although renal elimination of some drugs can be decreased by fasting, concentrations of free fatty acids in plasma rise dramatically binding with albumin, displacing the highly bound drugs. This makes them available for both metabolism and renal elimination.

DRUG METABOLISM AND DIET

Many drugs are completely absorbed from the gastrointestinal tract, but are then extensively metabolized in the small intestinal wall, or the liver, before reaching the general circulation. This process of "first-pass elimination" is known to reduce the systemic availability of many drugs. In rats the activities of drug oxidizing enzymes in the intestinal mucosa[47], placenta and liver[48], are increased by giving animals certain cruciferous vegetables, or benzo-(a)-pyrene, a constituent of both cigarette smoke and charcoal-grilled meat. Brassicas and some other vegetables markedly stimulate benzo-(a)-pyrene hydroxylase activity, as a result of the presence of indole compounds. For the same reason these vegetables stimulate the intestinal metabolism of phenacetin and 7-ethoxycoumarine[49]. Other important natural inducers of the cytochrome P-450 enzyme system include terpenes and flavones[50]. A rise in dietary fat, or protein, concentration up to the requirement for growth can stimulate induction of the P-450 system[47,51]. Miltenberger and Oltersdorf[52] demonstrated that deficiencies of riboflavin and, to a lesser extent, of thiamine or pyridoxine, reduce the activities of certain hepatic microsomal enzymes in rats - those particularly involved were hydroxylases. The microsomal drug metabolism system is also affected by deficiencies of ascorbic acid, alpha-tocopherol, riboflavin[53], vitamin A and folacin. The precise enzyme system depressed differs for each vitamin. Starvation and severe food restricition also influence the activity of these enzymes[54]. Dietary deficiencies of calcium, zinc, magnesium, iron, copper and potassium have been shown to impair the rate of drug metabolism in animals[54,55].

Wade and Norred[56] found that rat microsomes expressed a maximal rate of aniline and ethylmorphine metabolism with a diet containing 3% corn oil, whereas the maximal rate for hexobarbital occurred with a 10% corn oil diet. A fat-free diet depresses the metabolism of various drugs in rats[57], and Wade and Norred[56] suggest that a source of polyunsaturated fatty acids is necessary for their metabolism.

Kato et al.[58] demonstrated that the optimal dietary concentration of sulphur amino acids for rat growth was lower than the optimal level of these amino acids to induce maximal liver size, GSH conjugation and therefore maximal induction of metabolic processes in the presence of PCB. However, in general the relative biological value of proteins, as shown by gains in body weight of rats, is positively correlated with activity of the microsomal enzyme system, including aminopyrine N-demethylase, aniline hydroxylase, cytochrome P-450 and NADPH-cytochrome reductase[59]. Reduced energy intake also suppresses drug metabolism by creating competition for the use of tissue protein as a source of energy, and as a substrate for the synthesis of drug metabolizing enzymes[28]. Thus the effect can be similar to that induced by protein deficiency. It is not possible to give any general view as to whether drug metabolism is any more, or less, sensitive to nutrient status than other parameters of response. However, the relative nutrient status of laboratory animals and man, and their intake of dietary contaminants, is of considerable importance in the prediction of drug action. Hepatic drug metabolism is depressed by the presence of cadmium[60] and many other dietary contaminating poisons.

DIETARY FIBRE AND DRUGS

Sherrill et al.[61] demonstrated in F-344 rats that citrus pectin added to diet AIN-76A brought about an elevation of 2 to 3 fold in β-glucuronidase and nitro-reductase activity of caecal contents, and that at a 2% dietary level pectin resulted in a caecal bacterial population similar to that found in rats receiving a cereal based diet[62]. Previously these authors[63] had demonstrated that 5% dietary pectin enhanced the hepatic macromolecular binding of 2,6-dinitrotoluene, and proposed that microfloral enzymes were involved in the activation of this compound.

REFERENCES

1. Faloon, WW, Paes, IC, Woolfolk, D, Nankin, H, Wallace, K and Haro, EN (1966). Effect of neomycin and kanamycin upon intestinal absorption. Ann NY Acad Sci, 132, 879-87
2. Dobbins, WO III, Herrero, BA and Mansbach, CM (1968). Morphologic alterations associated with neomycin-induced malabsorption. Am J Med Sci, 255, 63-7
3. Roe, DA (1974). Minireview effects of drug on nutrition. Life Sci I, 15, 1219-34
4. Toskes, PP and Deren, JJ (1972). Selective inhibition of vitamin B_{12} absorption by para-aminosalicyclic acid. Gastroenterology, 62, 1232-7
5. Coronato, A and Glass, GBJ (1973). Depression of the intestinal uptake of radio-vitamin B_{12} by cholestyramine. Proc Soc Exp Biol Med, 142, 1341-4
6. Palva, IP, Salokannel, SJ, Timonen, T and Palva, HLA (1972). Drug-induced malabsorption of vitamin B_{12}. Acta Med Scand, 191, 355-7
7. Krondl, A (1970). Present understanding of the interaction of drugs and food during absorption. Can Med Assoc J, 103, 360-4
8. Streiff, RR (1970). Folate deficiency and oral contraceptives. J Am Med Assoc, 214, 105-8
9. Matsui, MS and Rozovski, SJ (1982). Drug-nutrient interaction. Clin Ther, 4, 423-40
10. Ellegaard, J, Esmann, V and Henriksen, L (1972). Deficient folate activity during treatment of psoriasis with methotrexate diagnosed by determination of serine synthesis in lymphocytes. Br J Dermatol, 87, 248-55
11. Vilter, RW (1964). The vitamin B_6 hydrazide relationship. Vit Horm, 22, 797-805
12. DaCosta, M and Rothenberg, SP (1974). Appearance of a fo-

late binder in leukocytes and serum of women who are pregnant or taking oral contraceptives. J Lab Clin Med, 83, 207-14

13. Doctor, MM, Sutowm, WW and Trunnell, JB (1973). Effect of steroid hormones on urinary excretion of citrovorum factor by patients with prostatic cancer or leukemia. Proc Soc Exp Biol Med, 113, 737-40

14. Wynn, V (1975). Vitamins and oral contraceptive use. Lancet, 1, 561

15. Lambert, MBT, Molloy, T and Wilson, CWM (1977). The effect of aspirin on the protein binding of ascorbic acid. Br J Pharmacol, 60, 300-1

16. Waxman, S, Corcino, JJ and Herbert, V (1970). Drugs, toxins and dietary amino acid absorption or utilization. Am J Med, 48, 599, 608

17. Jukes, TH and Broquist, HP (1963). In Hochsler, RM and Quartel, JH (eds) Metabolic Inhibitors. p.481 (New York: Academic Press)

18. England, JM and Coles, M (1972). Effects of co-trimoxazole on phenylalanine metabolism in man. Lancet, 2, 1341-3

19. Briggs, M and Briggs, M (1972). Vitamin C requirements and oral contraceptives. Nature, 238, 277

20. Bender, DA and Totoe, L (1984). Inhibitory of tryptophan metabolism by oestrogens in the rat: a factor in the aetiology of pellagra. Br J Nutr, 51, 219-24

21. Theuer, RC (1973). Effect of estrogens and oral contraceptive agents on vitamin and mineral needs. (Evansville: Mead Johnson)

22. Flower, RJ, Moncada, S and Vane, JR (1980). Analgesic-antipyretics and the anti-inflammatory agents. In Goodman, LS and Gilman, AG (eds) The Pharmacological Basis of Therapeutics. pp. 682-728. (New York: Macmillan)

23. Stamp, TCB, Round, JM, Rowe, DJF and Haddacl, JG (1972). Plasma levels and therapeutic effect of 25-hydroxycholecalciferol in epileptic patients taking anticonvulsant drugs. Br Med J, 4, 9-12

24. Hunter, J, Maxwell, JD, Stewart, DA, Parsons, V and Williams, R (1971). Altered calcium metabolism in epileptic children on anticonvulsants. Br Med J, 4, 202-4

25. Theuer, RC and Vitale, JJ (1977). Drug and nutrient interactions. In Schneider et al (eds) Nutritional Support of Medical Practice. (New York: Harper & Row)

26. Reid, C and Chanarin, I (1978). Effect of phenytoin on DNA synthesis by human bone marrow. Scand J Haematol, 20, 237-40

27. Bayliss, EM, Crowley, JM, Preece, JM, Sylvester, PE and Marks, V (1971). Influence of folic acid on blood-phenytoin levels. Lancet, 1, 62

28. Basu, TK (1977). Interaction of drugs and nutrition. J Hum Nutr, 31, 449-58

29. Ordonez, LA and Wurtman, RJ (1974). Folic acid deficiency and methyl group metabolism in rat brain: effects of L-dopa. Arch Biochem Biophys, 160, 372-6

30. Manner, RJ, Brechbill, DO and De Witt, K (1972).

Prevalance of hypokalemia in diuretic therapy. Clin Med, 79, 19-22

31. Seller, RH (1971). The role of magnesium in digitalis toxicity. Am Heart J, 82, 551-6

32. Vessell, ES (1984). Complex effects of diet and drug disposition. Clin Pharmacol Ther, 36, 285-96

33. Marcus, CS and Lengemann, FW (1962). Absorption of the ^{45}Ca and ^{85}Sr from solid and liquid food at various levels of the alimentary tract of the rat. J Nutr, 77, 155-60

34. Greenblatt, DJ, Allen, MD, MacLaughlin, DS, Harmatz, JS and Shader, RI (1978). Diazepam absorption: effects of antacids and food. Clin Pharmacol Ther, 24, 600-9

35. Welling, PG, Elliott, RL, Pitterle, ME, Corrick-West, HP and Lyons, LL (1979). Plasma levels following single and repeated doses of erythromysin estolate and erythromycin stearate. J Pharmaceut Sci, 68, 150-5

36. Toothaker, RD and Welling, PG (1980). The effect of food on drug bioavailability. Ann Rev Pharmacol Toxicol, 20, 173-99

37. Tenconi, LT, Buniva, G, Beretta, E and Pagani, V (1977). Influence of food intake on the absorption of diftalone in man. Int J Clin Pharmacol, 15, 485-91

38. Brandt, JL, Castleman, L, Ruskin, HD, Greenwald, J, Kelly, JJ and Jones, A (1955). The effect of oral protein and glucose feeding on splanchnic blood flow and oxygen utilization in normal and cirrhotic subjects. J Clin Invest, 34, 1017-25

39. Bates, TR and Gibaldi, M (1970). Gastrointestinal absorption of drugs. In Swarbrick, J (ed.) Current Concepts in the Pharmaceutical Sciences: Biopharmaceutics. (Philadelphia: Lea & Febiger)

40. Kohn, KW (1961). Mediation of divalent metal ions in the binding of tetracycline to macromolecules. Nature, 191, 1156-8

41. Svensson, CK, Mauriello, PM, Barde, SH, Middleton, E and Lalka, D (1983). Effect of carbohydrates on estimated hepatic blood flow: Implications in the "food effect" phenomenon. Clin Pharmacol, 34, 316-23

42. Daneshmend, TK and Roberts, CJC (1982). The influence of food on the oral and intravenous pharmacokinetics of a high clearance drug: a study with labetalol. Br J Clin Pharmacol, 14, 73-8

43. Awad, AG (1984). Diet and drug interactions in the treatment of mental illness - a review. Can J Psychiatry, 29, 609-13

44. Thomsen, K and Schou, M (1968). Renal lithium excretion in man. Am J Physiol, 215, 823-7

45. Zinn, MB (1970). Quinidine intoxication from alkali ingestion. Texas Med, 66, 64

46. Adithan, C, Gandhi, IS and Chandrasekar, S (1978). Pharmacokinetics of phenylbutazone in undernutrition. Ind J Pharmacol, 10, 301-8

47. Wattenberg, LW (1971). Studies of polycyclic hydrocarbon hydroxylases of the intestine, possibly related to cancer.

Cancer, 28, 99

48. Harrison, YE and West, WL (1971). Stimulatory effect of charcoal broiled ground beef on the hydroxylation of 3,4 benzpyrene by enzymes in rat liver and placenta. Biochem Pharmacol, 20, 2105-8

49. Pantuck, EJ, Hsiao, KC, Loub, WD, Wattenberg, LW, Kunkman, R and Conney, AH (1976). Stimulatory effect of vegetables on intestinal drug metabolism in the rat. J Pharmacol Exp Ther, 198, 278-83

50. McLean, AEM (1977). Diet, DDT, and the toxicity of drugs and chemicals. Fed Proc, 36, 1688-91

51. Wattenberg, LW (1972). In Cumley, RD (ed.) Environment and Cancer. pp. 241-55. (Baltimore: Williams & Wilkins)

52. Miltenberger, R and Oltersdorf, U (1978). The B-vitamin group and the activity of hepatic microsomal mixed-function oxidases of the growing Wistar rat. Br J Nutr, 39, 127

53. Zannoni, VG and Sato, PH (1976). The effect of certain vitamin deficiencies on hepatic drug metabolism. Fed Proc, 35, 2464

54. Oltersdorf, U, Miltenberger, R and Cremer, HD (1977). Interactions of non-nutrients with nutrients. World Rev Nutr Diet, 26, 41-134

55. Becking, GC (1976). Hepatic drug metabolism in iron-, magnesium- and potassium-deficient rats. Fed Proc, 35, 2480-5

56. Wade, AE and Norred, WP (1976). Effect of dietary lipid on drug metabolizing enzymes. Fed Proc, 35, 2475-9

57. Norred, WP and Wade, AE (1972). Dietary fatty-acid induced alterations of hepatic microsomal drug metabolism. Biochem Pharmacol, 21, 2887-97

58. Kato, N, Mochizuki, S, Kawai, K and Yoshida, A (1982). Effect of dietary level of sulfur-containing amino acids on liver drug-metabolizing enzymes, serum, cholesterol and urinary ascorbic acid in rats fed PCB. J Nutr, 112, 848-54

59. Kato, N, Takeshi, T and Yoshida, A (1981). Effect of dietary quality of protein on liver microsomal mixed function oxidase system, plasma cholesterol and urinary ascorbic acid in rats fed PCB. J Nutr, 111, 123-33

60. Schnell, RC (1978). Cadmium-induced alteration of drug action. Fed Proc, 37, 28

61. Sherrill, JM, Debethizy, JD and Hamm, TE Jr (1983). Influence of diet on gastrointestinal microfloral composition and metabolism in the rat. Proc Am Soc Microbiol, New Orleans

62. Sherrill, JM, Debethizy, JD and Hamm, TE Jr (1984). Dietary effects on the gastrointestinal microflora in the Fischer-344 rat. Proc Am Soc Microbiol, St Louis

63. Debethizy, JD, Sherrill, JM, Rickert, DE and Hamm, TE Jr (1983). Effects of pectin-containing diets on the hepatic macromolecular covalent binding of 2,6-dinitro-(^{3}H)toluene in Fischer-344 rats. Toxicol Appl Pharmacol, 69, 369-76

9.3 IMMUNE FUNCTION AND DIET

D. L. FRAPE

Immunity to infection results from the combined activities of several independent bodily functions, prominent amongst which are antibody formation, the activity of macrophages, the integrity of barriers formed by the superficial epithelial tissues and several other less prominent bodily functions. Antibodies are of two basic origins - those derived in secretory immunity and those in cell-mediated immunity. In this discussion the relationship of diet to antibody formation is of prime concern.

DIETARY PROTEIN

Of the dietary factors considered to influence disease resistance probably the greatest amount of both epidemiological and experimental information has been accumulated on the relationship between protein intake and immunity. Diet, and in particular protein, could exert its influence on immune reaction either at the level of the primary lymphoid organs, principally the thymus and bone marrow, or at the level of secondary lymphoid organs, including widely distributed lymph nodes and the spleen.

Earlier studies clearly demonstrated that dietary protein deficiency of rats is a cause of smaller spleens containing fewer cells, less RNA and more DNA per cell than is found in the spleens of rats given an adequate protein diet[1]. The number of specific antibody-forming cells and the amount of circulating antibody were about one-third normal in depleted animals, whilst the plasma concentration of gamma globulin was about two-thirds normal. The depression in antibody titre in protein deficiency could be attributed largely to a reduction in the number of antibody-forming cells in the spleen.

Whether both humoral and cell-mediated immune responses are reduced in experimental protein-energy malnutrition may depend upon both the length of time over which the malnutrition is imposed and the extent of depletion. Gebhardt and Newberne[2] and Chandra[3] reported that both types of immune response are adversely affected by protein-energy malnutrition, whereas Vijayalnaxmi[4] observed that 90 g of protein per kg diet of rats was sufficient to maximize both antibody response and rosette-forming T-lymphocyte response. On the other hand Bounous and Kongshaven[5] reported that protein source influenced humoral immune response in mice without influencing cell-mediated immunity, as measured by delayed type hypersensitivity, splenic cell mitogen response to phytohaemagglutinin and concanavalin A, and resistance to S. typhimurium. Lactalbumin as a protein led to greater humoral responses than casein, soya or wheat proteins and the response seemed to occur only in the peripheral lymphoid tissue. Bounous et al.[6] proposed that the effect was mediated by differences in plasma amino acid composition. The dietary level of protein at which immune response is maximized seems to differ between animal species as a greater cell-mediated immune response was detected with a purified diet containing 30% casein than with one containing 20% in the guinea pig[7].

Humoral immune responses have been observed in severely malnourished, moderately malnourished and control Ghanaian children[8], whereas cutaneous delayed hypersensitivity was decreased in both malnourished groups, and severely malnourished groups revealed a reduced in vitro lymphocyte response to phytohaemagglutinin. The stress of protein deprivation is thought to induce an increased corticosterone release and suppression of thymosin secretion necessary for the production of functionally mature T-lymphocytes[9]. Protein malnutrition appears to be a cause of atrophy of thymus tissue. Chandra[10] concluded that protein-energy malnutrition is associated with a consistent decrease in the number of circulating thymus-dependent T-lymphocytes, probably caused by an impairment of the differentiation of T-cell precursors, as a direct result of reduced thymic hormone activity, whereas the number of antibody - producing B-lymphocytes was unchanged by protein-energy malnutrition.

Experimental animals tend to be subjected to protein deprivation for a shorter period than human subjects experiencing chronic malnutrition. The reason that some animal experiments have failed to show an effect of dietary protein intake on cell-mediated immunity may depend upon the length of the experiment. Long-lived T-cells are relatively unaffected by temporary protein deprivation and in mice they are reduced only after a protracted protein deficiency[11], whereas there is a much earlier decrease in the number of short-lived rapidly dividing B-lymphocytes[12]. If nutritional deprivation occurs during the critical early stages of immunological development in intrauterine life depression of cell-mediated immunity is more profound and longer-lasting, both in infants[13] and animals[14].

Functionally different subpopulations of lymphocytes may be affected to different degrees by malnutrition. For example, Malave and Layrisse[15] demonstrated a reduction in the total number of spleen cells and in IgG antibody-forming lymphocytes in protein-deprived mice, whereas the proportion of IgM antibody-forming cells was increased. A complicating factor previously referred to is differences in half-lives of the various lymphocyte populations. Chronic protein deficiency seems to reduce the incidence of spontaneous tumours[16], to increase the resistance to transplantable tumours[17] and to be associated with enhanced tumour-specific cytotoxity in mice, explained as a preferential suppression of tumour-specific "blocking" antibody, when protein intakes are low or moderate, thereby resulting in heightened cell-mediated immune responses against tumour antigens[18,19]. In so far as the relationship between nutritional status and the function of other leucocytes is concerned the observations of Moriguchi et al.[20] and the earlier evidence of Benacerraf and his colleagues[21] indicate that dietary protein deficiency of young rats depresses macrophage numbers and their phagocytic function.

DIETARY LIPIDS

There is a complex interrelationship between dietary fat, serum lipids and immune response. Hyperlipidaemia is associated with an aberration in immune function. Obese mice express a reduced cell-mediated immune response although this appears not to be caused by any inherent defect in T-lymphocytes[10]. On the other hand it has been recognised that dietary polyunsaturated fatty acids[22] and alteration to plasma lipoprotein composition[23] can modify the fatty acid composition of the membranes of immunocompetent cells, which may influence their function. It has also been suggested that immune response may be affected by changes in blood cholesterol concentration[23]. An elevation of plasma cholesterol tends to increase the cholesterol:phospholipid value of blood cell membranes, leading to altered function of lymphocytes. Using female rats weaned at 14 days Carlomagno and co-workers[24] observed that while dietary vegetable oil had no effect on their measurements, and although a positive correlation occurred between serum HDL cholesterol and both serum antibody titre and plaque-forming cells (secretory immunity), cholesterol-enriched animal fat profoundly impaired cell-mediated immune response. The early introduction of the animal fat diet suppressed T-lymphocyte function as measured by the T-cell mitogen, phytohaemagglutinin.

Humoral immune response seems to be decreased by high levels of dietary polyunsaturated fat[25] and because of their interrelationship it would be surprising if there were a major nutritional difference in the effects on B- and T-cells. Several studies indicate that the feeding of polyunsaturated fat depresses the response of spleen cells to mitogens. It is possible that there is a low requirement for EFA in cytotoxic activity, and that a depressed response occurs both in deficiency and excess[23]. The scientific community was probably first alerted to the relationship between dietary fat and immune response by the observation that essential fatty acid deficiency could significantly accelerate the rejection of skin allografts in mice[26]. More recently Boyssonneault and Johnston[27] found that essential fatty acid-deficient rats and mice expressed an increased plaque-forming cell response when administered antigen by i.v. injection. Large amounts of polyunsaturated fats suppress delayed hypersensitivity reactions, delay skin graft rejection and reduce response to mitogens. Lymphocytes from corn oil-fed monkeys express a depressed blastogenic response as measured by the haemagglutination inhibition assay (humoral response) compared to monkeys given coconut oil[28]. Similarly Locniskar et al.[29] demonstrated a decreased lymphocyte transformation response for the splenocytes from rats given 24% polyunsaturated fat in their diet in comparison with those given 24% of partially saturated, or entirely saturated fat; and Olson et al.[30] observed a lower response to phytohaemagglutinin (T-cell activator) in mice given a diet containing 20% soya bean oil.

Several reports indicate that increased tumorigenesis is associated with high levels of dietary fat per se[31,32]. Fatty acids of different degrees of saturation have been shown to modify rosetting of sheep erythrocytes to human T-lymphocytes[33]. Clifford et al.[34] concluded that mitogen-induced lymphocyte transformation is unrelated to the degree of saturation of dietary lipids, and Thomas and Erickson[35] found that high levels of both saturated and unsaturated oils, as well as diets deficient in essential fatty acids, depressed T-cell-mediated delayed-type hypersensitivity in comparison to the response of mice receiving a minimum amount of essential fatty acids. A diet containing a high level of polyunsaturated fat increased the linoleic acid content of lymphocytes and depressed graft versus host reactions. Linoleic acid therefore appears to play a pivotal role in varying cellular immune response, in that there is an optimum intermediate cellular level for maximum response. Whether excessive dietary saturated fat contributes to a depression of the linoleate content below the optimum is not established. A minimum adequate level of essential fatty acids seems also to be necessary for B-lymphocyte response in mice[36].

The influence of dietary fat may be mediated in part through its modulating effect on prostaglandin synthesis[10], which in turn is thought to influence the activity of a suppressor T-cell subset[25]. Diets enriched in evening primrose oil (rich in gamma-linolenic acid, C18 : 3n-6) have been shown to inhibit chronic adjuvant-induced polyarthritis in rats[37]. Gamma-linolenic acid is metabolized to C20 : 3n-6 (DGLA) from which PGE_1 is synthesized. This in turn suppresses the formation of PGE_2 by raising cellular cyclic AMP activity[38]. However, further evidence indicates that PGE_1 synthesis suppresses TXB_2 synthesis from arachidonic acid and not PGE_2. PGE_2 is the prostaglandin that is most active in regulating immune response, and it has been found to act as a negative feedback inhibitor of T-cell response[23,39]. PGE_2 may enhance humoral immune response and it appears to inhibit T-cell suppression of B-cell function[4]. Oils rich in fatty acids of the n-3 series depress the level of arachidonic acid in phosphoglycerides of tissue membranes, including those of lymphocytes[22,23] and they probably depress the activity of phospholipases releasing arachidonic acid, reducing the level of 2-series prostaglandins (derived from arachidonic acid) and increase the formation of 3-series prostaglandins (derived from PUFA of the n-3 series). Dietary linseed oil (rich in C18 : 3n-3) has been shown to reduce prostaglandin production by the spleen and by peritoneal macrophages, but the consequential effects on immune function have not been established[22,40].

Dietary fats, both in quantity and fatty acid constitution, clearly influence immune response, but it is not yet possible to predict reliably most types of response or to formulate detailed mechanisms.

Administration of fatty acids by mouth may not be equivalent in effect to dietary supplementation in so far as immune response is concerned[41].

VITAMINS AND MINERALS

In addition to the general effects of protein-energy malnutrition and of fat on immune response, the specific deficiencies of zinc, vitamin A and pyridoxine each demonstrably impair cell-mediated immunity[10]. Recently Nauss and Newberne[42] concluded that no single defect in immune response can account for the increased susceptibility of vitamin A-deficient rats to ocular herpes simplex virus infection. These workers found that the splenic natural killer cell response was depressed in vitamin A-deficient rats, as was splenic mitogen-induced transformation response. On the other hand cervical lymphoid natural killer response was unaffected by diet. Zinc deficiency causes a rapid atrophy of the thymus and interferes with T-cell helper function in young adult mice, but has little effect on B-cells[43] and zinc-deficient mice possess a much lower resistance to Trypanosoma cruzi[44]. De Pasquale-Jardieu and Fraker[45] concluded that zinc deficiency may destroy a substantial portion of the memory cells in mice for sheep red blood cells.

A number of experiments have demonstrated that vitamin E is required for the functioning of both B- and T-lymphocytes. Vitamin E-deficient diets were shown to depress both T- and B-cell splenic mitogen responses in rats[46] and in guinea pigs[47]. Nevertheless excessive intakes of vitamin E (80 i.u. per kg by injection daily) seem to inhibit lymphoproliferative responses in mice compared with lower doses[48].

Insufficient evidence is available to indicate whether vitamin and mineral requirements in terms of dietary concentration for normal immune response are any different from those for other bodily functions. In accordance with the evidence in respect of these other functions vitamin E seems to invoke its influence on immune response more effectively at low concentrations of dietary polyunsaturated fatty acids.

Folic acid and vitamin B_{12} are essential for protein and nucleic acid biosynthesis and deficiencies of both depress immune function in laboratory animals and patients[49]. Biotin-deficient rats express a reduced immune response to sheep red cells accompanied by a decreased thymus size and cellularity[50]. Pyridoxine deficiency significantly reduces immune response in a variety of laboratory animal species. The mechanism by which vitamin B_6 deficiency affects the function of both B- and T-cells is related to its influence on cell transformation and multiplication.

Ascorbic acid is essential for immune function as measured by humoral and cell-mediated responses, and it is also required for both neutrophil and monocyte chemotaxis. The glycolytic and hexose monophosphate shunt activities of leucocytes increase during phagocytosis. These activities are depressed in the leucocytes of ascorbic acid-deficient guinea pigs. There is nevertheless no good evidence to recommend the consumption of massive doses of vitamin C with the hope of enhancing immune response and, in particular, with the objective of preventing viral infections of humans.

A knowledge of the undoubted impact of diet on resistance to infection has three possible and primary implications:

(1)   It may facilitate the formulation of diets for lifespan experiments in which the onset of spontaneous tumours is delayed and their incidence decreased.

(2)   The development of drugs for use in the treatment of disease should be assisted. Both the development and application of techniques employed in organ transplants may be made more successful.

(3)   The evidence in respect of lipids and immunity is perhaps a salutary reminder of the risks that may attend the promulgation of an untarnished image of linoleic acid as both a "cure-all" and a nutrient for "all seasons".

REFERENCES

1.   Kenney, MA, Roderuck, CE, Arnrich, L and Piedad, F (1968). Effect of protein deficiency on the spleen and antibody formation in rats. J Nutr, 95, 173-8

2.   Gebhardt, BM and Newberne, PB (1974). T-cell function in the offspring of lipotrope- and protein-deficient rats. Immunology, 26, 489

3.   Chandra, RK (1975). Antibody formation in first and second generation offspring of nutritionally deprived rats. Science, 190, 289

4.   Vijayalaxmi, G (1978). Immune response in rats given irradiated wheat. Br J Nutr, 40, 535-41

5.   Bounous, G and Kongshaven, PAL (1985). Differential effect of dietary protein type on the B-cell and T-cell immune response in mice. J Nutr, 115, 1403-8

6.   Bounous, G, Shenouda, N, Kongshaven, PAL and Osmond, DG (1985). Mechanism of altered B-cell response induced by changes in dietary protein type in mice. J Nutr, 115, 1409-17

7.   McMurray, DN and Yetley, EA (1982). Immune responses in malnourished guinea pigs. J Nutr, 112, 167-74

8.   Neumann, CG, Lawlor, GJ, Stiehn, ER, Swendseid, ME, Newton, C, Herbert, J, Ammann, AJ and Jacob, M (1975). Immunologic responses in malnourished children. Am J Clin Nutr, 28, 89-104

9.   Watson, RR, Chien, G and Chung, C (1983). Thymosin treatment: serum corticosterone and lymphocyte mitogenesis in moderately and severely protein-malnourished mice. J Nutr, 113, 483-93

10.   Chandra, RK (1980). Cell-mediated immunity in nutritional imbalance. Fed Proc, 39, 3088-92

11. Aschkenasy, A (1965). Influence of alimentary proteins on the size of blood lymphocytes in the rat. The role of the thymus in this effect. Israel J Med Sci, 1, 552-62

12. Bell, RG and Hazell, LA (1975). Influence of dietary protein restriction on immune competence. 1. Effect on the capacity of cells from various lymphoid organs to induce graft-vs-host reactions. J Exp Med, 141, 127-37

13. Chandra, RK, Ali, SK, Kutty, KM and Chandra, A (1977). Thymus-dependent T lymphocytes and delayed hypersensitivity in low birthweight infants. Biol Neonate, 31, 15-18

14. Gross, RL and Newberne, PM (1980). Role of nutrition in immunologic function. Physiol Rev, 60, 188-302

15. Malave, I and Layrisse, M (1976). Immune response in malnutrition. Differential effect of dietary protein restriction on the IgM and IgG response to alloantigens. Cell Immunol, 21, 337-43

16. Rous, P (1914). The influence of diet on transplanted and spontaneous mouse tumours. J Exp Med, 20, 433-51

17. Theuer, RC (1971). Effect of essential amino acid restriction on the growth of female C57BL mice and their implanted BW10232 adenocarcinomas. J Nutr, 101, 223-32

18. Jose, DG and Good, RA (1971). Absence of enhancing antibody in cell mediated immunity to tumour heterografts in protein deficient rats. Nature, 231, 323-5

19. Good, RA, Jose, D, Cooper, WC, Fernandes, G, Kramer, T and Yunis, EJ (1971). Influence of nutrition on antibody production and cellular immune responses in man, rats, mice and guinea pigs. In: Suskind, RM (ed.) Malnutrition and the Immune Response, pp. 169-85 (New York: Raven Press)

20. Moriguchi, S, Sore, S and Kishino, Y (1983). Changes of alveolar macrophages in protein-deficient rats. J Nutr, 113, 40-6

21. Benacerraf, B, Sebestyen, MM and Schlossman, A (1959). A quantitative study of the kinetics of blood clearance of ^{32}P-labeled Escherichia coli and Staphylococci by the reticuloendothelial system. J Exp Med, 110, 27

22. Marshall, LA and Johnston, PV (1983). The effect of dietary alpha-linoleic acid in the rat on fatty acid profiles of immunocompetent cell populations. Lipids, 18, 737-42

23. Smith, AD, Conroy, DM and Belin, J (1985). Membrane lipid modification and immune function. Proc Nutr Soc, 44, 201-9

24. Carlomagno, MA, O'Brien, BC and McMurray, DN (1983). Influence of early weaning and dietary fat on immune response in adult rats. J Nutr, 113, 610-17

25. Boissonneault, GA and Johnston, PV (1983). Essential fatty acid deficiency, prostaglandin synthesis and humoral immunity in Lewis rats. J Nutr, 113, 1187-94

26. Mertin, J and Hunt, R (1976). Influence of polyunsaturated fatty acids on survival of skin allografts and tumour incidence in mice. Proc Natl Acad Sci USA, 73, 928-31

27. Boissonneault, GA and Johnston, PV (1984). Humoral immunity in essential fatty acid-deficient rats and mice: effect of route of injection of antigen. J Nutr, 114, 89-94

28. Meydani, SN, Nicolosi, RJ, O'Connell, MJ and Hayes, KC

(1983). Immune response of Cebus and Squirrel monkeys fed saturated and polyunsaturated fat-containing diets. Fed Proc, 42, 1187

29. Locniskar, M, Nauss, KM and Newberne, PM (1983). The effect of quality and quantity of dietary fat on the immune system. J Nutr, 113, 951-61

30. Olson, LM, Clinton, SK and Visek, WJ (1983). Soyabean oil (SBO) and the immune response in C3H/OUJ mice. Fed Proc, 42, 1186

31. Broitman, SA, Vitale, JJ, Vavrousek-Jakuna, E and Gottlieb, LS (1977). Polyunsaturated fat, cholesterol and large bowel tumorigenesis. Cancer, 40, 2455-63

32. Kollmorgan, GM, Sansing, WA, Lehman, AA, Fischer, G, Langley, RE, Alexander, SS, King, MM and McCay, PB (1979). Inhibition of lymphocyte function in rats fed high-fat diets. Cancer Res, 39, 3458-62

33. Papamichail, M, Tsokos, G, Pepys, MB, Weyman, C, Berlin, J and Smith, AD (1979). Inhibition of complement-dependent rosette formation after lymphocyte incubation with fatty acids. Immunology, 38, 117-22

34. Clifford, CK et al. (1983). Effect of dietary triglycerides on lymphocyte transformation in rats. J Nutr, 113, 669-79

35. Thomas, IK and Erickson, KL (1985). Dietary fatty acid modulation of murine T-cell responses in vivo. J Nutr, 115, 1528-34

36. Erickson, KL and Adams, DA (1983). Dietary modulations of B-cell responses. Fed Proc, 42, 1187

37. Kunkel, SL, Ogawa, H, Ward, PA and Zurier, RB (1982). Suppression of chronic inflammation by evening primrose oil. Prog Lipid Res, 20, 885-8

38. Horrobin, DF (1983). The regulation of prostaglandin biosynthesis by the manipulation of essential fatty acid metabolism. Rev Pure Appl Pharmacol Sci, 4, 339-83

39. Goodwin, JS and Ceuppens, J (1983). Regulation of the immune response by prostaglandins. J Clin Immunol, 3, 295-315

40. Magrum, LJ and Johnston, PV (1983). Modulation of prostaglandin synthesis in rat peritoneal macrophages with Ω-3 fatty acids. Lipids, 18, 514-21

41. Sanders, TAB, Grahame, M and Mistry, M (1985). Influence of dietary eicosapentaenoic (20 : 5Ω3) and docosahexaenoic (22 : 6Ω3) acids on cell-mediated immunity in the mouse. Proc Nutr Soc, 44, 6A

42. Nauss, KM and Newberne, PM (1985). Local and regional immune function of vitamin A-deficient rats with ocular herpes simplex virus infections. J Nutr, 115, 1316-24

43. Fraker, PJ, Haas, SM and Luecke, RW (1977). Effect of zinc deficiency on the immune response of the young adult A/J mouse. J Nutr, 107, 1889-95

44. Fraker, PJ, Caruso, R and Kierszenbaum, F (1982). Alteration of the immune and nutritional status of mice by synergy between zinc deficiency and infection with Trypanosoma cruzi. J Nutr, 112, 1224-9

45. De Pasquale-Jardieu, P and Fraker, PJ (1984). Interference in the development of a secondary immune response in mice

by zinc deprivation: persistence of effects. J Nutr, 114, 1762-9

46. Bendich, A, Gabriel, E and Machlin, LJ (1983). Effect of dietary level of vitamin E on the immune system of the spontaneously hypertensive and normotensive Wistar Kyoto rat. J Nutr, 113, 1920-6

47. Bendich, A, D'Apoliti, P, Gabriel, E and Machline, LJ (1984). Interaction of dietary vitamin C and vitamin E on guinea pig immune responses to mitogens. J Nutr, 114, 1588-93

48. Yasunaga, T, Kato, H, Ohgaki, H, Inando, T and Hikasa, Y (1982). Effect of vitamin E as an immunopotentiation agent for mice at optimal dosage and its toxicity at high dosage. J Nutr, 112, 1075-84

49. Gross, RL, Reid, JVO, Newberne, PM, Burgess, B, Marston, R and Hilft, W (1975). Depressed cell-mediated immunity in megoblastic anemia due to folic acid deficiency. Am J Clin Nutr, 28, 225-32

50. Rabin, BS (1983). Inhibition of experimentally induced autoimmunity in rats by niotin deficiency. J Nutr, 113, 2316-22

9.4 CANCER AND DIET

D. L. FRAPE

A major problem of lifespan studies is the spontaneous incidence of tumours in experimental animals. It is clear that diet has a major impact on this incidence, so that it should be possible by dietary manipulation to reduce it. However, it is abundantly clear that not only may certain dietary factors have an inhibitory, or retarding influence on carcinogenesis but diet can also act as a cancer-promoter. By suppressing the background incidence of spontaneous tumours, the variability of response to potential carcinogens might be lowered. It should also be possible to formulate diets that increase the sensitivity of response to potential carcinogens, yet a conflict of interests is unlikely to be avoided. When a more profound understanding exists of the mechanisms of diet and oncogenetic interactions then a careful analysis of the objectives of each proposed experiment will be required before the most appropriate diet(s) to be used can be formulated.

DIETARY ENERGY RESTRICTION

A chronic restriction of dietary energy decreases the incidence of neoplasms and delays the time at which tumours appear[1]. Dietary restriction has been shown to reduce the incidence of pituitary[2-4], hepatic[5,6], mammary[2,7], lung, lymphoid and certain other tumours[6]. These effects in rats and mice have been observed following dietary or energy restrictions of as little as 20-25% of ad libitum intake[3,5], and the incidence of both spontaneous and chemically induced tumours seems to be affected[8]. Excessive food intake and growth rate, even in the early postnatal period of rats, seems to be associated with a higher incidence of spontaneous tumours[9]. The mechanisms by which dietary restriction mediates its protective effect have not been widely studied, although mitotic activity is inhibited by energy restriction, depressing the development of latent cancer cells[1] and a reduced rate of secretion of both oestrogen and pituitary hormones in rats and mice has been detected[7].

The author and his colleagues developed a feeder for the restricted feeding of rats in the 1960s that has been used in their lifespan studies and oncogenetic investigations in rats since that time, and Roe[10] proposed that there should be a widespread move from ad libitum to controlled feeding for laboratory animals subjected to lifespan investigations.

FAT CONSUMPTION

An increase in the fat content of the diet of laboratory animals from less than 5% to 20% or more seems to increase the incidence of spontaneous mammary carcinoma, skin neoplasms and probably of hepatic tumours[1,11]. Raised levels of dietary fat stimulate bile acid secretion, the microbial metabolism of which may be a cause of carcinoma of the colon as colonic and mammary tumours and possibly those of other types are associated with not only increased concentrations of dietary fat, but also with increasing unsaturation of dietary fat[1]. The observation that faecal bile acid concentration was higher when the source of fat was sunflower oil than when it was butter[12] may point to an explanation of the association of fat unsaturation with colonic cancer. Certain bile acids have been shown to be colon tumour promoters in both germ-free and conventional rats[13]. As promoters they seem to accelerate proliferation of colonic cells. Epidemiological evidence indicates that the effect of high dietary fat on the colon is counteracted to some extent by intake of cereal fibre[13,14].

High concentrations of dietary fat enhance both chemically induced and spontaneous carcinogenesis[7,15]. Weisburger concluded that excessive dietary fat is responsible for the endogenous production of a specific non-genotoxic, epigenetic, or promoting agent, associated with increased risk of cancers of the colon, breast and prostate[13].

Anaerobic bacteria are most active in steroid metabolism[16], and a survey and review[1] indicate that faecal steroids from individuals in high colonic cancer risk areas are far more extensively metabolized than those from low-risk areas and their faecal flora contains large numbers of Gram-negative non-sporing anaerobes and fewer enterococci than are found in people from areas of low incidence. Faecal clostridia capable of bile acid dehydrogenation are also found in a high proportion of patients with colonic cancer[16].

Excess dietary fat may stimulate the exocrine pancreas in a way comparable to that caused by protease inhibitors[17]. Concern has been expressed over the National Toxicology Programme, carcinogenicity bioassays, where oil gavage is used in rats and which demonstrates an increased frequency of proliferative lesions in the exocrine pancreas of male rats. It is speculated that corn oil gavage stimulates excessively gastrointestinal hormones and pancreatic enzyme secretion[18]. Sodium oleate added to the drinking water of male rats at concentrations of 2.5% and 5.0% for 108 weeks seemed to increase slightly the incidence of pancreatic tumours in Fischer rats[19].

LIPOTROPE DEFICIENCY

The hepatic microsomal mixed-function oxidase (MFO) system is active in the metabolism of many xenobiotes. A deficiency of dietary lipotropes - folic acid, vitamin B_{12}, choline and methionine - inhibits this metabolic system and enhances the chemical induction of tumours in the liver, colon and oesophagus[20]. For some chemicals, however, the metabolite is more toxic than the original chemical. Newberne and Rogers[21], for example, found fewer mammary tumours in Sprague-Dawley rats given N-2-fluorenylacetamide (FAA) in a low-lipotrope high-fat diet. They also suggested that a diet marginally deficient in lipotropes may interfere with the action of several hormones that control cell division in the liver, rendering hepatocytes more susceptible to chemical carcinogens.

Several other dietary nutrients and principal components, including dietary protein and fat, influence MFO activity and therefore the toxicity and genotoxicity of xenobiotes[22,23].

DIETARY PROTEIN

The activity of hepatic microsomal enzymes is influenced by the amount and quality of dietary protein. The induction of hepatic tumours by dimethylnitrosamine (DMN) was blocked by a dietary deficiency of protein and the induction of renal tumours enhanced, presumably because DMN was cleared from the blood less rapidly in deficient rats[24].

The effect of dietary protein concentration on oncogenesis is therefore seen to be complex. Decreased levels of dietary protein given before and after dosing rats with aflatoxin depressed the development of gamma-glutamyl transpeptidase-positive foci that are preneoplastic liver lesions[25,26], but chronic marginal protein deprivation predisposes rats to an early occurrence of tumours of the adrenal gland and lymphoid tissue. Increased amounts of dietary casein tended to inhibit the induction of malignant hepatic tumours induced by azo dyes[11]. On the other hand a high-protein diet subjects rats to the early appearance of mammary adenocarcinoma[27] and pituitary tumours[3] and subjects mice to both mammary and skin tumours[3]. Other types of tumour, principally those occurring in the pituitary, thyroid and pancreas, are apparently most prevalent when rats are given a diet adequate in protein content[28].

Source of dietary protein influences the development of Morris hepatoma 7800[29], and the results of a number of studies indicate that the amino acid composition of dietary protein is important. Low dietary cystine inhibits the induction of leukaemia in dba mice and spontaneous mammary carcinoma in C3H female mice is inhibited by lysine-deficient, or cystine-deficient, diets[11]. Dietary supplementation with arginine seems to decrease tumour induction in mammary cells caused by 7,10-dimethyl benzanthracene (DMBA)[30]. Cell-mediated immunity is probably a major defence against cancer, whereas humoral antibody formation may enhance tumour development by protecting the tumour from cell-mediated immune responses[31]. Cell-mediated immunity can be maintained intact during deficiencies of certain amino acids whilst antibody production is depressed[31].

DIETARY FIBRE

It has been widely reported that populations noted to suffer a high incidence of colonic cancer tend to consume diets rich in refined foods, low in fibre. These people yield higher than expected counts of anaerobic bacteria, lower counts of aerobic bacteria, higher concentrations of total neutral steroids and more degraded cholesterol and bile acids in their faeces[21]. The key dietary factor would appear to be fibre, and the mechanism by which it may promote its protective influence is by accelerating the passage of the contents of the large intestine, affording less time for bacteriological proliferation, for bacterial conversion of bile salts to potential carcinogens and for contact between carcinogens and the intestinal mucosa. Peristalsis is promoted by the water-binding property of fibre components and by the bacterial production of volatile fatty acids which exert a cathartic effect. Dietary fibre may also influence bile salt metabolism in a way that reduces the formation of potential carcinogens. This may be accomplished through a binding of bile salts, cholesterol and their degradation products, and through augmenting sterol excretion, or possibly through an inhibition of the 7-α-dehydroxylation process. Certain anaerobic bacteria carry out this reaction, converting the primary bile acids to deoxycholic acid and lithocholic acid that have been incriminated as carcinogens. Furthermore it has been shown that certain bacteria can introduce double bonds in the steroid nucleus by dehydrogenase reactions leading to full aromatization of the bile acid nucleus and yielding a family of potentially carcinogenic compounds[1]. As previously referred to, high-fat diets increase beta-glucuronidase activity of the faecal flora of rats[32], and this enzyme can convert procarcinogens into their active forms through the hydrolysis of the beta-glycolytic bond[33].

The influence of dietary fibre on faecal bile acid concentration depends on the balance between the acid-binding effect of lignin that increases faecal bile acids and the bulking effects of hemicellulose and cellulose that result in a reduction in faecal bile acid concentration by simple dilution. The precise significance of this is not entirely clear. However Frape et al.[34,35] reported that lignin residues of wheatbran significantly reduced the absorption of aflatoxin in rats, whereas sources of hemicellulose, cellulose or pectin were without influence. In this case the absorption of a fat-soluble toxin seems to be decreased by a reduction in the reabsorption of bile salts, whereas the dilution effect of the various fibre sources and the accelerated rate of passage through the intestinal tract were of little or no significance. A generally much greater toxicity of purified diets compared with commercial stock diets for laboratory animals, where these are used in studies of carcinogens, is in part at least attributed to differences in the chemical and physical structure of their fibre components.

RETINOIDS AND CANCER

As retinol is known to play a role in the differentiation of epithelial cells, it is not surprising that it also plays a role in the development of epithelial tumours. Many carcinogens are much more potent in animals with long-term vitamin A deficiency[36] and human cancer risks appear to be inversely correlated with blood retinol and dietary beta-carotene intake. Vitamin A deficiency has been related to the development of many types of epithelial tumour, including odontomas and salivary gland tumours[37], colonic tumours[21], precancerous lesions of the gastric mucosa[38], and gastric tumour growth[39]. High concentrations of dietary retinoids have some capacity to prevent chemical carcinogenesis in epithelial tissues; however the high toxicity of natural retinoids limits their usefulness for the prevention of cancer[40].

Several explanations have been advanced for the action of retinoids in cancer prevention:

1. Retinoids control the differentiation of basal cells to the specific mature cells that characterize the various epithelia of the body. These processes of differentiation are blocked, or altered, by the action of carcinogenic agents. Retinoids may arrest or reverse these pathological processes.
2. Retinoids may enhance immunological function[36].
3. Carotenoids, in particular, may function by quenching singlet oxygen[41].
4. Increased DNA synthetic and mitotic activity, which would enhance carcinogenesis occurs in retinoid-deficient epithelia[42].
5. The carcinogenic risk to the skin of actinic radiation may be reduced by vitamin A, or carotenoids, which absorb ultraviolet light[43].
6. The observation that carcinogens bind more tightly to DNA in cultured tracheas isolated from vitamin A-deficient hamsters than to the DNA in tracheas from healthy animals is important in the carcinogenic process[36].

NITRATE AND NITRITE AND CANCER

Gastric cancer is associated with the intake of nitrate, nitrite and other precursors of nitroso-compounds. From the nutritional standpoint the occurrence of precursors is of as much interest as N-nitroso compounds, because the acidic conditions of the stomach are suitable for nitrosation reactions. Nitrate is reduced to nitrite by oral and gastric bacteria[44], accounting for the relevance of both to gastric nitrosation[45]. Both are present in food, especially vegetable, and at low levels in most water supplies. Both are formed in the lungs on inhalation of nitrogen oxides in polluted atmospheres and in tobacco smoke[46]. As a nitrosating agent, nitrite probably acts similarly to many other dietary nitrogen-containing compounds - secondary and tertiary amines, amides, substituted urea and guanidine and also possibly proteins and peptides[45,47]. The formation of the carcinogen, which may be a nitrosamide or an aryldiazonium salt, is inhibited by the presence of vitamins C or E, certain phenolic antioxidants[21] and nitrite traps such as pyrogallol or tannins[48-50]. Ascorbic acid lowers the amount of available nitrate by reducing nitrites to nitrogen oxides[51]. The net result is a reduction in the amount of nitrosamine and nitrosamide formed. Ascorbic acid and the antioxidants BHA and BHT have also been shown to promote the induction of tumours[52,53].

Both riboflavin deficiency[54] and riboflavin-rich diets[38] have been shown to inhibit tumour growth, although riboflavin deficiency enhances the carcinogenicity of azo dyes in the liver[54]

Selenium at high dietary concentrations may be carcinogenic itself[55], but in addition there appears to be a relationship between the dietary concentration of selenium and the carcinogenicity of certain chemical carcinogens[56,57] in liver tissue.

ANTIOXIDANTS

BHA and BHT are phenolic antioxidants that have been shown to affect the microsomal mixed-function oxidase system of liver microsomes. These antioxidants can reduce gastric tumour incidence in mice[58], and DMBA-induced mammary tumours have been inhibited by BHA, BHT and ethoxyquin[58]. Dietary antioxidants may also act directly by combining with free radical carcinogens, thereby preventing their cellular reactions.

SODIUM CHLORIDE AND CANCER

Sodium chloride, particularly when given as a saturated solution weekly, and probably when administered continuously in water, or in the diet, has been demonstrated to increase the incidence of gastric carcinoma caused by either MNNG or N-nitrosoquinoline (NQO)[59]. Sodium chloride alone was not carcinogenic, and the authors suggested that salt may have modified the mucopolysaccharides of the mucosal barrier, rendering the stomach lining more permeable to the carcinogens.

NON-NUTRIENT CONSTITUENTS OF DIET

The inclusion of the vegetative parts of cruciferae in animal diets has been shown to influence the metabolism of drugs by promoting microsomal enzyme induction in hepatic and intestinal tissue, so stimulating a detoxification mechanism for food contaminants. Certain indigenous indoles of cruciferae may account for all or part of the effect. Three indoles with inducing activity have been identified in these vegetables[60]. Vegetable matter itself may also contain enzymes capable of modifying chemical carcinogens. Alfalfa apparently contains aryl hydrocarbon hydroxylase performing such an activity[21].

Beans and other seeds are rich in plant proteins called lectins (haemagglutinins) which are either toxic themselves or bound to natural toxins. This characteristic may be the explanation for their stimulation both of intestinal movements and the production of mucus and gas in the bowel. They have been found to protect animals against cancer, and they may also similarly protect humans by stimulating the growth of normal cells or by promoting white blood cells to attack cancer cells. Lectins have the ability to bind to the surface carbohydrates of many mammalian cells, and by this they are endowed with a multitude of characteristics:

1. agglutination of erythrocytes, bacteria and of neoplastic cells in preference to the normal adult equivalents;
2. induction of lymphocyte transformation;
3. stimulation of mast-cell degranulation.

Lectins may protect against intestinal cancer by a number of possible mechanisms:

1. mast-cell degranulation would cause inflammation and increase mucus production, increasing faecal bulk and tending to sweep away malignant cells and carcinogens;
2. by binding with mucosal cells, mytosis may be induced, increasing epithelial turnover and allowing less opportunity for neoplastic cells to become established;
3. a similar process would stimulate the cytotoxicity of lymphocytes;
4. the neoplastic cells themselves would be susceptible to direct damage by the lectin[61].

Protease inhibitors are widely distributed in vegetable matter and are considered to have anti-tumour properties[62]. However, it is well established that pancreatic enlargement occurs ultimately precipitating pancreatic cancer when significant amounts of protease inhibitors are present in the diet[17]. It is speculated that exposure of the pancreas to an initiating carcinogen following stimulation of the pancreas to regeneration, or stimulation to growth by protease inhibitors, is a cause of that cancer[63].

Autoclaving of a stock diet reduced the tumour incidence in mice given methylcholanthrene[64]. However, Frape et al.[34] found no difference in the protective action of wheatbran for aflatoxicosis in rats whether it was autoclaved or not. The mechanisms of action in the two situations, however, were considered to be quite different - in the first case essential fatty acid deficiency afforded protection and in the second autoclaving did not detract from the protective properties of the dietary fibre.

PURIFIED VERSUS COMMERCIAL STOCK DIETS

Many observations have demonstrated lower toxicity and lower carcinogenicity of chemicals when added to natural ingredient diets in comparison with the effects of their addition to purified diets. Some of these differences have been attributed to larger amounts of dietary fibre in natural diets[65]. Wise demonstrated quite different microbial enzyme activities of significance to toxin metabolism between the faecal micro-organisms of rats given natural ingredient diets in comparison with those given purified diets containing chemically similar mixtures of purified fibres[66]. The contrasting effects might be attributed in part to the differences in physical relationships between dietary fibre sources in the two types of diet, and possibly to the presence of a number of enzyme inducers found in natural ingredients and referred to in the previous section.

REFERENCES

1. Alcantara, EN and Speckman, EW (1976). Diet, nutrition and cancer. Am J Clin Nutr, 29, 1035-47
2. Tucker, MJ (1979). The effect of long term food restriction on tumours in rodents. Int J Cancer, 23, 803-7
3. Tucker, MJ (1986). Diet and disease in the rodent. ICLAS Bulletin, No.58
4. Pickering, RG and Pickering EC (1984). The effect of diet on the incidence of pituitary tumours in female Wistar rats. Lab Animals, 18, 298-314
5. Wostman, BS and Pollard, M (1983). Prevention of spontaneous hepatic neoplasms among aged germ-free Lobund Wistar rats by dietary restriction. Fed Proc, 4, 801
6. Conybeare, G (1980). Effect of quality and quantity of diet on survival and tumor incidence in outbred Swiss mice. Food Cosmet Toxicol, 18, 65-76
7. Newberne, PM, Gross, RL and Roe, DA (1978). Drug toxin and nutrient interactions. World Rev Nutr Diet, 29, 130-69
8. Gori, GB (1979). Food as a factor in the etiology of certain human cancers. Food Technol, 33, 48-56
9. Ross, MH, Lustbader, ED and Bras, G (1982). Dietary practices of early life and spontaneous tumours of the rat. Nutr Cancer, 3, 150-67
10. Roe, FJC (1982). Labsure Symposium, 19 October, Albany Hotel, Birmingham
11. Tannenbaum, A (1957). Nutrition and the Genesis of Tumours. (London: Butterworth), p. 306
12. Hill, MJ (1975). Metabolic epidemiology of dietary factors in large bowel cancer. Cancer Res, 35, 3398
13. Weisburger, JH (1985). Nutrition and carcinoma of the large intestine. Proc Nutr Soc, 44, 115-20
14. Reddy, BS, Hedges, AR, Laakso, K and Wynder, EL (1978). Metabolic epidemiology of large bowel cancer. Faecal bulk and constituents of high-risk North American and low-risk Finnish population. Cancer, 42, 2832-8
15. Rogers, AE and Newberne, PM (1973). Dietary enhancement of intestinal carcinogenesis by dimethylhydrazine in rats. Nature, 246, 491-2
16. Rowland, IR (1976). Diet and cancer of the colon. Food Cosmet Toxicol, 14, 209-12
17. McGuinness, EE, Morgan, RGH, Levison, DA, Frape, DL, Hopwood, D and Wormsley, RG (1980). The effects of long term feeding of soya flour on the rat pancreas. Scand J Gastroenterol, 15, 497-502

18. Beiber, MA (1985). Use of fat in formulating animal diets. Workshop XIII, Int Cong Nutr, 18-23 August, Brighton, UK

19. Haisa, Y, Konishi, N, Kitahori, Y and Shimoyama, T (1985). Carcinogenicity study of a commercial sodium oleate in Fischer Rats. Food Chem Toxicol, 23, 619-23

20. Rogers, AE (1975). Variable effects of a lipotrope-deficient, high fat diet on chemical carcinogens in rats. Cancer Res, 35, 2469

21. Newberne, PM and Rogers, AE (1976). Nutritional modulation of carcinogenesis. In: Magee, PN et al. (eds) Fundamentals of Cancer Prevention. (Baltimore: University of Tokyo Press), pp.15-40

22. MacLean, AEM (1977). Diet, DDT, and the toxicity of drugs and chemicals. Fed Proc, 36, 1688-91

23. Balakrishnan, G, Ramachandran, M, Banerjee, BD and Hussain, QZ (1985). Effect of dietary protein, dichlorodiphenyltrichloroethane (DDT) and hexachlorocyclohexane (HCH) on hepatic microsomal enzyme activity in rats. Br J Nutr, 54, 563-6

24. McLean, AEM and Magee, PN (1970). Increased renal carcinogenesis by dimethylnitrosamine in protein-deficient rats. Br J Exp Pathol, 51, 587-90

25. Campbell, TC and Dunaif, GE (1985). Relationship between dietary protein level and formulation of hepatic Y-glutamyl transpeptidase positive foci in rats following aflatoxin B1 administration. Fed Proc, 44, 1672

26. Dunaif, GE and Campbell, TC (1985). Decreasing dietary protein levels suppress preneoplastic liver lesion development despite increasing doses of aflatoxin B_1 (AFB_1). Fed Proc, 44, 938

27. McSheeh, TW (1974). The onset of mammary adenocarcinoma in mice: a possible correlation with nutrition. Ecol Food Nutr, 3, 147

28. Ross, MH and Bras, G (1973). Influence of protein under and overnutrition on spontaneous tumour prevalence in the rat. J Nutr, 103, 944

29. Okonkwo, CJ, Knight, EM, Adkins, JS and Criss, W (1984). The effect of dietary plant protein on tumor growth in tumor-bearing male buffalo rats. Fed Proc, 43, 854

30. Takeda, Y, Tominaga, T, Tei, N, Kitamura, M, Taga, S, Murase, J, Jaguchi, T and Miwatani, T (1975). Inhibitory effect of L-arginine on growth of rat mammary tumors induced by 7,12-dimethybenx(a) authracene. Cancer Res, 35, 2390-3

31. Worthington, BS (1974). Effect of nutritional status on immune phenomena. J Am Diet Assoc, 65, 123

32. Mallett and Rowland (personal communication)

33. Reddy, BS, Weisburger, JH and Wynder, EL (1974). Faecal bacterial B-glucuronidase: control by diet. Science, 183, 416

34. Frape, DL, Wayman, BJ, Tuck, MG and Jones, E (1982). The effects of gum arabic, wheat offal and various of its fractions on the metabolism of ^{14}C-labelled aflatoxin B_1 in the male weanling rat. Br J Nutr, 48, 97-110

35. Frape, DL, Wayman, BJ and Tuck, MG (1981). The effect of dietary fibre sources on aflatoxicosis in the weanling male

rat. Br J Nutr, 46, 315-26
36. Maugh, TH (1974). Vitamin A: potential protection from carcinogens. Science, 186, 1198
37. Shils, ME (1973). Nutrition and Neoplasia. In: Goodhart, RS and Shils, ME (eds) Modern Nutrition in Health and Disease. Dietotherapy. (Philadelphia: Lea & Febiger), pp.966-80
38. Kraybill, HF (1963). Carcinogenesis associated with foods, food additives, food degradation products, and related dietary factors. Clin Pharmacol Ther, 4, 73
39. Chu, EW and Malmgren, RA (1965). An inhibitory effect of vitamin A on the induction of tumors of forestomach and cervix in the Syrian hamster by carcinogenic polycyclic hydrocarbons. Cancer Res, 25, 884
40. Sporn, MB, Dunlop, NM, Newton, DL and Smith, JM (1976). Prevention of chemical carcinogenesis by vitamin A and its synthetic analogs (retinoids). Fed Proc, 35, 1332
41. Peto, R, Doll, R, Buckley, JD and Sporn, MB (1981). Can dietary beta-carotene materially reduce human cancer rates? Nature, 290, 201-8
42. Sporn, MB (1977). Retinoids and carcinogenesis. Nutr Rev, 35, 65-9
43. Newberne, PM, Chan, WCM and Rogers, AE (1974). Influence of light, fiboflavin and carotene on the response of rats to the acute toxicity of aflatoxin and monocrotaline. Toxicol Appl Pharmacol, 28, 200-8
44. Ralt, D and Tannenbaum, SR (1981). In: Scanlan, RA and Tannenbaum, SR (eds) N-Nitroso Compounds. ACS Symposium Series 174. (Washington, DC: American Chemical Society), pp.157-64
45. Challis, BC (1985). Nutrition and nitrosamine formation. Proc Nutr Soc, 44, 95-100
46. Goldstein, E, Goldstein, F, Peek, NF and Park, NJ (1980). In: Lee, SD (ed) Nitrogen Oxides and Their Effects on Health. (Ann Arbour, Michigan: Ann Arbor Science), pp.143-60
47. Mirvish, SS (1983). The etiology of gastric cancer. Intragastric nitrosamide formation and other theories. J Natl Cancer Inst, 71, 629-47
48. Correa, P, Haenszel, W and Tannenbaum, SR (1982). Epidemiology of gastric carcinoma: review and future prospects. Natl Cancer Inst Monogr, 62, 129-34
49. Weisburger, JH and Horn, CL (1983). Factors associated with esophageal and gastric cancer in man. In: Magee, PN (ed) Nitrosamines and Human Cancer, Banbury Report Vol.12. (New York: Cold Spring Harbour Laboratory), pp.523-8
50. Joosens, JV and Geboers, J (1983). Epidemiology of gastric cancer. A clue to etiology. In: Sherlock, P et al. (eds) Gastrointestinal Tract. (New York: Raven Press), pp.97-114
51. Clayson, DB (1975). Nutrition and experimental carcinogenesis: a review. Cancer Res, 35, 3292
52. Fukushima, S, Imaida, K, Sakata, T, Okamura, T, Shibata, M and Ito, N (1983). Promoting effects of sodium L-ascorbate on two-stage urinary bladder carcinogenesis in rats. Cancer Res, 43, 4454-7

53. Lok, E, Iverson, F, Nera, EA and Clayson, DB (1983). Studies on effect of butylated hydroxyanisole (BHA) on cell proliferation in rat forestomach. Report prepared for World Health Organization: Joint FAO-WHO Expert Committee on Food Additives

54. Rivlin, RS (1973). Riboflavin and cancer. A review. Cancer Res, 33, 1977

55. Sunderman, FW (1978). Carcinogenic effects of metals. Fed Proc, 37, 40

56. Chen, J, Goetchius, MP, Campbell, TS and Combs, GF Jr (1982). Effect of dietary selenium and vitamin E on hepatic mixed function oxidase activities and in vivo covalent binding of alfatoxin B in rats. J Nutr, 112, 324-31

57. Baldwin, S, Parker, RS and Misslbeck, N (1983). Effect of dietary fat and selenium on the development of preneoplastic lesions in rat liver. Fed Proc, 42, 1312

58. Wattenburg, L (1972). Dietary modification of intestinal and pulmonary aryl hydrocarbon hydroxylase activity. Toxicol Appl Pharmacol, 23, 741-8

59. Tatematsu, M, Takahashi, M, Fukushima, S, Hananouchi, M and Shirai, T (1985). Effects in rats of sodium chloride on experimental gastric cancers induced by N-methyl-J-nitro-N-nitrosoguanidine or 4-nitroquinoling-1-oxide. J Natl Cancer Inst, 55, 101-6

60. Wattenberg, LW (1975). Effects of dietary constituents on the metabolism of chemical carcinogens. Cancer Res, 35, 3326

61. Freed, DLJ and Green FHY (1975). Do dietary lectins protect against colonic cancer? Lancet, 2, 1261

62. Troll, W (1976). Blocking tumor promotion by protease inhibitors. In: Magee, P and Matsushima, P (eds) Fundamentals in Cancer Prevention. (Tokyo/Baltimore: University of Tokyo Press/University Park Press), p.41

63. Wormsley, KG (1985). Carcinoma of the pancreas. Proc Nutr Soc, 44, 113

64. Medawar, P, Hunt, R and Mertin, J (1979). An influence of diet on transplantation immunity. Proc R Soc Lond B, 206, 265-80

65. Ershoff, BH (1974). Antitoxic effects of plant fibre. Am J Clin Nutr, 27, 1395-8

66. Wise, A (1985). Evidence that different nutritionally satisfactory diets influence toxicological parameters. Medical Research Council Laboratories, Carshalton, Surrey

9.5 INFLUENCE OF DIET ON LONGEVITY

D. L. FRAPE

A number of dietary factors influences voluntary food intake. Three distinct and important factors are the effect of diet on blood glucose concentration, dietary bulk and the amino acid content of dietary proteins. The latter may suggest means of controlling food intake independently of energy status by adopting relatively minor adjustments to dietary composition that affect the post-prandial pattern of circulating amino acids.

Depressed food intake by rodents receiving imbalanced amino acid mixtures in their diet has been related to depletion of brain pools of individual amino acids[1]. A preference is shown for diets that will produce a balanced plasma amino acid pattern over one that will not. The effects do not appear to be associated with a depletion of any specific amino acid, although Anderson[2] has proposed that control of protein and energy intakes of rats is mediated by the changes that occur in response to dietary influences on the ratios of the plasma concentrations of tryptophan and other large neutral amino acids, affecting brain serotonin concentration and dietary ratios of tyrosine and phenylalanine affecting brain catecholamine content. However, these views are disputed, and although the results of recent studies in rats indicate effects of dietary protein level[3] and of amino acid analogues[1] on food intake and brain amino acid concentrations no influence on neurotransmitter concentrations has been revealed.

Bolze et al.[4] compared lysine-, methionine-, or histidine-deficient diets given to rats ad libitum with a control diet given in varying amounts daily. All amino acid-deficient rats had lost more weight than the control rats fed at comparable energy levels. Although serum somatomedin and growth hormone activities were reduced in rats given the amino acid-deficient diets ad libitum and in those given restricted amounts of the control diet, the effects were not caused by reductions in plasma levels of any of the three test amino acids. Thus the mechanisms by which abnormal dietary amino acid concentrations exert their influence on appetite remain unclear.

Nevertheless enzymatic adaptation decreases the effect on

food intake of imbalanced dietary amino acids. Peters and Harper[3] showed that a gradual improvement in growth and food intake of rats fed diets containing more than 35% casein was accompanied by dramatic increases in the activities of hepatic SDH and GPT, promoting amino acid catabolism and decreases in the concentrations of most amino acids in plasma and brain.

DIET AND LONGEVITY

The most striking influence of diet on lifespan of laboratory animals is the extension brought about by a reduction in the daily rate of energy intake throughout life, and more particularly in the phase following the early growth spurt. There is considerable circumstantial evidence that cancer incidence increases, and longevity is prejudiced, by excessive energy intake. Pickering and Pickering[5] compared the effects of several commercial rodent diets given to Wistar rats. The rate of energy intake and consequential geriatric body weight seemed to impart an overriding influence on longevity and the incidence of pituitary tumours. Energy intake can be reduced by a restricted access to diet or by a reduction in the energy density of diet. Although dietary protein concentration had little impact on longevity in the study of Pickering and Pickering a complex analysis by Ross et al.[6] on dietary practice up to 200 days of age amongst Charles River rats indicated there may be a slight positive correlation between protein intake to 105 days and tumour incidence. However, the impact of dietary protein concentrations on longevity would seem to be far less than that of energy.

A reduction in metabolizable energy intake brought about by decreasing energy density of diet has two principal disadvantages:

1. The introduction of water-soluble, or water-insoluble fibre to the diet may influence the incidence of certain metabolic disorders; it may affect drug metabolism and the sensitivity of response of test animals to test substances. Frequently the effect is to decrease the sensitivity of response, counteracting the advantages achieved by a reduction in background incidence of spontaneous metabolic disorders.

2. Most laboratory animal species achieve partial compensation for reduced energy density by eating more where they are given ad libitum access to feed. Alternatively, increased energy density of diets leads to lower ad libitum intakes, but the reduction seems not to be sufficient to prevent energy intake of rats increasing, especially that of males, when either purified or natural ingredients are used[7,8].

The many effects of dietary energy dilution imposed by the introduction of fibre on the initiation and progression of various metabolic disorders, including cancer, are discussed in other sections of this chapter. The imposition of dietary restriction by daily rationing of laboratory animals has been tested by a number of research workers. A reduction of the food intake of mice to 60% of ad libitum intake was shown to improve the accelerated senescence score, and a reduction to 60% and 80% of ad libitum intake was shown to decrease ageing score[9]. Food restriction has also been demonstrated to reduce slightly the incidence of cystic thyroids[10], but to have no influence on pulmonary mineralization[11] amongst virgin females of a fat sub-line of mice. Food restriction of breeding male and female rats[12] brought about a marked and reversible improvement in their breeding performance and it is clear that test chemicals that cause a depression in appetite will introduce confounding effects on many response parameters of both growing and breeding rodents unless pair feeding is practised.

Where rodents are given ad libitum access to their diet for a very restricted period of time, such as 1 hour, food wastage can be considerably reduced, so that the measurement of intake is more accurate and any circadian rhythm in metabolism and post-prandial changes in metabolism are more uniform between individual animals. James et al.[13] reported that the majority of their rats could be trained to a regime of meal feeding during 1 hour at night, achieving an adequate intake as shown by protein mass of liver cells. Nevertheless ad libitum access for a restricted period of time inevitably leads to variable daily intakes and the author routinely used a system in which weanling rats were trained to consume a fixed allowance of diet between 0800 and 1000 hours daily from the year 1970 onwards, in order that treatment differences were not confounded with variation in intake, and so that measurement of that intake was accurate. The adaptation of rats to access to their feed for say 2 hours daily leads to a more rapid stomach emptying and differences in metabolism in comparison with nibble feeders. For example, Buraczewski et al.[14] observed somewhat higher concentrations in the systemic plasma of several amino acids. Dietary composition also influences the rate of post-prandial stomach emptying, and the author observed differences between dietary structural carbohydrates in this characteristic in meal-fed rats[15]. Readers are referred to a review by Fabry[16] for a detailed discussion of the effects of feeding patterns on metabolism in rats.

Much speculation exists on the mechanism by which dietary restriction has such a wide spectrum of effects resulting in increased longevity. Chipalkatti et al.[17] proposed that the improvement in longevity brought about by a restriction could be related to a reduction in lipoperoxidation and a reduced accumulation of lipofuscins in tissues, implying that the effects are mediated through a reduction of free radical-mediated cellular damage.

REFERENCES

1. Tews, JK and Harper, AE (1985). Food intake, growth and tissue amino acids in rats fed amino acid analogues. J Nutr, 115, 1180-95

2. Anderson, GH (1979). Control of protein and energy intake: role of plasma amino acids, and brain neurotransmitters. Can J Physiol Pharmacol, 57, 1043-57

3. Peters, JC and Harper, AE (1985). Adaption of rats to diets containing different levels of protein: effects on food intake, plasma and brain amino acid concentrations and brain

neurotransmitter metabolism. J Nutr, 115, 382-98

4. Bolze, MS, Reeves, RD, Lindbeck, FE and Elders, MJ (1985). Influence of selected amino acid deficiencies on somatomedin, growth and glycosaminoglucan metabolism in weanling rats. J Nutr, 115, 782-7

5. Pickering, RG and Pickering, CE (1984). The effect of diet on the incidence of pituitary tumours in female Wistar rats. Lab Animals, 18, 298-314

6. Ross, MH, Lustbader, ED and Bras, G (1982). Dietary practices of early life and spontaneous tumors of the rat. Nutr Cancer, 3, 150, 167

7. Edwards, DG and Dean, J (1985). The responses of rats to various combinations of energy and protein II. Diets made from natural ingredients. Lab Animals, 19, 336

8. Edwards, DG, Porter, PD and Dean, J (1985). The responses of rats to various combinations of energy and protein I. Diets made from purified ingredients. Lab Animals, 19, 328-35

9. Kohno, A, Yonezu, T, Matsushita, M, Irino, M, Higuchi, K, Takeshita, S, Hosokawa, M and Takeda, T (1985). Chronic food restricting modulates the advance of senescence in the senescence accelerated mouse. J Nutr, 115, 1259-66

10. Rehm, S, Hitsche, B and Deerberg, F (1985). Non-neoplastic lesions of female virgin Han:NMRI mice, incidence and influence of food restriction throughout life span I: Thyroid. Lab Animals, 19, 214-23

11. Rehm, S, Wcislo, A and Deerberg, F (1985). Non-neoplastic lesions of female virgin Han: MNRI mice, incidence and influence of food restriction throughout life span II: Respiratory tract. Lab Animals, 19, 224-35

12. Hamm, TE Jr, Working, PK and Raynor, TH (1983). The effect of restricted diet on respiration in F-344 rats. Lab Animals, 19, 505

13. James, J, Fronik, GM and Hesseling, JMG (1985). Experiences with standardized feeding of rats with an automatic food dispensing apparatus. Lab Animals, 19, 255-7

14. Buraczewski, S, Geoffrey Porter, JW, Rolls, BA and Zebrowska, T (1979). Sources of variability in rat feeding trials with single meal tests. J Sci Food Agric, 30, 47-52

15. Frape, DL, Wayman, BJ and Tuck, MG (1981). The effect of dietary fibre sources on aflatoxicosis in the weanling male rat. Br J Nutr, 46, 315-25

16. Fabry, P (1967). Metabolic consequences of the pattern of food intake. In: Handbook of Physiology, Vol.1. American Physiological Society

17. Chipalkatti, S, De Ajit, K and Aiyar, AS (1983). Effect of diet restriction on some biochemical parameters related to ageing in mice. J Nutr, 113, 944-50

9.6 ESSENTIAL FATTY ACIDS, PROSTAGLANDINS AND ANTI-INFLAMMATORY DRUGS

D. L. FRAPE

The activity of both non-steroidal and steroidal anti-inflammatory drugs is influenced by dietary composition, and the need for such drugs could be affected by that composition.

Both glucocorticoids and non-steroidal anti-inflammatory drugs function by blocking different steps in the intermediary production of endoperoxides from essential fatty acids (EFA). Prostaglandins (PG), thromboxanes, prostacyclins and leukotrienes are formed by a short sequence of reactions from dietary EFA. It would seem that their synthesis can be influenced by the modulation of dietary fat composition as well as by drugs, and Figure 9.1 outlines the reactions occurring in their formation by the intermediary metabolism of dietary fatty acids.

There are two naturally occurring groups of EFAs derived from (1) the n-6 series and (2) the n-3 series. The principal fatty acid source of the first of these is linoleic acid (18:2 n-6) and for the second alpha-linolenic acid (18:3 n-3). Another unsaturated dietary fatty acid (oleic acid 18:1 n-9) corresponds to the other two but it is readily synthesized in mammals from simple precursors. Nevertheless it seems that the n-3, n-6 and n-9 series are all metabolized by the same sequence of desaturases and elongases. The enzymes seem to have the highest affinity for the n-3 series and least for the n-9 series, indicating that the rate of metabolism of n-6 fatty acids is decreased by an increase in the concentration of members of the n-3 series. The metabolism of EFA is uniquely different in cats from other mammals studied, as this species apparently lacks the first enzyme in the sequence, Δ-6-desaturase (D-6-D) (see Figure 9.1).

Most vegetable oils are rich in linoleic acid and contain very little or no C20 acids. On the other hand, fats of animal origin contain important quantities of the C20 acids of the n-6 series. Fish oils are rich in acids of the n-3 series and some are found in certain vegetable oils, for example linseed and soya oil contain C18:3 n-3 (alpha-linolenic acid). The n-3 series is relatively less stable than the n-6, and some stabilization of vegetable oils is

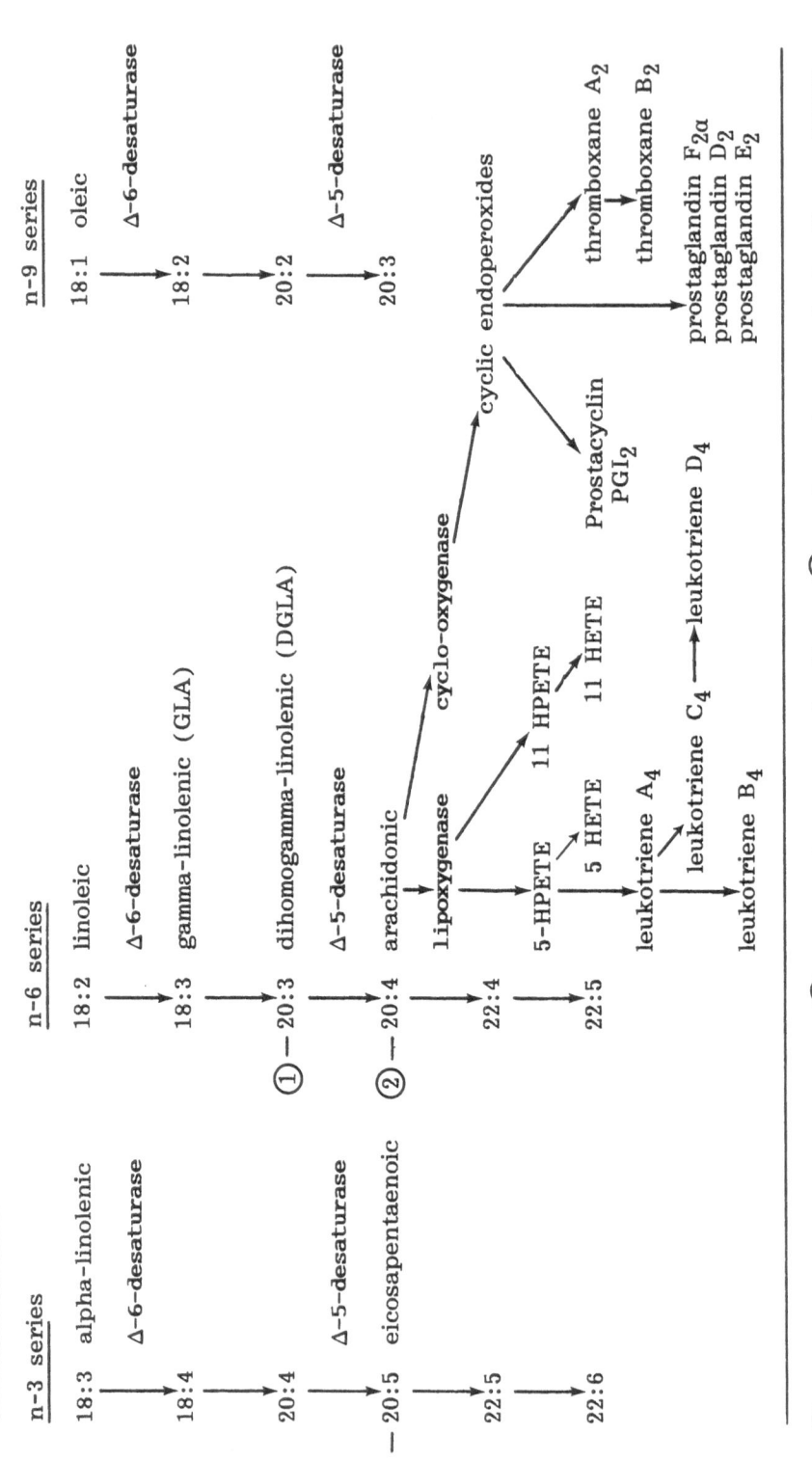

Figure 9.1 Desaturation and elongation pathways for essential fatty acids and oleic acid series, giving only the enzymes and the 2 series prostaglandins and thromboxanes for which considerable data have been accumulated

① = 1 series prostaglandins; ② = 2 series prostaglandins; ③ = 3 series prostaglandins; HPETE = hydroperoxy-eicosatetraenoic acid; HETE = hydroxy-eicosatetrenoic acid.

202

achieved by food processors through hydrogenation, leading to a loss of activity of the n-3 series in particular.

PROSTAGLANDINS

The metabolism of n-6 EFAs entails desaturation and elongation and the formation of C20:3 from C18:3 is efficient[1]. Elongation appears to be less affected than is desaturation by nutrient deficiencies and by diabetes. The dietary requirement for EFAs is increased in diabetes and in the presence of dietary trans fatty acid isomers[2]. Amongst the fat-soluble vitamins the absence of vitamin E leads to the production of toxic lipoxygenase products in greater quantities[3].

Raised cholesterol can rapidly lower the EFA content of plasma[4], and both dietary cholesterol and saturated fats were observed to reduce arachidonic acid in monkey retina, suggesting that they may suppress the conversion of linoleic acid to arachidonic acid[5].

D-6-D is responsible for the desaturation of linoleic acid. In the rat this occurs readily but the activity of the enzyme varies considerably between tissues[6]. Fasting and protein deficiency reduces its activity[7-9] whereas a protein-rich diet activates linoleic acid desaturation and a glucose-rich diet inhibits desaturation[7,9].

Insulin seems to be important in the activity of D-6-D and diabetic rats are depleted of arachidonic acid and 22-carbon acids with the development of skin abnormalities, testicular atrophy, renal necrosis and cataracts[10]. Glucagon, as might be anticipated, inhibits D-6-D[11]. Microvascular disease, a complication of diabetes, is closely associated with the suppression of the conversion of linoleic acid to arachidonic acid[12] and, in fact, linoleate supplementation of the diet of diabetics has been shown to decrease the incidence of cardiovascular events and retinopathy[13]. There is, however, evidence which contrasts with this, and perfused hearts from diabetic animals have been shown to release more PGI_2 than controls, and diabetic platelets are excessively susceptible to aggregation with thrombin[14]. It seems that where levels of all D-6-D metabolites are decreased, the conversion of arachidonic acid to the 2 series PGs (see Figure 9.1) is increased, possibly as a consequence of a fall in the concentration of cyclic AMP which inhibits the mobilization of arachidonic acid from phospholipid reserves[15].

Prostaglandins are synthesized from EFA by the cyclo-oxygenase pathway. There is a high degree of substrate specificity for this enzyme, which has a considerable affinity for C20 unsaturated fatty acids and a greater affinity for C20:4 than for C20:3 or C20:5[16]. The prostaglandins synthesized are respectively E2, E1 and E3. Cyclic endoperoxides produced as intermediate products are transformed into different end-products in different tissues. In platelets and neutrophils thromboxane is generated from endoperoxides[17], while in blood vessels the major cyclo-oxygenase product is prostacyclin[18]. Thromboxane A2 (TXA_2) is produced by platelets, has potent vasoconstrictor properties and is a potent platelet-aggregating agent[17]. A further unstable product derived from cyclic endoperoxides of the vascular endothelial cells, prostacyclin, prevents platelet aggregation and is a potent vasodilator. The homeostatic balance between the hormones is important, as prostacyclin probably protects blood vessel walls from the deposition of platelet thrombi induced by thromboxane.

A series of hydroxy acids is produced by alternative pathways of fatty acid peroxidation in the presence of lipoxygenase and absence of cyclo-oxygenase. The products of this pathway are known as leukotrienes because of their structure and leucocytic origin.

A major component of fish oil is a member of the n-3 series, C20:5 n3, eicosapentaenoic acid (EPA). Present in platelets, this acid is converted to a prostacyclin-like substance and has a similar anti-aggregating potency to prostacyclin itself[19]. Some epidemiological evidence exists to support the hypothesis that EPA-rich diets protect against thrombosis, and may explain why Eskimos have a lower incidence of acute myocardial infarction and an increased tendency to bleed[20]. Volunteer studies support this view[21]. This n-3 fatty acid may also compete effectively with the formation of series 2 prostaglandins from arachidonic acid (C20:4 n-6)[22,23]. This competition is thought to selectively enhance the synthesis of 1 series prostaglandins from dihomo-γ-linolenic acid (DGLA C20:3 n-6)[24]. Although linolenic acid is a precursor of arachidonic acid, it may similarly displace the latter from phospholipids, competitively inhibit access of arachidonic acid to cyclo-oxygenase and also stimulate 1 series prostaglandin formation from C20:3n-6[25].

Prostaglandins derived from arachidonic acid, principally 2 series (PGE_2), always accompany the inflammatory response. PGE_2 and prostacyclin have potent vasodilator properties and they are present in acute inflammation in sufficient amounts to account for the characteristic erythema. Vasodilatation of peripheral arterioles increases the blood supply to postcapillary venules, and enhances the effects of mediators which increase vascular permeability[26]. Non-steroidal anti-inflammatory drugs are selective inhibitors of cyclo-oxygenase[27-29]. This explains the anti-oedema, anti-pyretic and analgesic properties of aspirin-like drugs. Similarly the reduction of platelet aggregation by aspirin can be accounted for by inhibition of thromboxane production[21]. Polymorphonuclear leucocytes contribute to cyclo-oxygenase activity in inflammation but they are also a major source of leukotriene B_4, a potent chemotactic factor[30]. Non-steroidal anti-inflammatory drugs that inhibit cyclo-oxygenase do not prevent leukotriene production, which probably explains why they do little to modulate leucocyte-mediated aspects of inflammatory diseases.

Substantial amounts of arachidonic acid are present in the average human diet - 100-200 mg per day. As the total daily production of PGE is of the order of 1 mg per day, the amounts of arachidonic acid in food might meet the demand for series 2 prostaglandins. Very little EFA, as components of cell structural phospholipids, appears to be utilized in PGE synthesis[31], and so the relationship between dietary EFA and PG has major implications for the control of PG synthesis by dietary means with the possibility of regulating the balance between 1 and 2 series PGs without using drugs[2]. It must be emphasized that PG synthesis is not a function of the concentration in tissues of various members of the n-3 or n-6 series of fatty acids. The phospholipids of platelets contain enormously greater amounts of arachidonic acid than of DGLA, but their amounts in the free fatty acid fraction are almost equal (2:1). The esterified form of EFA in the platelets is not accessible to cyclo-oxygenase or lipoxygenase, and hydrolysis of the ester by phospholipase releases massive amounts of arachidonic acid with a surge in synthesis of the 2 series PGs. A rise in dietary linoleic acid content by 1% may inhibit PG formation in laboratory animals[32,33].

Unsaturated fatty acids in natural foods have their double bonds characteristically in the cis configuration. The proportion of unsaturated fats with this configuration is decreased in the human diet by the introduction of trans double bonds in dairy products, as a result of the activity of rumen bacteria of dairy cows, and in the processing of much vegetable oil to increase its stability and shelf-life. Trans acids interfere with D-6-D activity and have no EFA activity[34]. Furthermore ageing both in rats and man is seemingly correlated with a decrease in the tissue activity of D-6-D[2]. Thus the deterioration in cardiovascular function may in part be associated with a loss of metabolites of C18:3n-6, in particular by loss of PGE_1[35].

The enzyme D-5-D (Δ-5-desaturase) converts DGLA to arachidonic acid. In the rat both D-6-D and D-5-D are relatively slow and rate-limiting. D-5-D is highly active in the mouse, has intermediate activity in the rat, but only minimal activity in humans, guinea-pigs and rabbits[36]. Dietary composition has been shown to influence the activities of these desaturases. Signs of zinc deficiency are similar to those of EFA deficiency and would seem to be associated with inhibition of D-6-D function[37]. High sucrose intakes[38] and low protein intakes[39] may suppress D-5-D activity. Glucocorticoids inhibit D-5-D, indicating a possible mechanism for their anti-inflammatory effect[40].

REFERENCES

1. Garcia, PT and Holman, RT (1965). Competitive inhibitions in the metabolism of polyunsaturated fatty acids studied via the composition of the phospholipids, triglycerides and cholesteryl esters of rat tissues. J Am Oil Chem Soc, 42, 1137-41

2. Horrobin, DF (1983). The regulation of prostaglandin biosynthesis by the manipulation of essential fatty acid metabolism. Rev Pure Appl Pharmacol Sci, 4, 339-83

3. Panganamala, RV, Miller, JS, Gwebu, ET, Sharma, HM and Cornwell, DG (1977). Differential effects of vitamin E and other anti-oxidants on prostaglandin synthetase, platelet aggregation and lipoxidase. Prostaglandins, 14, 261-70

4. Portman, OW, Pinter, K and Hayashida, T (1959). Dietary fat and hypercholesterolemia in the cebus monkey. III Serum polyunsaturated fatty acids. Am J Clin Nutr, 7, 63-9

5. Hyman, BT, Haimann, MH, Armstrong, ML and Spector, AA (1981). Fatty acid and lipid composition of the monkey retina

in diet-involved hypercholesterolemia. Atherosclerosis, 40, 321-8

6. Brenner, RR (1971). The desaturation step in the animal biosynthesis of polyunsaturated fatty acids. Lipids, 6, 567-75

7. Brenner, RR (1982). Nutritional and hormonal factors influencing desaturation of essential fatty acids. Prog Lipid Res, 20, 41-8

8. De Thomas, ME, Mercuri, O and Rodrigo, A (1980). Effects of dietary protein and EFA deficiency on liver delta, 5, 6 and 9 desaturase activities in the early developing rat. J Nutr, 110, 595-9

9. De Gomez Dumm, INT, De Alaniz, MJT and Brenner, RR (1970). Effect of diet on linoleic acid desaturation and on some enzymes of carbohydrate metabolism. J Lipid Res, 11, 96-101

10. Brenner, RR (1974). The oxidative desaturation of unsaturated fatty acids in animals. Molec Cell Biochem, 3, 41-52

11. De Gomez Dumm, INT, De Alaniz, MJT and Brenner, RR (1975). Effects of glucagon and dibutyryl cAMP on oxidative desaturation of fatty acids in the rat. J Lipid Res, 16, 264-7

12. Jones, DB, Carter, RD, Haitas, B and Mann, JI (1983). Low phospholipid arachidonic acid values in diabetic platelets. Br Med J, 286, 173-5

13. Houtsmiller, AJ, van Hal-Ferwerda, J, Zahn, KJ and Henkes, HE (1982). Favorable influences of linoleic acid on the progression of diabetic micro and macro-angiopathy in adult onset diabetes mellitus. Prog Lipid Res, 20, 377-86

14. Largarde, M, Burtin, M and Berciaud, P (1980). Increase of platelet thromboxane A2 formation and of its plasmatic half life in diabetes mellitus. Thromb Res, 19, 823-30

15. Minkes, M, Stanford, N, Chi, MMY, Roth, GJ, Raz, A, Needleman, P and Majerus, PW (1977). Cyclic adenosine monophosphate inhibits the availability of arachidonate to prostaglandin synthetase in human platelets suspension. J Clin Invest, 59, 449-54

16. van Dorp, DA (1967). Prog Biochem Pharmacol, 3, 71-82

17. Hamberg, M, Svensson, J and Samuelsson, B (1975). Thromboxanes: a new group of biologically-active compounds derived from prostaglandin endoperoxides. Proc Natl Acad Sci USA, 72, 2994-8

18. Monacada, S, Gryglewski, RJ, Bunting, S and Vane, JR (1976). An enzyme isolated from arteries transforms prostaglandin endoperoxides to an instable substance that inhibits platelet aggregation. Nature, 263, 663-5

19. Gryglewski, RJ, Salmon, JA, Ubatuba, FB, Weatherley, BC, Moncada, S and Vane, JR (1979). Effects of all cis-5,8,11,14,17 eicosapentaenoic acid and pGH on platelet aggregation. Prostaglandins, 18, 453-78

20. Dyerberg, J and Bang, HO (1979). Haemostatic function and platelet polyunsaturated fatty acids in Eskimos. Lancet, 2, 433-5

21. Higgs, GA (1985). The effects of dietary intake of essential fatty acids on prostaglandin and leukotriene synthesis. Proc Nutr Soc, 44, 181-7

22. Hwang, DH and Carroll, AE (1980). Decreased formation of prostaglandins derived from arachidonic acid by dietary linolenate in rats. J Clin Nutr, 33, 590-7

23. Lands, WEM (1982). Biochemical observations on dietary long chain fatty acids from fish oil and their effect on prostaglandin synthesis in animals and humans. In Barlow, SM and Stansby, ME (eds) Nutritional Evaluation of Long Chain Fatty Acids in Fish Oil. (New York: Academic Press), pp. 267-82

24. Boukhchache, D and Lagarde, M (1982). Simultaneous utilization of prostaglandin precursors by human platelet prostaglandin synthetase and lipoxygenase. 5th International Conference on Prostaglandins, Florence. Abstract book, p. 692

25. Horrobin, DF (1980). The regulation of prostaglandin biosynthesis: negative feedback mechanisms and the selective control of formation of 1 and 2 series prostaglandins: relevance to inflammation and immunity. Med Hypotheses, 6, 687-709

26. Williams, TJ and Peck, MJ (1977). Role of prostaglandin-mediated vasodilatation in inflammation. Nature, 270, 530-2

27. Ferreira, SH, Moncada, S and Vane, JR (1971). Indomethacin and aspirin abolish prostaglandin release from the spleen. Nature, 231, 237-9

28. Smith, JB and Willis, AL (1971). Aspirin selectively inhibits prostaglandin production in human platelets. Nature, 231, 235-7

29. Vane, JR (1971). Inhibition of prostaglandin synthesis as a mechanism of action for aspirin-like drugs. Nature, 231, 232-235

30. Ford-Hutchinson, AW, Bray, MA, Doig, MV, Shipley, ME and Smith, MJH (1980). Leukotriene B, a potent kimokinetic and aggregating substance released from polymorphonuclear leukocytes. Nature, 286, 264-5

31. Hassam, AG, Willis, AL, Denton, JP, Stevens, P and Crawford, MA (1979). The effect of essential fatty acid deficient diet on the levels of prostaglandins and their fatty acid precursors in the rabbit brain. Lipids, 14, 78-83

32. Hwang, DH, Mathias, MM, Dupont, J and Meyer, DL (1975). Linoleate enrichment of diet and prostaglandin metabolism in rats. J Nutr, 105, 995-1002

33. Galli, C, Agradi, E, Petroni, A and Tremoli, E (1981). Differential effects of dietary fatty acids on the accumulation of arachidonic acid and its metabolic conversion through the cyclo-oxygenase and lipoxygenase in the platelets and vascular tissue. Lipids, 16, 165-72

34. Kinsella, JE, Hwang, DH, Yu, P, Mai, J and Shimp, J (1981). Metabolism of trans fatty acids with emphasis on the effects of trans, trans-octa-decadienoate on lipid composition, essential fatty acid and prostaglandins: an overview. Am J Clin Nutr, 34, 2307-18

35. Horrobin, DF (1981). Loss of delta-6-desaturase activity as a key factor in ageing. Med Hypotheses, 7, 1211-20

36. Blond, JP, Lemarchal, P and Spielman, D (1981). Desaturation of linoleic and dihomogammalinoleic acids by human liver in vitro. CR Acad Sci, 292, 911-4

37. Huang, YS, Cunnane, SC, Horrobin, DF and Davignon, L (1982). Most biological effects of zinc deficiency corrected by gamma-linolenic acid but not by linoleic acid. Atherosclerosis, 41, 193-207

38. Abrahamsson, H, Gustafson, A and Ohlson, R (1974). Polyunsaturated fatty acids in hyperlipoproteinemia. 1. Influence of a sucrose-rich diet on fatty acid composition of serum lipoprotein lipids. Nutr Metab, 17, 329-37

39. Mercuri, O, De Thomas, ME and Itarte, H (1979). Prenatal protein depletion and delta 9, delta 6 and delta 5 desaturases in the rat. Lipids, 14, 822-5

40. De Gomez Dumm, INT, De Alaniz, MJT and Brenner, RR (1979). Effect of glucocorticoids on the oxidative desaturation of fatty acids by rat liver microsomes. J Lipid Res, 20, 834-9

9.7 INFLUENCE OF DIET ON VARIOUS DISORDERS

D. L. FRAPE

CORONARY HEART DISEASE AND DIET

High-fat diets, particularly those rich in saturated fats, may increase the risk of coronary heart disease in man through their influence on serum cholesterol concentration, endothelial cell integrity, platelet aggregability, clotting tendency, fibrinolytic activity, and red blood cell agglutination[1]. Epidemiological evidence has revealed an association between a reduction of blood cholesterol in men previously having high blood levels, and a decreased incidence of coronary heart disease (CHD)[2].

Plant sterols seem to compete with cholesterol at sites of intestinal absorption, and Bhattachargya and Eggen[3], working with rhesus monkeys, observed that plant sterols decreased serum cholesterol concentration by 53% when they were included in a high-cholesterol diet. An effect of plant sterols may partly explain the observations of Jenkins et al.[4], who replaced starch with kidney beans (pinto), chick peas and green and red lentils in the diet of human subjects, bringing about a lowering of fasting cholesterol and triglycerides without influencing either LDL or HDL plasma levels. Moreover Liebman and Bazzarre[5] found that neither egg nor egg cholesterol influenced total plasma lipids in vegetarian males, but a comparison of vegetarian with non-vegetarian diets showed that the former produced lower total cholesterol, LDL and fasting triglycerides. Peas and beans, however, are also rich in certain non-starch water-soluble carbohydrates. These have been described as water-soluble plant fibres that seem to have distinct benefits in both human subjects and experimental animals. These substances exert their greatest influence on plasma cholesterol when added to cholesterol-containing diets. Pectin[6,7], guargum, oatbran[6], wheat bran[8], high molecular weight pectin[9], gum arabic and agar[7] lower plasma total cholesterol under these conditions and generally lower plasma and hepatic triglycerides and raise plasma HDL cholesterol in rats, in comparison with the effects of cellulose. HDL probably binds cholesterol released from peripheral tissues, including blood vessels, transporting it to the liver for metabolism, and it may counteract the passage of LDL into endothelial cells. Raised concentrations of plasma HDL protect against atherosclerosis and carry 70-80% of plasma cholesterol in rats, whereas in man only 20-30% is transported by this fraction[8]. Nevertheless it has been asserted[7] that elevated plasma HDL cholesterol is associated with a lower incidence of CHD in man.

Both dietary wheat bran and pectin reduce the concentration of cholesterol in the bile of rats receiving a high-fat, high-cholesterol diet, without affecting bile phospholipids[10]. The evidence supports the hypothesis that pectin and plant sterols lower plasma cholesterol by interfering with cholesterol absorption and reabsorption, increasing cholesterol turnover. Pectin may both interfere with micelle formation, essential in cholesterol absorption, and decrease hepatic fatty acid synthesis[11]. Thomas et al.[12] concluded that dietary pectin lowers plasma and hepatic cholesterol in rats and humans by altering the identity of bile acids synthesized in favour of chenodeoxycholic acid and its metabolites (dihydroxy bile acids). Dihydroxy bile acids decrease cholesterol absorption, they are less efficiently reabsorbed than trihydroxy bile acids, and also they are adsorbed by pectin, promoting their faecal excretion. Pectin thus increases the flux of steroid through the bile and out of the body. Bile salts are also adsorbed onto lignin and wheat bran[13], but the adsorption of sodium taurocholate by dietary lignin appears to be less than that achieved with cellulose[14], although cellulose does not adsorb bile lipids, and has little influence on bile cholesterol, or other aspects of cholesterol metabolism[10]. The modified acid detergent fibre fraction of wheat bran rich in lignin, and wheat bran itself, lowered plasma triglycerides in both fasted rats and rats receiving a cholesterol-free diet, but failed to reduce total plasma cholesterol concentration[15], and wheat bran seems to have little effect on plasma cholesterol concentration in man[16], although Story and Kritchevsky[17] had previously shown lignin to be more effective than other fibre sources tested in the in vitro binding of sodium salts of bile acids. Several fibre sources may reduce the lymphatic absorption of cholesterol and triglycerides in the rat[18], but the effects on bile acids and plasma lipids may depend upon the presence of saponins in the fractions[19,20]. These substances are absent from wheat bran. An influence of certain dietary fibre sources on plasma lipids has been clearly demonstrated in normal laboratory rodents, but under clinical conditions a definite effect of acceptable dietary fibre levels in humans may rely on the existence of hyperlipidaemia. Recent carefully controlled studies in healthy normolipidaemic male and female subjects failed to demonstrate any effect of adding 12 g pectin, 15 g cellulose, or 12 g lignin, to the daily diet[21].

The enterohepatic cycle in rats seems to be influenced not only by dietary fibre, but also by the type of dietary starch. Riottot and Sacquet[22] demonstrated that amylomaize starch increased the ileal absorption of sodium taurocholate in rats when it was substituted in the diet for normal maize starch. Digestible carbohydrates interact with dietary fibre in terms of their effect on the shape and amplitude of the glucose tolerance curve, which is recognized as influencing fat metabolism. Dietary soluble fibre influences the rate of glucose absorption from digested starch.

Sambrook and Rainbird[23] observed that peak post-prandial plasma glucose and insulin levels were lowered in pigs given a low-fat diet to which 4% guar gum had been added. Starches of different origins, and foods given in different physical forms, also led to differing glucose tolerance curves in animals and man[24].

Dietary saturated fat appears to be more lipogenic than polyunsaturated fat, for the reason that to a greater extent the latter suppresses hepatic fatty acid synthesis and lipogenic enzyme activity in rats, by reducing acetyl-CoA carboxylase and fatty acid synthetase[25]. Wolf and Grundy[26] found that by replacing 10% of saturated fats with 10% glucose in the diets of their patients they were able to reduce fasting triglycerides, total cholesterol and LDL and HDL cholesterol. On the contrary, Grande et al.[27] could not demonstrate that the oleic acid, or even the stearic acid component, of fats in the diet of middle-aged men had any influence on serum cholesterol concentration, supporting the earlier evidence of Hegsted's group[28,29] that the saturated fatty acid, myristic acid, was the only dietary fatty acid in fat capable of significantly elevating serum cholesterol in male volunteers. No specific effect on serum cholesterol could be detected with sources of stearic, lauric, or shorter chain saturated fatty acids, or with monounsaturated acids. Polyunsaturated fatty acids, on the other hand, had a cholesterol-lowering effect. Their work furthermore demonstrated that diet relatively rich in total fat could have a cholesterol-lowering effect in man if the total energy intake is not increased and the proportion of fat represented by polyunsaturated fatty acids is raised whilst those of myristic and palmitic acids and of cholesterol are lowered. These workers also suggested that not only was the chain length and degree of saturation of fatty acids important in determining blood lipid responses, but the position of the fatty acid on the glycerol molecule also influences its metabolism. Recently Reiser et al.[30] compared beef fat, coconut oil and safflower oil in the diet of healthy male volunteers, and revealed only small differences in their serum lipids. Plasma total cholesterol, HDL cholesterol and LDL cholesterol responses to beef fat were lower, and triglyceride responses higher, than to coconut oil. Beef fat produced similar responses to those of safflower oil except for marginally higher total cholesterol values. Thus from this evidence it seems that the effects of different dietary fats in healthy individuals are quite small, and that they may have minimal effects on health.

At least in susceptible individuals dietary fat type has a considerable influence not only on the incidence and extent of atherosclerosis but also on the incidence of arterial thrombosis - saturated fatty acids are pro-thrombic, whereas polyunsaturated fatty acids have an anti-thrombotic effect. Monounsaturated fatty acids behave neutrally in this respect. A close relationship exists between the effect of a fat on arterial thrombosis and its influence on platelet aggregability. Human studies[31] have shown that whereas diets rich in linoleic acid lower platelet aggregability, certain oils, including linseed oil and some of the marine oils, have a definite anti-thrombotic effect, probably mediated by their content of n-3 polyunsaturated fatty acids reducing the tissue content of free arachidonic acid. This reduction changes the thromboxane-prostacyclin balance towards the latter. Nevertheless, linoleic acid itself has an anti-thrombotic effect, it lowers plasma cholesterol, slightly decreases elevated blood pressure and stimulates cardiac contractility[32]. Beynen and Katan[33] concluded that the replacement of saturated, by polyunsaturated, fatty acids in the diet may lower serum VLDL lipoprotein concentrations because the liver preferentially converts polyunsaturated fatty acids to ketones instead of to VLDL triglycerides. Thus the polyunsaturated fatty acids are transported to tissues for oxidation without leaving lipoprotein remnants in the form of LDL.

The prostaglandins, thromboxanes, prostacyclins and leukotrienes are derived from both the n-6 and n-3 series of polyunsaturated fatty acids, and are collectively referred to as the eicosanoids. They are responsible in very low concentrations for a wide variety of effects in the body. Prostaglandins control smooth muscle contraction and relaxation, whilst thromboxanes and prostacyclins are involved in the aggregation and disaggregation of blood platelets. Leukotrienes, the production of which occurs in response to hypersensitivity reactions, play a general role in the control of vascular permeability. The n-6 fatty acid linoleic, and to a lesser extent the n-3 fatty acid alpha-linolenic acid, constitute more than 50% of the fatty acids esterified to cholesterol and 20% of those present in the phospholipids of lipoproteins. In the form of lipoproteins essential fatty acids (EFA) are delivered to all tissues, and in combination with EFA excess cholesterol is transported to the liver for oxidation. High-density lipoproteins (HDL) transport cholesterol mainly as cholesteryl linoleate, and supply EFA to tissue phospholipids. A relative deficiency of EFA causes an increase in plasma cholesterol and aggregation of platelets. Atherosclerosis is probably associated with a relative deficiency of EFA in the intima of blood vessels leading to an accumulation there of cholesteryl oleate and of LDL[34]. Oh and Monaco[35] demonstrated that by increasing the polyunsaturated to saturated fat ratio (P/S) in the diet of men, there was a reduction in plasma cholesterol, lipids and apoproteins of LDL regardless of the dietary level of cholesterol. The plasma levels of HDL depended on both the concentration of dietary cholesterol and on the dietary ratio of polyunsaturated to saturated fatty acids. An elevated P/S ratio increased faecal bile acid excretion. These workers concluded that dietary EFA lowered plasma cholesterol concentration without reducting HDL. A relative deficiency of dietary EFA brings about a reduction in HDL and a consequential decrease in the removal of cholesteryl fatty acid esters and their accumulation in fatty streaks. This deficient diet also increases the plasma concentration of LDL and of cholesterol, contributing to the accumulation of saturated fatty acids in atheroma.

The eicosanoids derived from n-6 polyunsaturated fatty acids would seem, on some evidence, to be greater stimulants to platelet aggregation and thrombosis than the eicosanoids derived from the n-3 fatty acids, which do not seem to stimulate platelet aggregation. Nevertheless Sanders and Hochland[36] found that platelet aggregation was similarly reduced by supplements of n-3 or n-6 polyunsaturated fatty acids, although the n-3 source (fish oil) lowered plasma triglycerides and increased the plasma concentration of HDL cholesterol. The effect on HDL depended entirely on the C20 and C22 n-3 fatty acids, whereas the C18 n-3 fatty acid had no effect.

A major function of the n-3 EFA seems to be the suppression of eicosanoid formation from arachidonic acid. Certain fish oils are rich in eicosapentaenoic acid and decosahexaenoic acid, respectively C20 and C22, n-3. Both these marine fatty acids competitively inhibit the metabolism of arachidonic acid by cyclo-oxygenase; and the prostaglandin endoperoxides and thromboxane A_3 derived from eicosapentaenoic acid have attenuated platelet aggregating ability as compared with the arachidonic acid-derived products. Eskimos have prolonged bleeding times, and this has been attributed to changes in the composition of platelet lipids that cause a diminished response to agonists such as collagen. These agonists normally stimulate the release of arachidonic acids from platelet-membrane phospholipids. This acid is then rapidly converted to thromboxane A_2, a highly potent inducer of platelet aggregation and secretion[36,37]. Diets rich in fish-oil fatty acids appear to decrease the content of arachidonic acid and increase the content of eicosapentaenoic acid in platelet membrane. Furthermore, platelet membrane eicosapentaenoic acid, released in response to agonists, inhibits the metabolism of arachidonic acid, and is converted to metabolic products that themselves inhibit platelet function. Platelets have a key role in thrombosis and are thought to promote the proliferation of arterial smooth muscle cells during atherogenesis[37]. Fenn and Littleton[38] described how a meal containing saturated fat affected the fatty acid composition of plasma of volunteers and led to increased saturation of platelet membrane fat and a greater tendency to aggregation under the influence of collagen. A diet containing fish oil polyunsaturated fatty acids seems also to alter the function of monocytes[39]. Monocytes adhere to the arterial endothelium and migrate into the intima at early stages of hypercholesteraemia-induced atherosclerosis. They are then transformed into macrophages which not only act as scavengers of plasma lipoprotein and lesion cholesterol, but also probably release growth factors that stimulate the proliferation of arterial smooth muscle cells. If leukotriene B_4 influences the adherence of monocytes to the arterial endothelium, as it does the adherence of neutrophils, then monocytes that contain increased amounts of eicosapentaenoic acid and reveal decreased production of leukotriene B_4 may not express this behaviour[37]. Lee et al.[39] concluded that diets enriched with fish oil-derived fatty acids may express anti-inflammatory effects by inhibiting the 5-lipoxygenase pathway in neutrophils and monocytes, reducing the leukotriene B_4 mediated functions of neutrophils.

It has been known for some time that rapeseed oil is a cause of myocardial lesions in rats, and the effect has been attributed to its erucic acid content. High erucic acid rapeseed oil was shown to induce a high frequency of degenerative focal myocardial lesions, whereas the oil of rape selected for low erucic acid content produces less severe lesions[40]. Nevertheless the incidence of these lesions is not eliminated, and Hulan et al.[41] suggested that rapeseed oil contains some other factors that also induce cardiac lesions in male rats. Aherne et al.[42] could find no difference between rapeseed oils of high and low erucic acid contents on cardiac lipidosis and myopathies in castrate and female pigs, and the addition of choline and inositol to the diet of rats seems to decrease the incidence of so-called degenerative myocardial lesions induced by rapeseed oil[40].

It has long been suggested that garlic contains some valuable properties in respect of plasma lipids and the petroleum-methanol-water extract of garlic[43], or garlic oil[44], has been shown to lower total plasma cholesterol, fasting trigylcerides and plasma and hepatic LDL. On the other hand, Arora et al.[45] could demonstrate only a transient increase in the fibrinolytic activity of blood by providing IHD patients with a garlic supplement to their diet.

At specified concentrations, dietary protein may also influence plasma lipid composition. Portman et al.[46] gave monkeys a diet in which the protein represented only 3.8% of the dietary energy, and this led to an increase in plasma VLDL plus HDL concentrations when compared with monkeys receiving a diet in which the protein content was 13.9% of the energy. The amino acid content of protein may also be significant. A comparison in rats between soya protein and casein revealed that the former decreased total plasma cholesterol and had marginal lowering effects on plasma LDL and HDL[47], although presumably an effect of contaminants cannot be ruled out. The addition of lysine to the soya had no effect in this experiment, but it has been suggested that the lysine to arginine ratio of protein in the diet is of significance[48].

A number of other normal dietary constituents has also been shown to influence plasma lipids. Chick pea isoflavones and p-coumaric acid appear to lower fasting total plasma cholesterol[49]. The supplementation of a vitamin E-depleted diet with vitamin E lowers plasma cholesterol in rats proportionately to the level of vitamin E added[50]. Nevertheless there is no evidence that high levels of dietary supplementation with vitamin E have any effect on plasma cholesterol, triglycerides, or HDL in normal healthy subjects. Copper deficiency, or high dietary zinc to copper ratios, has been found to raise total plasma cholesterol in rats[51].

Whereas a number of similarities exist between species in pathogenic lipid metabolism, many differences exist not only between, but even within, species. For example, dietary orotic acid increases total plasma cholesterol in mice, but is without effect on hamsters and is hypocholesterolaemic in rats[52]. Within species, enzyme patterns may vary. The neonatal exposure of rats to high cholesterol diets lowers their response to dietary cholesterol as adults through the imprint of cholesterol-metabolizing enzyme patterns[53].

HYPERTENSION

The relationship of the consumption of fluid and its excretion by the kidneys with chronic arterial pressure is expressed by an S-shaped curve. An increase in fluid intake brings about an increase in arterial pressure, a decrease in renin and aldosterone secretion and an increased renal output of water and salt. On the other hand increase in renin-angiotensin production and secretion increases total peripheral resistance, cardiac output and arterial pressure, and increases aldosterone secretion with a consequential retention of salt and water. There is an increase in extracellular fluid volume and the renal function curve is shifted to the right, or to a higher pressure range. The shape and position of this curve is changed in hypertension.

Renin is secreted by the juxtaglomerular apparatus in hypotension increasing constriction of the efferent arterioles, thus increasing glomerular filtration pressure allowing wastes to be disposed of effectively but stimulating the reabsorption of water, and sodium and potassium ions. This mechanism undoubtedly has a survival value. If there is a fall in the chloride, or sodium, ion content of the macula densa, afferent arterioles are dilated again, increasing glomerular pressure and filtration.

The blood pressure in any particular subject, or animal, at which the input-output relationship of body fluid stabilizes, may result from some innate discordance in the physiological mechanisms described, from reduced kidney mass, or from pathological ageing of the nephrons. The composition of diet nevertheless can influence arterial pressure in each of these situations.

Renin acts in the blood on a protein synthesized by the liver releasing angiotensin I. On passing through the pulmonary circulation angiotensin II is released from this molecule. Angiotensin II constricts arteriolar smooth muscle, raising arterial pressure and stimulating the release of catecholamines and aldosterone. The latter stimulates the distal tubule of the kidney to retain sodium and water, also increasing extracellular fluid volume and arterial pressure. Potassium excretion is increased, and in the extreme this can lead to hypokalaemia. Angiotensin II also acts in the brain to increase the outflow of sympathetic impulses, further elevating arterial pressure and promoting thirst, ensuring greater fluid intake and volume retention.

Norepinephrine is released from post-ganglionic sympathetic nerve endings and stimulates cardiovascular adrenergic receptors. Dietary sodium excess may increase the number of myocardial beta receptors[54] which increase the rate and vigour of contraction of the heart muscles when they are stimulated. The release of norepinephrine under the influence of angiotensin II is apparently depressed by low-sodium diets[55].

The view is generally held that dietary salt precipitates hypertension in all individuals, but those genetically resistant to hypertension may ingest as much as 200 mEq of salt per day without developing elevated blood pressure. Those genetically susceptible to hypertension may avoid it by restricting salt intake to less than 60 mEq per day in adults. This view has recently been challenged[56] by the results of a study on adults who were the offspring of parents in the top and bottom thirds of the blood pressure distribution. A restriction of the sodium intake, when urinary sodium excretion was below 50 mmol per day, had no effect on blood pressure in comparison with a control period, during which sodium excretion exceeded 120 mmol per day. However, the general view is that there seems only to be a difference in the salt threshold between resistant and sensitive individuals reflecting a difference in the position, or shape, of the renal function curve.

A comparable situation exists in rats sensitive to hypertension, in which kidneys secrete only half as much sodium as do those which are resistant at equal inflow pressures in vitro[57]. Thus in a sensitive strain a higher inflow pressure is needed to achieve a given sodium excretion, reflecting a change of the pressure natriuresis curve. This evidence would point to a rise in arterial pressure in sensitive rats given a high-sodium diet, and sodium balance would be achieved at a raised arterial pressure. A drug such as chlorothiazide may shift the natriuresis curve of the sensitive kidney to the left, increasing sodium excretion for a given pressure. Tobian et al.[58] demonstrated that a diuretic agent permits isolated kidneys of sensitive rats to excrete 60% more sodium per minute when perfused at normotensive inflow pressures.

The introduction of hypotension in normotensive animals and a reduction in blood pressure in hypertensive animals and humans receiving a potassium depleted diet, may result from a decrease in aldosterone concentration, a decrease in vasopressin, or decreased responsiveness to the pressor effects of angiotensin II. A high potassium intake has no effect on blood pressure of normotensive animals and humans, but it lowers blood pressure in those with hypertension. Several alternative mechanisms for this effect have been proposed[59]. Natriuresis leads to sodium depletion, and a decrease in plasma renin activity, or an alteration in the neurogenic components of blood pressure regulation and possibly a decrease in the number of angiotensin II receptors. A high potassium intake increases plasma aldosterone activity by a direct effect on the adrenal cortex. Although high potassium consumption induces natriuresis the associated increase in aldosterone serves to minimize the degree of sodium depletion, and so acts to protect the individual from an excessive decline in blood pressure[60]. The chronic intake of a diet rich in potassium frequently depresses the plasma activity of renin, although the effect is variable[59]. This variability may be the result of two opposing effects: (1) natriuresis and volume contraction that stimulates renin release, and (2) a direct inhibitory effect of potassium on renin release[61].

Whereas the inhibition of renin release by sodium chloride has been attributed to sodium, the contribution of chloride to this response has not been widely considered. Kotchen et al.[62] demonstrated that the chronic administration of sodium salts, other than sodium chloride, failed to suppress plasma renin activity in Sprague-Dawley rats. Alternatively, plasma renin activity was stimulated by selective chloride depletion. In humans, plasma renin activity was suppressed by sodium chloride, but not by sodium bicarbonate infusion. Similarly in the Dahl salt-sensitive rat, sodium bicarbonate loading failed to induce hypertension.

A characteristic manifestation of hypertension is an increase in peripheral vascular resistance. There is an increased resting tension and increased contractility of vascular smooth muscle in response to agonists such as norepinephrine and angiotensin II. A rise in intracellular free calcium ion concentration is the immediate trigger for contraction of muscle. The metabolism of sodium and calcium is linked by a counter-transport system in which the movements of the two ions across cell membranes are coupled. Similarly an increased filtered load of calcium facilitates renal sodium excretion[63], and increased sodium excretion by the kidney will cause a rise in urinary calcium excretion[64]. The restriction of dietary calcium increases, and supplementation with calcium lowers, the blood pressure of both normal and hypertensive rats[65]. Magnesium is also vital to many vascular-tissue-related processes that are functionally important for normal blood pressure regulation[66]. Calcium and magnesium ions are synergistic in many of their cardiovascular actions potentiating each other's roles, and reduced consumption of either is associated with increased risk of developing hypertension[65]. Johnson et al.[67] were unable to demonstrate a relationship between blood pressure and total calcium intake in normotensive women, but a decrease in systolic pressure was demonstrated in hypertensive women supplemented with dietary calcium. The exposure of vascular tissue preparations to increased calcium concentrations has been shown to relax vascular smooth muscle cells[68] and cellular depletion of magnesium increases vascular smooth muscle tone[66]. Although it is unlikely that a high-calcium diet would counteract the adverse effect of a high-sodium diet because of the constraints on calcium absorption, vitamin D supplementation in women receiving marginal amounts of the vitamin decreases systolic blood pressure, probably through stimulation of calcium absorption from the gut, or interaction with parathyroid hormone maintaining plasma calcium homeostasis[69].

A natriuretic hormone secreted by the hypothalamus, or whose secretion is controlled by the hypothalamus, appears to be involved in hypertension. This agent promotes sodium excretion by inhibiting transport from the renal tubular epithelial cell cytoplasm into the interstitial fluid in exchange for potassium. As a consequence more sodium will then remain in the tubular lumen and be excreted.

Studies both in animals and humans suggest that blood pressure can be lowered during high salt feeding by dietary supplementation with polyunsaturated fatty acids that are precursors of prostaglandins involved in blood pressure regulation[70]. Hoffman et al.[71] demonstrated that male Wistar rats given a diet containing 7% sunflower seed oil for 4 weeks, in conjunction with a sodium chloride solution to drink, developed lower systolic blood pressures than comparable rats receiving a diet containing 7% hydrogenated palm kernel oil. Fat-enriched diets have been shown to increase blood pressure in rabbits[72]; but an oil rich in linoleic acid causes a lower increase in blood pressure than does one containing much less[73]. The greatest change in serum lipid values resulted in the greatest change in blood pressure in rabbits. The hypertensive effect of fat is partly counteracted by the addition of cellulose to the diet of rabbits[72], or by the inclusion of fibre in the diet of human volunteers[74]. The mechanism by which polyunsaturated fats, rich in linoleic acid, may mediate a protective or neutral effect in hypertension may be to stimulate the synthesis of the series I prostaglandins derived from dihomo-gamma-linolenic acid (C20:3 n-6), as recent evidence[75] indicates that dietary cod liver oil incorporated eicosapentaenoic acid into tissue stores of the rat with a corresponding decrease in the release of arachidonic acid from phospholipids, impaired ability to generate tissue thromboxane B_2 and prostaglandins $F_{1\alpha}$ and E_2 and prevention of glucocorticoid (dexamethasone)-induced hypertension. (For further details see section on prostaglandin metabolism.)

Dietary sucrose decreases sodium excretion in the urine of both rats[76] and humans[77], in whom sucrose and fructose cause different degrees of fasting salt retention. The response to sugar may be a consequence of increased circulating levels of catecholamines, or of increased sympathetic nervous system activity that is capable of enhancing sodium reabsorption by the kidney. An explanation of lower average blood pressures in diabetic men given a high-fibre diet[78] may be related to the effect of fibre on the shape of the glucose absorption curve and on insulin response. It has been suggested that insulin increases the renal reabsorption of sodium[79].

Diets rich in protein are accompanied by sustained increases in glomerular capillary pressures and flows. Intrarenal hypertension, associated with protein, may eventually cause glomerular sclerosis and account for decreased renal function seen with ageing. Further elevation of glomerular capillary pressures and flows contributes to progressive glomerular destruction and loss of renal function[80]. This gradual loss of functional renal mass eventually may lead to an increase in systemic blood pressure, especially when dietary sodium is elevated for the reasons previously given.

Animal studies in which the relationship between drugs and blood pressure are being considered must take into account the dietary concentration of a number of nutrients. It has been demonstrated that sodium, potassium and chloride can have a major impact on blood pressure. Dietary calcium, magnesium and vitamin D seem also to influence blood pressure, and smaller effects have been demonstrated by variation in the level and composition of dietary fats and dietary fibre. In the longer term, dietary protein level may indirectly influence systemic blood pressure. Depending on the objectives of dietary manipulation, the need for drugs, or the sensitivity of response of both humans and laboratory animals to drugs, can be increased or lowered.

DIABETES

Functions of insulin

Insulin serves a number of functions that modulate the metabolism of cells. One of its actions in the liver is to decrease the concentration of cyclic AMP. In a deficiency of insulin cAMP is formed promoting the activity of fat cell lipases and therefore stimulating lipolysis. Insulin functions by increasing glucose uptake of adipose tissue cells, increasing fatty acid synthesis, glucose conversion into α-glycerophosphate and the lipoprotein-lipase activity of fat cells, so that more fatty acid uptake may occur from various circulating lipoproteins, particularly from chylomicrons and very low-density lipoproteins. Thus insulin stimulates the storage of both dietary fat and carbohydrates as fat in adipose tissue, inhibiting its breakdown.

The greater part of the pathology of diabetes mellitus (type

I) can be attributed to decreased uptake of glucose by tissue cells with the resultant increase in blood glucose concentration. An increased mobilization of storage fat occurs accompanied by abnormal rates of fat and protein catabolism[81]. However, as the metabolic derangements that characterize insulin deficiency can be overcome, the major threat of both types I and II diabetes is atherosclerosis, in the development of which diet plays a crucial role both in inducing and in controlling hypertriglyceridaemia and hypercholesterolaemia[82].

It has been recommended that, in the absence of functional insulin, diets should contain minimal amounts of digestible carbohydrate, whereas such diets aggravate abnormal fat metabolism, promoting fat mobilization, and hepatic fat deposition, and stimulating the metabolic pathways accelerating phospholipid and cholesterol synthesis. Conversely, more normal levels of dietary carbohydrate depress fat metabolism and tend to lower blood cholesterol.

There is a general consensus of opinion that both type I and type II diabetics should restrict their intake of dietary fat, although it has been established that arachidonic acid incorporation into pancreatic islet phospholipid is an important step in the initiation of insulin secretion[83]. The concentration of this acid is reduced in various tissues of diabetics and the provision of increased amounts of linoleic acid for adult onset diabetics decreases retinal angiopathy[84]. In rat models of insulin-dependent diabetes the desaturation of linoleic acid is depressed in various tissues. Insulin would seem to be required for the desaturation of polyunsaturated fatty acids, in particular that of linoleic acid. Nevertheless, Cunnane et al.[85] found that plasma glucose concentrations were higher in type II genetic diabetic mice supplemented with PUFA, compared with unsupplemented mice, but the arachidonic acid content of pancreatic phospholipids was proportionally decreased in the diabetic mice, a characteristic rectified by supplementation with essential fatty acids.

Adult-onset diabetes (type II) is characterized by high circulating insulin levels, functionally inadequate for normalization of blood sugar but apparently sufficient for fat deposition. Hypertriglyceridaemia occurs in patients with this form of diabetes causing severe atherosclerosis, as insulin stimulates incorporation of fat precursors into the arterial wall. Nevertheless a suppression of insulin function occurs, described as insulin resistance and decreased insulin responsiveness. These consequences are probably a result of obesity, and in fact nutritional alterations that depress insulin action in both rats and humans are high-fat diets, obesity and starvation[86]. Excessive dietary fat, especially hydrogenated fat, decreases the binding of insulin to plasma membranes and results in hyperinsulinaemia. Insulin binding is increased in diabetic rat liver membranes but depressed when high-fat diets are given to rats[86] and nutritionally induced changes in insulin binding, and in glucose transport capacity could contribute to insulin resistance in man. Starvation causes increased insulin binding but decreased glucose tolerance and decreased activity of glycogen synthetase. High-carbohydrate diets increase insulin sensitivity, but increase circulating insulin, even when total food intake is reduced[87], and the consumption of a glucose solution by mice with their diet increases the frequency of polyploid beta-cells independently of genotype, probably accelerating premature ageing[88]. Certain amino acids, in particular lysine and arginine, are also potent stimulators of insulin secretion when administered in the presence of elevated blood glucose.

The rise in fasting triglycerides that occurs within a few days of instituting a very high-carbohydrate diet is observed in hyperlipidaemic patients, in diabetics and in normal persons. This lipaemia is thought to be linked to the high insulin levels stimulated by the high-carbohydrate diet[89]. As insulin resistance is promoted by excessive fat, weight reduction leads to a decrease in circulating insulin in normal obese patients and a normalization of circulating insulin in obese diabetics[90]. Cunnane et al.[85] concluded that genetically obese and type II genetically diabetic mice are phenotypically similar, in that there are increases in plasma glucose and circulating insulin, and liver phospholipids are deficient in several polyunsaturated fatty acids, namely C18:3 n-6, C22:5 n-6 and C18:3 n-3. Other similarities were observed in tissue PUFA. Nevertheless, differences were detected after essential fatty acid supplementation. There was proportionately a slight decline in the C20:4 n-6 acid in the phospholipids of obese mice, whereas this fatty acid was significantly increased in the phospholipids of diabetic mice and differences occurred in the fatty acid composition of triglycerides. Furthermore, essential fatty acid supplementation of the diet failed to overcome two major pathological features of the diabetic mice, namely obesity and elevated blood glucose. The possible relation between essential fatty acids and genetic diabetes in mice therefore remains unclear.

The principal role for diet in the control of diabetes is to minimize post-prandial elevation in blood glucose and in circulating insulin. It has become clear that glycaemic propensity of individual dietary components is blurred by several associative effects in mixed diets, which include interactions of the energy yielding sources and associative effects of dietary processing and physical characteristics. Such effects have been observed for sucrose in mixed diets[91], sucrose in the presence or absence of dietary fat, and the degree of unsaturation of that fat[92]. The characteristic of fructose that it is only partly converted to glucose, resulting in a flattened glycaemic response, and that it does not require insulin for cellular uptake, is also relevant. Glucose causes four times the insulin stimulation of fructose[93].

Although carbohydrates stimulate insulin secretion, they also increase insulin sensitivity of plasma membranes and increase glucose tolerance. Thus diabetic prevalence declines as the dietary percentage of energy derived from carbohydrates is increased[94]. The introduction of carbohydrate-rich diets therefore does not increase insulin requirements of diabetics if the change is introduced gradually, but of considerable import is the total daily energy intake and the extent of the post-prandial glycaemic response.

Blood glucose response to various complex and simple carbohydrate foods varies so greatly that the two groups cannot in general be distinguished on the basis of post-ingestion glycaemic excursion. For example, the blood glucose rise after the consumption of pasta (spaghetti) is less than that which occurs after the consumption of a similar amount of starch in the form of bread[82]. Furthermore, potato starch elicits a similar blood glucose response to an equivalent amount of glucose, whereas rice generally causes a flattened glycaemic response. Grinding, cooking and the rate of meal consumption also influence blood glucose concentration[24].

Several workers have observed that high-fibre diets reduce insulin response and blood lipids in healthy young adults. Albrink et al.[95] demonstrated that dietary fibre could halve the insulin response and lower blood cholesterol and triglycerides in healthy young adults given a high-carbohydrate diet. Lousley et al.[96] demonstrated that a diet rich in complex carbohydrates and fibre, and low in fat, greatly benefited poorly controlled type II diabetic patients when compared with the effects of a low-carbohydrate, high-fat diet of approximately the same energy content and the same polyunsaturated to saturated fat ratio.

Dietary fibre may be divided for convenience into water-soluble and water-insoluble groups. Insoluble fibre such as cellulose, lignin and most hemicelluloses appears to have a major impact on gastrointestinal transit times and faecal bulk, but less influence on plasma glucose and insulin levels, or cholesterol metabolism. In contrast, the water-soluble fibres - pectins, gums and a few hemicelluloses and the starches - have little effect on faecal bulk, but may influence glucose and insulin responses. The soluble fibres are the predominant type in seeds of the legume family eliciting exceptionally low glycaemic responses, and the rate of intestinal hydrolysis of starch is an important determinant of the metabolic response.

Williams and MacDonald[97] concluded that the viscosity of a carbohydrate meal, a property of the polymer length of the starch, can alter the serum insulin but not serum glucose response in healthy adults; but one would nevertheless expect it to reduce the fat storage effect of insulin in diabetics that have not completely lost the ability to synthesize insulin. The viscosity of a meal is also increased by the addition of guar, or other, gum leading to a slower rate of glucose absorption. It is possible that this is due to a guar-containing meal maintaining its viscosity in the duodenum and jejunum, whereas the viscosity of starch would be expected to fall owing to the hydrolytic action of amylase. Rainbird et al.[98] demonstrated that guar gum significantly reduced the net absorption of both glucose and water from perfusates with glucose and maltose in the jejunum of pigs. Furthermore the peak post-prandial plasma glucose and plasma insulin concentrations were reduced in pigs given a semi-purified diet containing guar and moderate amounts of fat, but not when given a diet containing 16% fat[23]. Gums and viscous-type fibre seem to be more effective than other fibres in slowing carbohydrate absorption, reducing post-prandial rise in serum glucose and insulin, and in delaying the post-prandial fall in serum glucose - thus extending the satiety effect of food in humans[99,100]. Xanthan gum given to patients managing without insulin has also been shown to reduce both fasting and post-load blood glucose and total cholesterol[101], and Jenkins[100] concluded that gums and viscous fibres had a general capacity to lower the glycaemic index of diet.

Diets that are moderately rich in fat will alleviate some diabetic disturbances in rats, including elevated plasma glucose, glycosuria and hyperphagia[102]. Such diets can, however, lead to the development of other diabetic sequelae, including hypertriglyceridaemia[103] and severe ketosis[104]. Schmidt et al.[104] demonstrated that diets containing little carbohydrate but that are rich in fat and protein (6% carbohydrate, 30% fat and 63% protein) may be beneficial in reducing hyperglycaemia, polyuria, polydipsia, glucosuria and hypertriglyceridaemia, and may limit the development of diabetic cataract. On the other hand, Lousley et al.[96] reported that a high-carbohydrate, high-fibre, low-fat diet was more successful in lowering pre-prandial blood glucose, VLDL cholesterol and mean 24-hour triglyceride in type II diabetic patients, with persistently elevated blood glucose, than was a diet of similar energy content and polyunsaturated to saturated fatty acid ratio of fat (0.8), but containing low concentrations of carbohydrate and fibre and high levels of fat. The explanation of the beneficial effect of excessive dietary protein in the work of Schmidt et al.[104] requires further elucidation, as recent evidence has demonstrated that diabetic rats, given the choice, consume more protein and less carbohydrate than non-diabetic rats, with the consequence that there is an absence of hyperphagia, fat stores are not depleted, and polyuria, polydipsia and glycosuria are reduced in comparison with diabetic rats given a normal diet[105].

It is apparent that the distinction between complex and simple carbohydrates is blurred in so far as their glycaemic effect is concerned, and it is no longer necessary to restrict disproportionately the carbohydrate content of diets for diabetics. Birdsall[94] recommends diets rich in carbohydrates, including simple sugars for patients with both types I and II diabetes.

It is clear that further work is required in laboratory animals concerning the metabolic pathways interrupted in diabetes, and the specific effects on it of dietary protein and amino acids and on the role of fat and its component essential fatty acids in insulin function and fatty degeneration.

NEPHROCALCINOSIS

Nephrocalcinosis is a debilitating condition of renal insufficiency, owing to the bilateral and diffuse precipitation of calcium phosphate together with small amounts of other salts in the lumen of the kidney tubules, their walls and surrounding tissues. The condition is distinguishable from dystrophic focal calcification of local origin, which may be irregular and unilateral.

Nephrocalcinosis develops in man and many animal species under conditions in which the weight of dietary phosphorus (P) exceeds that of dietary calcium (Ca). Clapp et al.[106] reduced the incidence (predominantly in female as opposed to male rats) by increasing the calcium to phosphorus ratio of the diet from 0.8 to 1.2. Mice are much less prone to the condition.

The parathyroid gland

The secretion of parathyroid hormone (PTH) responds to variation in dietary Ca and P contents, and it is accepted that its renal effects are mediated via an adenylate cyclase-cyclic AMP (cAMP) system. Raised urinary concentrations of cAMP derived from the kidney are detected both in man and animals following a PTH response. PTH functions by decreasing the tubular reabsorption of inorganic phosphate and increasing that of ionized Ca. It also stimulates the conversion of 25-hydroxycholecalciferol to 1,25-dihydroxycholecalciferol. This hormone, produced in extremely small quantities, not only stimulates the small intestinal absorption of Ca, Mg and possibly of P, but it also stimulates the mobilization of bone Ca salts. This series of events, initiated by PTH, is triggered by a slight fall in the concentration of plasma Ca ions. An above-normal rise in blood Ca suppresses PTH release and stimulates the release of calcitonin from the thyroid gland. The precipitation of calcium salts in renal tissue is probably caused by elevated levels of circulating PTH and not directly by a rise in plasma phosphate[107,108] as nephrocalcinosis does not occur when the concentration of plasma phosphate is elevated and the activity of PTH is severely depressed[109]. Moreover plasma concentrations of Ca and phosphate are too low to exceed the solubility product of Ca and phosphate with a K of 4.3 mmol/l in neutral solutions. On the assumption that ionized Ca represents 50% of total plasma Ca, and on the evidence that the K value in rats given normal diets is 3.1, in rats given high-phosphate diets 3.01, in parathyroidectomized (PTX) rats fed normal diets 3.76, and in PTX rats given a high phosphate diet 2.98[110], then precipitation cannot simply arise from excessive concentrations. On the other hand the greater the deviation of the diet from normal the more intense is the pathological effect, although the initiating dietary progenitors can be decreasingly extreme as the amount of healthy renal mass is reduced by ageing or for other reasons[111].

Dietary magnesium

Parathyroid activity is influenced not only by the concentration of plasma Ca but also by that of plasma Mg[112], and earlier evidence[113,114] suggested that PTH induces a similar retention of both Ca and Mg. The severity of a Mg deficiency is accentuated[115] by a high level of dietary Ca, thus the dietary requirement for Mg is partly a function of the level of dietary Ca. Increments in dietary Mg bring about a proportional increase in the urinary excretion of Ca, so the urinary Ca to Mg ratio remains more or less constant over a wide range of Mg intakes, despite a constancy[116] of dietary Ca.

Prostaglandins

Prostaglandins may play a role in intranephronic calcification, as they behave as Ca ionophores and facilitate the movement of Ca into and out of cell membranes[117]. Moreover prostaglandin synthetase inhibitors inhibit cortical nephrocalcinosis in rats[118] and the intra-arterial infusion of prostaglandin E_2 causes a marked calciuresis[119]. Prostaglandins are synthesized in both the renal cortex and medulla by a Ca ion-dependent process in which arachidonic acid is released from tissue phospholipid stores by activation of phospholipase. Cellular injury associated with renal stones, together with a secondary inflammation, could be the challenging event stimulating the synthesis and release of prostaglandins giving rise to associated intracellular and interstitial Ca precipitation.

Oxalosis

Crystals of Ca oxalate are freqently involved in urolithiasis and have been observed in nephrocalcinosis. Magnesium ions have been shown to increase the solubility of Ca oxalate and phosphate, and the addition of Mg to calcifying urine rendered it non-calcifying[120]. Progressive renal insufficiency, renal nephrocalcinosis and stone formation occur, as a consequence of primary oxalosis in man, caused by an inherited enzyme defect in organic acid metabolism, leading to oxalate accumulation[121,122]. A comparable situation exists in pyridoxine deficiency which has been reproduced in rats[123]. Hyperoxaluria occurs in patients with ileal bypass and in those with digestive and absorptive disorders, including chronic pancreatitis and coeliac disease[124]. In these conditions there is decreased fat digestion leading to the formation of Ca soaps, "mopping up" most of the available soluble Ca in the intestinal lumen. Soluble Ca has, for example, a greater affinity for oleate ions than for oxalate ions, freeing the oxalate for absorption, and indicating that patients with ileal resection should be given a low-fat high-Ca diet[124].

Metabolic alkalosis and acidosis

Infants and rats given chloride-deficient batches of milk develop hypochloraemia and consequent metabolic acidosis, associated with raised serum concentrations of Ca and inorganic phosphate and the development of nephrocalcinosis[125]. The elevated serum Ca and associated hypercalciuria may be a cause of a decrease in the serum concentration of Mg and related hypermagnesiuria[126].

Alkaline urine and nephrocalcinosis are common features of distal renal tubular acidosis (dRTA), an autosomal dominant condition occurring in both complete and incomplete forms. Patients suffering from this ailment are unable to lower urine pH below 5.5, owing to an inability to secrete H^+ ions and reabsorb Na^+, HCO_3^- and Ca^{2+} in the distal renal tubules. It would seem that the metabolic acidosis induces proximal tubular reabsorption of citrate, considerably reducing its urinary concentration, and therefore depleting urine of an entity which normally binds Ca in a soluble complex[127]. Despite the formation of alkaline urine the appropriate therapy is to correct acidaemia by alkali therapy, inhibiting the reabsorption of citrate, and so promoting urinary Ca solubility[128]. The failure of H^+ ion secretion in dRTA inhibits normal reabsorption of Ca stimulated by PTH, which in turn exerts a calciuric effect and accounts for hyperparathyroidism in the patients.

Primary dRTA normally initiates hypercalcaemia and hypercalciuria as a consequence of the mobilization of bone buffer in an endeavour to counteract metabolic acidosis[129]. Bone is a significant extrarenal buffer in man, and can provide the equivalent of 35,000 mmol/l buffer - more than any other tissue. Each molecule of tricalcium phosphate neutralizes two atoms of hydrogen and each molecule of calcium carbonate neutralizes one atom of hydrogen with a production of monohydrogen phosphate and bicarbonate. Hypercalcaemia, hypercalciuria and nephrocalcinosis can also arise from an excessive consumption of calcium[130] in, for example, Ca-containing antacids and from excessive vitamin D intake. The renal tubular damage caused by these events can precipitate a defect in H^+ ion secretion, renal tubular acidosis and its consequences. Thus calcification of cells may simply be a function of damage and not of Ca intake, rather than the reverse.

Dietary protein

There is a rapid rise in urinary Ca within 2-4 hours of a high-protein meal. A substantial cohort of the population may be subject to such a cause of Ca loss, as Linksweiler and co-workers[131] demonstrated that subjects ingesting 142 g protein daily were in negative Ca balance. As a smaller fraction of endogenous Ca is excreted in the urine of rodents, the effect of dietary protein is less in rats[132,133], and in mice[134]. The increment in urinary Ca is largely accounted for by a decrease in fractional tubular reabsorption of Ca, offset by a decrease in endogenous faecal Ca and the maintenance of Ca balance in rodents. There is substantial evidence that the decrease in renal reabsorption is caused by an increase in endogenous acid production generated from the catabolism of excess dietary protein. Dietary acidity induces urinary cAMP excretion - a measure of PTH activity, and elevates urinary Ca and Mg[135]. The net renal acid excretion can be accounted for mainly by the oxidation of the sulphur amino acids, methionine and cysteine-producing sulphate and H^+ ions that are excreted in the urine[132,136]. The tendency of a particular diet to cause calciuria can be estimated from the difference in the sums of the total dietary fixed cations and anions[137,138]. The addition of sodium bicarbonate, or sodium citrate, to diets containing excessive acid, or protein, partially inhibits metabolic acidosis and a calciuretic effect. The acidotic effect caused by many proteins may be counteracted by the P in phosphoproteins when the P content of those proteins has not been allowed for in diet formulation. The additional P stimulates Ca reabsorption by triggering PTH secretion.

Humans appear to maintain Ca balance at relatively higher intakes of P than do rodents, indicating that bone formation remains closely coupled to bone resorption in the human. It is not entirely clear why Meyer et al.[139] observed nephrocalcinosis in rats given casein, but not in those given lactalbumin when P-intakes were equalized, even though Whiting and Draper[133] detected double the amount of urinary Ca in rats given lactalbumin compared with those given casein. On the other hand, it has been suggested[140] that casein interferes with the intestinal absorption of Ca, stimulating PTH secretion, precipitating nephrocalcinosis and accounting for greater amounts of urinary Ca in the rats given lactalbumin.

Evidence that PTH and the vitamin D hormone may not be involved in protein induced hypercalciuria has been put forward by Kim and Linksweiler[141], who could detect no influence on PTH activity, and Schuette et al.[142], who found no influence on circulating 1,25-dihydroxyvitamin D following elevated dietary protein intakes. Allen et al.[143] suggest that a rise in serum insulin which follows an influx of amino acids is a possible cause of the calciuretic effect of high-protein diets.

Carbohydrates

A higher incidence of nephrocalcinosis, and of renal Ca accumulation, has been observed amongst rats given sucrose compared with those receiving starch, glucose or fructose[144]; although no influence of carbohydrate on the renal concentration of Mg was detected. The differences might in part be explained by the much greater absorption of fructose from dietary sucrose than from an equimolar mixture of glucose and fructose (I. MacDonald, personal communication).

Hodgkinson and colleagues[145] reported that dietary lactose increased intestinal absorption and urinary excretion of Ca, enhanced renal calcification and induced medullary and pelvic nephrocalcinosis in rats in comparison with pre-gelatinized waxy maize starch, acetylated distarch phosphate, and acetylated distarch adipate. Lactose is known to reduce urinary pH. There was no treatment-related hyperparathyroidism to account for any of the kidney pathology.

The effects of certain carbohydrates and of polyols on Ca metabolism are probably related to their stimulation of intestinal Ca absorption, although no definitive conclusions have yet been reached. Differences between dietary carbohydrates in their effects on intestinal microflora, and on the rates of monosaccharide absorption, subsequent metabolic pathways and consequential endocrine stimulation, may be significant. Sucrose increases plasma insulin:glucagon ratio[146] and fructose increases plasma growth hormone activity. Furthermore Ribaya-Mercado[123] observed that rats given galactose, or lactose, excreted larger amounts of oxalate in their urine and faeces.

Dietary fat

Kang et al.[147] observed the highest renal Ca concentration and most intense nephrocalcinosis amongst rats given sucrose in conjunction with fat. Although polyunsaturated margarine caused no greater effect than butter, it is tempting to conclude that the greater calcification induced by maize oil than by medium-chain triglycerides, observed by Kaunitz and Johnson[148], was a consequence of the stimulation to renal synthesis of prostaglandin by maize oil.

Conclusions

The important predisposing dietary factors to nephrocalcinosis are:

1. a low Ca : P ratio;
2. excess Ca;
3. Mg deficiency;
4. excess vitamin D;
5. certain carbohydrates and polyols, in particular lactose and sucrose;
6. oxalate and its precursors, especially in conjunction with excessive fat and insufficient Ca, or pyridoxine deficiency;
7. polyunsaturated fatty acids, although further evidence is required to confirm their significance.

The roles of dietary acidifying agents and anion : cation imbalances require clarification. Important mediating factors are:

1. parathyroid hormone;
2. certain prostaglandins;
3. plasma pH;
4. urinary pH;
5. renal damage.

Each of these factors is inoperative in all types of nephrocalcinosis. Factors which appear not to be instrumental in the syndrome except under very abnormal conditions include:

1. urinary Ca concentration;
2. plasma P (except indirectly);
3. plasma (Ca) x (P).

REFERENCES

1. Hopkins, PN and Williams, RR (1981). A survey of 246 suggested coronary risk factors. Atherosclerosis, 40, 1-52
2. Cottrell, RC (1984). Coronary prevention trial in USA. Nutr Bull 41, The British Nutrition Foundation, 9 (2), 105-6
3. Bhattachargya, AK and Eggan, DA (1984). Effects of feeding cholesterol and mixed sterols on the fecal excretion of acidic steroids in Rhesus monkeys. Atherosclerosis, 53, 225-32
4. Jenkins, DJ, Wong, GS, Patten, R, Bird, J, Hall, M, Buckley, GC, McGuire, V, Reichert, R and Little, JA (1983). Leguminous seeds in the dietary management of hyperlipidemia. Am J Clin Nutr, 38, 567-73
5. Liebman, M and Bazzarre, TL (1983). Plasma lipids of

vegetarian and non-vegetarian males: effects of egg consumption. Am J Clin Nutr, 38, 612-19

6. Chen, WL and Anderson, JW (1979). Effects of plant fibre in decreasing plasma total cholesterol and increasing high-density lipoprotein cholesterol (40671). Proc Soc Exp Biol Med, 162, 310-3

7. Brown, WV and Karmally, W (1985). Coronary heart disease and the consumption of diets high in wheat and other grains. Am J Clin Nutr, 41, 1163-71

8. Asp, NG, Bauer, HG, Nilsson-Ehle, P, Nyman, M and Roste, R (1981). Wheat bran increases high-density-lipoprotein cholesterol in the rat. Br J Nutr, 46, 385-93

9. Judd, PA and Truswell, AS (1985). The hypocholesterolaemic effects of pectins in rats. Br J Nutr, 53, 409-25

10. Lafont, H, Lairon, D, Vigne, JL, Chanussot, F, Chabert, C, Portugal, H, Pauli, AM, Crotte, C and Hauton, JC (1985). Effect of wheat bran pectin and cellulose on the secretion of bile lipids in rats. J Nutr, 115, 849-55

11. Kelly, JJ and Tsai, AC (1978). Effect of pectin, gum arabic and agar on cholesterol absorption, synthesis and turnover in rats. J Nutr, 108, 630-9

12. Thomas, JN, Kelly, MJ and Story, JA (1984). Alteration of regression of cholesterol accumulation in rats by dietary pectin. Br J Nutr, 51, 339-45

13. Calvert, GD and Yeates, RA (1982). Adsorption of bile salts by soya-bean flour, wheat bran, lucerne (Medicago sativa), sawdust and lignin; the effect of saponins and other plant constituents. Br J Nutr, 47, 45

14. Chang, MLW and Johnson, MA (1980). Effects of lignin versus cellulose on the adsorption of taurocholate and lipid metabolism in rats fed cholesterol diet. Nutr Rep Int, 21 (4), 513-8

15. Frape, DL, Wayman, BJ and Tuck, MG (1982). The effects of gum arable, wheat offal and various of its fractions on the metabolism of ^{14}C-labelled alfatoxin B, in the male weanling rat. Br J Nutr, 48, 97-110

16. Truswell, AS and Kay, RM (1976). Brain and blood lipids. Lancet, 1, 367

17. Story, JA and Kritchevsky, D (1976). Comparison of the binding of various bile acids and bile salts in vitro by several types of fibre. J Nutr, 106, 1292-4

18. Vahouny, GV, Roy, T, Gallo, LL, Story, JA, Kritchevsky, D and Cassidy, M (1980). Dietary fibres III. Effects of chronic intake of cholesterol absorption and metabolism in the rat. Am J Clin Nutr, 33, 2182-91

19. Oakenfull, DG, Fenwick, DE, Hood, RL, Topping, DL, Illman, RL and Storer, GB (1979). Effects of saponins on bile acids and plasma lipids in the rat. Br J Nutr, 42, 209

20. Oakenfull, DG and Fenwick, DE (1978). Adsorption of bile salts from aqueous solution by plant fibre and cholestyramine. Br J Nutr, 40, 299-309

21. Hillman, LC, Peters, SG, Fisher, CA and Pomare, EW (1985). The effect of the fibre components pectin, cellulose and lignin on serum cholesterol levels. Am J Clin Nutr, 42,

207-13
22. Riottot, M and Sacquet, E (1985). Increase in the ileal absorption rate of sodium taurocholate in germ-free or conventional rats given an amlyomaize-starch diet. Br J Nutr, 53, 307-10
23. Sambrook, IE and Rainbird, AL (1985). The effect of guar gum and level and source of dietary fat on glucose tolerance in growing pigs. Br J Nutr, 54, 27-35
24. Crapo, PA (1985). Simple versus complex carbohydrate use in the diabetic diet. Ann Rev Nutr, 5, 95-114
25. Toussant, MJ, Wilson, MD and Clarke, SD (1981). Coordinate suppression of liver acetyl CoA carboxylase and fatty acid synthetase by polyunsaturated fat. J Nutr, 111, 146-53
26. Wolf, RN and Grundy, SM (1983). Influence of exchanging carbohydrate for saturated fatty acids on plasma lipids and lipoproteins in men. J Nutr, 113, 1521-8
27. Grande, F, Anderson, JT and Keys, A (1970). Comparison of effects of palmitic and stearic acid in the diet on serum cholesterol in man. Am J Clin Nutr, 23 (9), 1184-93
28. Hegsted, DM, McGandy, RB, Myers, ML and Stare, FJ (1965). Quantitative effects of dietary fat on serum cholesterol in man. Am J Clin Nutr, 17, 281-95
29. McGandy, RB, Hegsted, DM and Myers, ML (1970). Use of semisynthetic fats in determining effects of specific dietary fatty acids on serum lipids in man. Am J Clin Nutr, 23, 1288-98
30. Reiser, R, Probstfield, JL, Silvers, A, Scott, LW, Shorney, ML, Wood, RD, O'Brien, BC, Gotto, AM Jr and Insell, W Jr (1985). Plasma lipid and lipoprotein response of humans to beef fat, coconut oil and safflower oil. Am J Clin Nutr, 42, 190-7
31. Hornstra, G (1985). Dietary lipids, platelet function and arterial thrombosis in animals and man. Proc Nutr Soc, 44, 371-8
32. Hornstra, G (1979). Effect of dietary fats on arterial thrombosis: Rationale for dietary primary prevention of coronary artery disease. In, Symposium on "Dietary Prevention of Coronary Heart Disease", 29-30 November. Zoological Society, Regent's Park, London
33. Beynan, AC and Katan, MB (1985). Why do polyunsaturated fatty acids lower serum cholesterol? Am J Clin Nutr, 42, 560-3
34. Sinclair, HM (1979). Perspectives on the role of fats in heart disease. Symposium on "Dietary Prevention of Coronary Heart Disease", 29-30 November. Zoological Society, London
35. Oh, SY and Monaco, PA (1985). Effect of dietary cholesterol and degree of fat unsaturated on plasma lipid levels, lipoprotein composition and fecal steroid excretion in normal young adult men. Am J Clin Nutr, 42, 399-413
36. Sanders, TAB and Hochland, MC (1983). A comparison of the influence of plasma lipids and platelet function of supplements of W3 and W6 polyunsaturated fatty acids. Br J Nutr, 50, 521-9
37. Glosmet, JA (1985). Fish, fatty acids and human health. N

Engl J Med, 312, 1253-4

38. Fenn, CG and Littleton, JM (1984). Interactions between ethanol and dietary fat in determining human platelet function. Thromb Haemostas, 51, 50-3

39. Lee, TH, Hoover, RL, Williams, JD, Sperling, RI, Ravalses, J III, Spur, BW, Robinson, DR, Corey, EJ, Lewis, RA and Austin, KF (1985). Effect of dietary enrichment with eicosapentaenoic and decosahexaenoic acids on in vitro neutrophil and monocyte leukotriene generation and neutrophil function. N Engl J Med, 312, 1217-24

40. Clandinin, MT and Yamashiro, S (1982). Dietary factors affecting the incidence of dietary fat-induced myocardial lesions. J Nutr, 112, 825-8

41. Hulan, HW, Kramer, JKG, Mahadevan, S and Sauer, FD (1975). Relationship between erucic acid and myocardial changes in male rats. Lipids, 11, 9

42. Aherne, FX, Bowland, JP, Christian, RG and Hardin, RT (1976). Performance of myocardial and blood seral changes in pigs fed diets containing high or low erucic acid rapeseed oils. Can J Animal Sci, 56, 275-84

43. Qureshi, AA, Din, ZZ, Abuirmeileh, N, Burger, WC, Ahmad, Y and Elson, CE (1983). Suppression of avian hepatic lipid metabolism by solvent extracts of garlic: Impact on serum lipids. J Nutr, 113, 1746-55

44. Shoetan, A, Augusti, KT and Joseph, PK (1984). Hypolipidemic effects of garlic oil in rats fed ethanol and a high lipid diet. Experientia, 40, 261-3

45. Arora, RC, Arora, A and Gupta, RK (1981). The long-term use of garlic in ischemic heart disease. Atherosclerosis, 40, 175-9

46. Portman, OW, Alexander, M and Neuringer, M (1985). Dietary protein effects on lipoproteins and on sex and thyroid hormones in blood of Rhesus monkeys. J Nutr, 115, 425-35

47. Nagata, Y, Tanaka, K and Sugano, M (1981). Further studies on the hypocholesterolaemic effect of soya bean protein in rats. Br J Nutr, 45, 233

48. Park, M-SL and Liepa, GU (1982). Effects of dietary protein and amino acids on the metabolism of cholesterol-carrying lipoproteins in rats. J Nutr, 112, 1892-8

49. Siddiqui, MT and Siddiqui, M (1976). Hypolipidemic principles of Cicer arietinum. Biochanin-A and formononetin. Lipids, 11, 243-6

50. Chen, LH, Liao, S and Packett, LV (1972). Interaction of dietary vitamin E and protein level or lipid source with serum cholesterol level in rats. J Nutr, 102, 729-32

51. Croswell, SC and Lei, KY (1985). Effect of copper deficiency on the apolipoprotein E-rich high density lipoproteins in rats. J Nutr, 115, 473-82

52. Harden, KK and Robinson, JL (1984). Hypocholesteremia induced by orotic acid: dietary effects on species specificity. J Nutr, 114, 411-21

53. Coates, PM, Brown, SA, Sonawane, BR and Koldovsky, O (1983). Effect of early nutrition on serum cholesterol levels

in adult rats challenged with high fat diet. J Nutr, 113, 1046-50

54. Frohlich, ED (1983). Mechanisms contributing to high blood pressure. Ann Intern Med, 98, 709-14

55. Meldrum, MJ, Xue, CS, Badino, L and Westfall, TC (1984). Angiotensin facilitation of noradrenergic neurotransmission in central tissues of the rat: effects of sodium restriction. J Cardiovasc Pharmacol, 6, 989-95

56. Watt, GCM, Foy, CJW, Hart, JT, Bingham, G, Edwards, C, Hart, M, Thomas, E and Walton, P (1985). Dietary sodium and arterial blood pressure: evidence against genetic suscep-tibility. Br Med J, 291, 1525-8

57. Tobian, L (1983). Human essential hypertension: implications of animal studies. Ann Intern Med, 98, 729-34

58. Tobian, L, Johnson, MA, Ganguli, M, Lange, J, Kartheiser, K, Iwai, J (1982). Effect of a high linoleic diet and thiazide in rats. Clin Sci, 63, 239-41

59. Tannen, RL (1983). Effects of potassium on blood pressure control. Ann Intern Med, 98, 773-80

60. Young, DB, McCaa, RE, Pan, Y and Guyton, AC (1976). The natriuretic and hypotensive effects of potassium. Cir-culation Res, 38, 84-9

61. Sealey, JE, Clark, I, Bull, MB and Laragh, JH (1970). Potassium balance and the control of renin secretion. J Clin Invest, 49, 2119-27

62. Kotchen, TA, Luke, RG, Ott, CE, Calla, JH and Whitescar-ver, S (1983). Effect of chloride on renin and blood pres-sure responses to sodium chloride. Ann Intern Med, 98, 817-22

63. Lindenmayer, GE and Schwartz, A (1975). A kinetic charac-terization of calcium on $(Na^+ + K^+)$- ATPase and its potential role as a link between extracellular and intracellular events: hypothesis for digitalis-induced inotropism. J Molec Cell Car-diol, 7, 591-612

64. Suki, WN (1979). Calcium transport in the nephron. Am J Physiol, 237, F1-6

65. McCarron, DA (1983). Calcium and magnesium nutrition in human hypertension. Ann Intern Med, 98, 800-5

66. Altura, BM and Altura, BT (1981). Magnesium ions and con-traction of vascular smooth muscles: relationship to some vascular diseases. Fed Proc, 40, 2672-9

67. Johnson, NE, Smith, EL and Frendenheim, JoL (1985). Ef-fects on blood pressure of calcium supplementation of women. Am J Clin Nutr, 42, 12-17

68. Bohr, DF (1963). Vascular smooth muscle: dual effect of cal-cium. Science, 139, 597-9

69. Sowers, MR, Wallace, RB and Lemke, JH (1985). The as-sociation of intakes of vitamin D and calcium with blood pres-sure among women. Am J Clin Nutr, 42, 135-42

70. Smith-Barbaro, PA and Pucak, GJ (1983). Dietary fat and blood pressure. Ann Intern Med, 98, 828-31

71. Hoffman, P, Taube, H, Forster, K, Samova, L, Obertoza, V and Davidson, F (1978). Influence of linoleic acid content on arterial blood pressure of salt loaded rats. Acta Biol Med

German, 37, 863-7

72.   Gardey, T, Burstyn, PG and Taylor, TG (1978). Fat in-
       duced hypertension in rabbits. 1. The effects of fibre on the
       blood pressure increase induced by coconut oil. Proc Nutr
       Soc, 37, 97A

73.   Kennedy, M, Burstyn, PG and Husbands, DR (1978). Fat
       induced hypertension in rabbits. 2. The effect of feeding
       diets containing high concentrations of safflower oil and palm
       oil. Proc Nutr Soc, 37, 98A

74.   Wright, A, Burstyn, PG and Gibney, MJ (1980). Dietary
       fibre and blood pressure. Proc Nutr Soc, 39, 3A

75.   Codde, JP and Beilin, LJ (1985). Dietary fibre fish oil
       prevents dexamethasone induced hypertension in the rat.
       Clin Sci, 69, 691-9

76.   Ahrens, RA, Demuth, P, Lee, MK and Majkowski, JW (1980).
       Moderate sucrose ingesting and blood pressure in the rat. J
       Nutr, 110, 725-31

77.   Hodges, RE and Rebello, T (1983). Carbohydrates and blood
       pressure. Ann Intern Med, 98, 838-41

78.   ʻndaerson, JW (1984). Plant fibre and blood pressure. Ann
       intern Med, 98, 842-6

79.   Defronzo, RA, Cooke, RA, Andres, R, Faloon, GR and
       Davis, PJ (1975). The effect of insulin on renal handling of
       sodium, potassium, calcium and phosphate in man. J Clin In-
       vest, 55, 845-55

80.   Meyer, TW, Anderson, S and Brenner, BM (1983). Dietary
       protein and progressive glomerular sclerosis: the role of
       capillary hypertension and hyperfusion in the progression of
       renal disease. Ann Intern Med, 98, 832-7

81.   Houtsmuller, AJ (1966). The influence of carbohydrates and
       disturbances   in   carbohydrate   metabolism   upon   the
       lipoidspectrum in the serum of patients with atherosclerosis;
       results of some investigations on atherosclerosis. Eds. van
       den Bergh and Jurgens, p20, Rotterdam

82.   Bierman, EL (1985). Diet and diabetes. Am J Clin Nutr, 41,
       1113-6

83.   Laychock, S (1983). Fatty acid incorporation into phos-
       pholipids of isolated pancreatic islets of the rat. Relationship
       to insulin release. Diabetes, 32, 6-13

84.   Poisson, JP, Le Marchal, P, Blond, JP, Lecerf, J and
       Mendy, F (1978). Effect of alloxan diabetes upon the in vivo
       conversion of (1 sup 4C) linoeic and gamma-linoleic acids into
       arachidonate in rats. Diabetes Metab, 4, 39-45

85.   Cunnane, SC, Manku, MS and Horrobin, DF (1985). Abnor-
       mal essential fatty acid composition of tissue lipids in geneti-
       cally diabetic mice is partially correct by dietary linoleic and
       Y-linoleic acids. Br J Nutr, 53, 449-58

86.   Tepperman, HM and Tepperman, J (1985). Membranes and
       the response to insulin. Proc Nutr Soc, 44, 211-20

87.   Salans, LB, Horton, E and Sims, E (1976). Influence of fat
       cell size and dietary carbohydrate intake on adipose tissue
       insulin sensitivity in adult onset obesity. Clin Res, 18, 463

88.   White, JW, Swartz, FJ and Schwartz, AF (1985). Excess
       glucose intake induces acceletayed B-cell polyploidization in

normal mice: a possible deleterious effect. J Nutr, 115, 271-8

89. Farquhar, JW, Frank, A, Gross, RC and Reaven, M (1966). Glucose, insulin and triglyceride response to high and low carbohydrate diets in man. J Clin Invest, 45, 1648

90. Karam, JH, Grodsky, GM, Pavlatos, FCh and Forsham, PH (1965). Critical factors in excessive serum-insulin response to glucose. Obesity in maturity-onset diabetes and growth hormone in acromegaly. Lancet, 1, 286

91. Slama, G, Jean-Joseph, P, Goicolea, I, Elgrably, F, Haardt, MJ, Costagliola, D, Bornet, F and Tchobroutsky, G (1984). Sucrose taken during mixed meal has no additional hyperglycaemic action over isocaloric amounts of starch in well-controlled diabetes. Lancet, 2, 122-4

92. Nestel, PJ, Carroll, KF and Havenstein, N (1970). Plasma triglyceride response to carbohydrates, fats and caloric intake. Metabolism, 19, 1

93. Rozen, P and Shafrir, E (1972). Comparison of changes in plasma free fatty acids, glycerol and insulin following glucose and fructose loads. Israel J Med Sci, 8, 75

94. Birdsall, JJ (1985). Summary and areas for future research. Am J Clin Nutr, 41, 1172-6

95. Albrink, MJ, Newman, T and Davidson, PC (1979). Effect of high- and low-fibre diets on plasma lipids and insulin. Am J Clin Nutr, 32, 1486-91

96. Lousley, SE, Jones, DB, Slaughter, RD, Carter, RD, Jelfs, R and Mann, JI (1984). High carbohydrate-high fibre diets in poorly controlled diabetes. Diabetc Med, 1, 21-5

97. Williams, and MacDonald (1982). Serum glucose and insulin responses in man after varying the viscosity of starch. Proc Nutr Soc, 41, 47A

98. Rainbird, AL, Low, AG and Zebrowska, T (1982). Effect of guar gum on glucose absorption from isolated loops of jejunum in conscious growing pigs. Proc Nutr Soc, 41, 48A

99. Haber, GB, Heaton, KW, Murphy, D and Burroughs, LF (1977). Depletion and disruption of dietary fibre. Effects on satiety, plasma-glucose, and serum-insulin. Lancet, 2, 8040

100. Jenkins, DJA (1979). Dietary fibre, diabetes and hyperlipidaemia. Lancet, 2, 1287

101. Osilesi, O, Trout, DL, Glover, EE, Harper, SM, Koh, ET, Behall, KM, O'Dorisio, TM and Tartt, J (1985). Use of xanthan gum in dietary management of diabetes mellitus. Am J Clin Nutr, 42, 597-603

102. Baxter, LCA and Schofield, PJ (1980). The effects of a high-fat diet on chronic streptozotocin-diabetic rats. Diabetologica, 18, 161-8

103. Reaven, EP and Reaven, GM (1974). Mechanisms for development of diabetic hypertriglyceridemia in streptozotocin-treated rats: effect of diet and duration of insulin deficiency. J Clin Invest, 54, 1167-78

104. Schmidt, FH, Siegel, EG and Trapp, VE (1980). Metabolic and hormonal investigations in long-term streptozotocin diabetic rats on different dietary regimens. Diabetologica, 18, 161-8

105. Tepper, BJ and Kanarek, RB (1985). Dietary self-selection

patterns of rats with mild diabetes. J Nutr, 15, 699-709

106. Clapp, MJL, Wade, JD and Samuels, DM (1982). Control of nephrocalcinosis by manipulating the calcium: phosphorus in commercial rodent diets. Lab Animals, 16, 130-2

107. Jowsey, J, Reiss, E and Canterbury, JM (1974). Long-term effects of high phosphate intake on parathyroid hormone levels and bone metabolism. Acta Orthopaed Scand, 45, 801-8

108. Hitchman, AJ, Hasany, SA, Hitchman, S, Harrison, JE and Tam, C (1979). Phosphate-induced renal calcification in the rat. Can J Physiol Pharmacol, 57, 92-7

109. Borle, AB and Uchikawa, T (1978). Effects of parathyroid hormone on the distribution and transport of calcium in cultured kidney cells. Endocrinology, 102, 1725-32

110. Borle, AB and Clarke, I (1981). Effects of phosphate-induced hyperparathyroidism and parathyroidectomy on rat kidney calcium in vivo. Am J Physiol, 241, E136-41

111. Haut, LL, Alfrey, AC, Guggenheim, S, Buddington, B and Schrier, N (1980). Renal toxicity of phosphate in rats. Kidney Int, 17, 722-31

112. Clarke, I (1969). Metabolic interrelations of calcium, magnesium and phosphate. Am J Physiol, 217, 871-7

113. Alcock, N and MacIntyre, I (1960). Interrelation of calcium and magnesium absorption. Biochem J, 76, 19p

114. MacIntyre, I, Boss, S and Troughten, VA (1963). Parathyroid hormone and magnesium homoeostasis. Nature, 198, 1058-60

115. Hegsted, DM, Vitale, JJ and McGrath, H (1956). The effect of low temperature and dietary calcium upon magnesium requirement. J Nutr, 58, 175-88

116. Harwood, EJ (1982). The influence of dietary magnesium on reduction of nephrocalcinosis in rats fed purified diet. Lab Animals, 16, 314-8

117. Reed, PW (1977). Calcium ionophore activity of prostaglandin endoperoxides and stabilised analogues pGH2. Fed Proc, 36, 673

118. Buck, AC, Davies, RL, Leaker, B and Moffat, DB (1983). Inhibition of experimental nephrocalcinosis with a prostaglandin synthetase inhibitor. Br J Urol, 55, 603-8

119. Thompson, RB, Kauffman, CE and Di Scala, VA (1971). Effect of renal vasodilation on divalent excretion and TmpAH in anesthetised dogs. Am J Physiol, 221, 1097-104

120. Goulding, A and Malthus, RS (1969). Effect of dietary magnesium on the development of nephrocalcinosis in rats. J Nutr, 97, 353-8

121. Hockaday, TDR, Clayton, JE, Frederick, EW and Smith, LH Jr (1964). Primary hyperoxaluria. Medicine, 43, 315-45

122. Morris, MC, Chambers, TL, Evans, PWG, Malleson, PN, Pincott, JR and Rose, GA (1982). Oxalosis in infancy. Arch Dis Childh, 57, 224-8

123. Ribaya-Mercado, JD and Gershoff, SN (1984). Effects of sugars and vitamin B-6 deficiency on oxalate synthesis in rats. J Nutr, 114, 1447-53

124. Andersson, H (1984). Dietary treatment of hyperoxaluria in malabsorptive states. Nutr Abstr Rev, 54, 329-37

125. Rodriguez-Soriano, J, Vallo, A, Castillo, G, Oliveros, R, Cea, JM and Balzategui, MJ (1983). Biochemical features of dietary chloride deficiency syndrome: a comparative study of 30 cases. J Pediat, 103, 209-14

126. Eliel, P, Smith, WO and Thomsen, C (1960). Magnesium and calcium interrelationships. J Oklahoma State Med Assoc, 53, 359

127. Norman, ME, Feldman, NI, Cohn, RM, Roth, KS and McCurdy, DK (1978). Urinary citrate excretion in the diagnosis of distal renal tubular acidosis. J Pediat, 92, 394-400

128. Rodriguez-Soriano, J, Vallo, A, Castillo, G and Oliveros, R (1982). Natural history of primary distal renal tubular acidosis treated since infancy. J Paediat, 101, 669-76

129. Hamed, IA, Czerwinski, AW, Coats, B, Kaufman, C and Altmiller, DH (1979). Familial absorptive hypercalciuria and renal tubular acidosis. Am J Med, 67, 385-91

130. Cremin, B, Wiggelinkhuizen, J and Bonnici, F (1982). Nephrocalcinosis in children. Br J Radiol, 55, 413-18

131. Linksweiler, HM, Joyce, CL and Anand, CR (1974). Calcium retention of adult males as affected by level of protein and of calcium intake. Trans NY Acad Sci, Ser II, 36, 333-40

132. Whiting, SJ, Draper, HH and Hadley, M (1981). Protein induced calciuria in diabetic rats. Nutr Res, 1, 581-7

133. Whiting, SJ and Draper, HH (1980). The role of sulfate in calciuria of high protein in adult rats. J Nutr, 110, 212-22

134. Yuen, DE and Draper, HH (1983). Long term effects of excess protein and phosphorus on bone homeostasis in adult mice. J Nutr, 113, 1374-80

135. Petito, SL and Evans, JL (1984). Calcium status of the growing rat as affected by diet acidity from ammonium chloride, phosphate and protein. J Nutr, 114, 1049

136. Hunt, JN (1956). The influence of dietary sulfur on the urinary output of acid in man. Clin Sci, 5, 119-34

137. McCance, RA and Widdowson, EM (1978). The composition of foods. (4th rev, edn, by Paul, AA and Southgate, DAT). (London: HMSO)

138. McCance, RA, Widdowson, EM and Lehmann, H (1942). The effect of protein intake on the absorption of calcium and magnesium. Biochem J, 36, 686-91

139. Meyer, O, Blom, L and Sondergaard, D (1982). The influence of minerals and protein on the nephrocalcinosis potential for rats of semisynthetic diets. Lab Animals, 16, 271-3

140. Howe, JC and Beecher, GR (1981). Effect of dietary protein and phosphorus levels on calcium and phosphorus metabolism of the young, fast growing rat. J Nutr, 111, 708-20

141. Kim, Y and Linksweiler, HM (1979). Effect of level of protein intake on calcium metabolism and on parathyroid and renal function in adult human male. J Nutr, 109, 1399-1404

142. Schuette, SA, Zemel, MB and Linksweiler, HM (1981). Renal acid, urinary cyclic AMP, and hydroxyproline excretion as affected by level of protein, sulfur-amino acid and phosphorus intake. J Nutr, 111, 2106-16

143. Allen, LH, Geoffrey, D, Block, MS, Richard, J, Wood, MS

and Graeme, FB (1981). The role of insulin and parathyroid hormone in the protein induced calciuria of man. Nutr Res, 1, 3-11

144. Oxley, JA and Bruckdorfer, KR (1979). The effect of dietary carbohydrates and other diet constituents on nephrocalcinosis in the rat. Proc Nutr Soc, 38, 85A

145. Hodgkinson, A, Davis, D, Fourman, J, Robertson, WG and Roe, FJC (1982). A comparison of the effects of lactose and of two chemically modified waxy maize starches on mineral metabolism in the rat. Food Chem Toxicol, 20, 371-82

146. Gardner, LB, Spannhake, B, Keeney, M and Reiser, S (1977). Effect of dietary carbohydrate on serum insulin and glucagon in two strains of rats. Nutr Rep Int, 15, 361-6

147. Kang, SS, Price, RG, Yudkin, J, Worcester, NA and Bruckdorfer, KR (1979). The influence of dietary carbohydrate and fat on kidney calcification and the urinary excretion of N-acetyl-B-glucosamidase (EC 3.2.1.30). Br J Nutr, 41, 65-71

148. Kaunitz, H and Johnson, RE (1976). Dietary protein, fat and minerals in nephrocalcinosis in female rats. Metabolism, 25, 69-77

9.8 GENERAL CONCLUSIONS – DIETARY CONSIDERATIONS RELATIVE TO FUTURE TOXICOLOGY

D. L. FRAPE

Disorders in five areas of metabolism that afflict a substantial proportion of the population, and that can be reproduced in laboratory animals, have been chosen for detailed consideration and analysis. The purpose of this analysis has been to determine whether, by manipulation of laboratory animal diets, a greater rate of progress can be achieved not only in the development of drugs, but also in a successful and predictable application of new drugs and therapeutic diets in clinical practice.

METABOLIC, SHORT- AND MEDIUM-TERM STUDIES

1. In metabolic short- and medium-term studies using laboratory animals for drug development, it is concluded that diet should be used as a tool and not simply as a means of sustaining animals for general use in that development. It is relatively unimportant to know the level of performance achieved by a particular group of animals given a known diet, or a nutrient at a known level, but it is unarguably more important to know what effect variation in the intake of a particular nutrient, or group of nutrients, has on the response, and mechanism of response, of a given test substance.

Where a given pattern of diets is repeatedly used the perennial problem of instability of components of the lipid or other fraction may be minimized by serial analysis of diet, which should facilitate the prediction of dietary composition at the time of consumption by test animals.

It has been noted that both in laboratory animals and human subjects most drugs interact in some way with diet, and either influence the requirement for particular vitamins, trace elements, minerals and other nutrients, or the potency of the drug is influenced in some specific fashion. Similar statements can be made for the effect on drug potency of a variety of dietary contaminants, including heavy metals and pesticides. Therefore particular attention must be paid to the concentrations of dietary con-

237

stituents known to induce variation in response of laboratory animals, and the dietary level sought for each nutrient and energy-yielding component must depend upon the objective of the experiment. The composition of diets derived should take into consideration the range of dietary habits to be expected of the ultimate patients. Moreover, dosage rates should be combined with more specific dietary advice, so that both the desired potency is achieved and nutrient deficiencies are avoided during chronic treatment.

The young, and geriatrics, are likely to be at greatest risk as a consequence, particularly, of high nutrient requirements and misguided diets amongst the young, and insufficient food and poor utilization amongst the elderly. A greater interest in dietary effects of drugs during their development should preclude the occurrence of many episodes of malnutrition in the early clinical use of those drugs.

2. Knowledge of the interrelationships that exist between the metabolism of dietary nutrients, or other components, and drugs should facilitate a more calculated clinical application of drugs with improved precision of, and lower, dosages. For example, many drugs designed to modulate PG synthesis should be examined to determine their interaction with dietary EFA. Dietary manipulation can, it is clear, reduce 2 series lipoxygenase and cyclo-oxygenase products, especially thromboxane A_2, while increasing the synthesis of PGE_1 formed from DGLA. Raised intakes of linoleic acid, C20 acids of the n-3 series found in fish oils, or oleic acid found in olive oil and glucocorticoids may all have this effect. As animal, protein and fat sources contain arachidonic acid, it is clear that any variation in these sources should also influence the synthesis of 2 series PGs.

Dietary manipulation may accommodate lower dosage rates, or even the avoidance of drugs, for mild forms of certain disorders. The control of the metabolism of diabetics by drugs is being, and can be, reduced by research into the mechanism of insulin action and the complementary role that diet can play in limiting pathological metabolic developments. A number of measurements of glycaemic and lipidaemic responses to mixed diets has been reported both in healthy volunteers and in diabetics. More data of this kind on the interactive effects of various components of natural diets are required, so that greater control of post-prandial blood glucose and blood lipid concentrations can be achieved.

Several disorders, including diabetes (type II), are associated with obesity, and may be partly a result of this condition. Nevertheless both similarities and dissimilarities in metabolism have been detected between obese and genetically diabetic rodents.

3. Of considerable importance during drug development is the modulating effect that can be achieved on the metabolic disorder under study by varying the intake of several major dietary components. The dietary concentrations of these are very rarely used as controlled variables in routine work, and frequently these concentrations are incompletely known. For example, the intensity of all five disorders was shown to be markedly influenced by the dietary concentration, or rate of intake, of various components of

the lipid fraction of diet - particularly the sterols, polyun-saturated, monounsaturated, and saturated fatty acids. Four of the disorders were shown to be influenced by protein and amino acid variation; three were shown to be influenced by various com-ponents of structural carbohydrates, composed of water-soluble and water-insoluble fibres; three were shown to be influenced by dif-ferent forms of digestible carbohydrate; and one was particularly influenced by the electrolyte composition of diet. These major dietary components should play the role of controlled variables in drug development.

4. The adoption of major energy-yielding and some other com-ponents of diet as controlled variables is more readily achieved by resort to purified diets. A greater understanding, however, is necessary concerning the role of the three-dimensional structure of the fibre fraction of diet before realistic widespread adoption of purified diets can be entertained. Nevertheless, these diets will play increasing roles in metabolic, short- and medium-term studies.

LIFESPAN STUDIES

Many lifespan studies are dogged by spontaneous metabolic disor-ders.

1. Immune response, and therefore susceptibility, to spontaneous tumours is influenced by diet. Thus appropriate dietary formulation may delay the onset, and incidence, of spontaneous tumours. However, a conflict may exist, for example, between nutrient requirements for the appropriate immune response and those required for delaying the development of atherosclerosis.

2. Decline of the functional integrity of the nephron in ageing animals is an example of an important characteristic that influences lifespan. The rate of this decline can in part be controlled by diet, and particular attention should be paid to those factors re-lated to Ca and Mg metabolism, fat quantity and composition, cation-anion balance and carbohydrate source, in the formulation of diets. Where the use of purified and semi-purified diets is invoked for extended experiments great care should be exercised in the selection of carbohydrate source; but much is yet to be learned about this particular aspect of diet formulation.

3. An increasing quantity of reliable evidence indicates that exces-sive dietary energy intake, and obesity, amongst rodents are fac-tors associated with a higher incidence of several disorders and a reduced life expectancy. It has been asserted, and some evidence supports the view, that a reduction in the energy density of the diet, achieved by the introduction of fibre, can reduce the in-cidence of several degenerative disorders and tumours. However, the fibre component of diet frequently interacts with the test sub-stance, reducing the sensitivity of response to that substance, and an added fibre source may camouflage an oncogenic propensity. Such compositional adjustment of the diet of rabbits can reduce the

severity of atherosclerosis and influence longevity, but it can exert a complementary, or antagonistic, effect on drug action. Both these roles are necessary in drug development, requiring detailed lipid and carbohydrate analysis of diet. The interactions revealed should provide a better insight into mechanisms of drug action.

4. As energy intake per se, as well as its form, seems to have an impact on coronary heart disease, the frequent confounding of these determinants can be avoided by restricting the amounts of food consumed, so that energy intake is reduced independently of a reduction in the energy density of diet.

5. Where rodents and other laboratory animals are meal-fed, the confounding effect on response caused by a drug-induced reduction in appetite can be largely overcome. Intake control might be achieved by the introduction of specific dietary amino acid imbalances. Much more work in this area is nevertheless necessary before any routine and reliable guidelines can be provided for such an approach.

6. The nutrient composition of diets for long-term studies must be addressed with the objectives of the study clearly stated. Several compositional characteristics have been noted to influence longevity; however there seems to be a conflict between the specific requirement for certain nutrients, or groups of nutrients, and the metabolic reliability of various bodily functions. This seems to apply, for example, both to amino acids and lipids. Some intermediate dietary level of protein might best serve the interests of several bodily functions for lifespan studies. A restriction of dietary intake may allow greater freedom to be exercised in terms of the lipid content of laboratory diets. Nevertheless an excessive intake of total fat and of polyunsaturated fats is undesirable for maximum lifespan. Attention should be paid to the calcium : phosphorus ratio and the magnesium content of diets, in particular, to reduce the incidence of nephropathy. Hypertension is subject to comparable dietary control through modulation of electrolyte, and possibly vitamin D, lipid and fibre composition of diet.

7. Where purified diets are introduced careful attention should be paid to anion : cation balance, acid : base balance and carbohydrate source. Generally speaking, metabolic disorders are less frequent amongst animals given natural diets than amongst those given purified diets. Nevertheless the amount of information that may be accumulated concerning the test substance is unlikely to be greater where natural diets are used, owing to a probable reduction in the sensitivity of response to the test substance. Moreover, there is an increasing case to be made for the adoption of purified diets in lifespan studies, as nutritional knowledge is accumulated. This practice would allow the interfering effects that may be caused by a number of variable non-nutrient components (indoles, lectins, antiproteases, nitrates, etc.) to be eliminated, and it would ensure greater nutrient control. Careful consideration should be given to the carbohydrate component of diet in respect of the

accumulated evidence that various sources of digestible carbohydrate influence the incidence and severity on nephrocalcinosis and atherosclerosis.

8. Where a reduction of energy intake and obesity are desired an unwanted interaction of dietary fibre, or some other component, with drug action may be avoided by controlling the daily intake of a diet. Such a practice could frequently extend lifespan, reduce the incidence of spontaneous neoplasms and allow the diet to be formulated from nutrient sources achieving a desired relationship of test substances and diet.

9. Little has been said about in vitro studies. However, tissues derived from animals provided with diets over which proper control has been achieved must be tools that provide more predictable results than can be attained with tissues of unknown nutritional background. Therefore similar arguments apply as for in vivo studies.

10. The dietary variables that have been discussed are likely to be of much greater significance in predictive safety evaluation than are the many contaminants of diets which have preoccupied the attention of many scientists and introduced considerable analytical costs in the control of standard laboratory diets during the past 15 years. Evidence indicates that these contaminants are today under much better control than was the case during the early part of that time. Now is the time to use diet as a biological tool in the modelling process.

PART 4
Applied Aspects

10

Toxicology for Pharmaceutical Substances: The Needs

J. MARKS

INTRODUCTION

In the Introduction to this book (Volume 1, pp 1 to 12) it was noted that a general knowledge about substance toxicity was nothing new, and that most of the early controls concentrated on substances that were to be deliberately administered to the human subject in the form of medicines. Indeed regulations relating to what we would now call pharmaceutical substances were first established in the United Kingdom when the Royal College of Physicians was established in 1518 to control the activities of physicians within London. The controls were, however, poor; for they were based on hearsay evidence of toxicity. For many centuries no means existed for the accurate determination of toxicity.

Formal recognition of the subject of toxicology appeared about the middle of the 19th century, but even then the number of substances in use as therapeutic agents was small and most were derived from natural substances whose toxicity had been assessed over the intervening years by use in practice. Testing as a scientific discipline did not exist, and the use of some of the substances which we still regard as valuable in medicine (e.g. digitalis) might well not have been permitted had current tests and standards been applied in those days.

The availability of medicinal substances increased sharply about the turn of the century, with intensive developments in the field of organic chemistry. Even then the extent of the toxicological testing was small, and in a large number of countries it was possible for a physician or pharmacist to take an unknown substance off the shelf and use it as a therapeutic agent without any tests, within a wide framework of claims of therapeutic benefit. For example legislation only came in the UK and many other developed countries in the early 1960s. An international programme of coordination came in 1962/3 and in several developing countries controls only came into being several years later[1].

However, though legislation arrived late in the scene, most of the innovative pharmaceutical organizations have for the major part of this century undertaken tests to attempt to define the toxicity of the substances which they have developed, though with the wisdom of hindsight it is clear that the tests which they were using lacked precision and were inadequate. Nevertheless they were attempting such studies, largely ahead of the requirements imposed by governments.

The most important single factor which led to a change in the whole concept of the testing of pharmaceuticals was the thalidomide disaster. Not only did this indicate the terrible effects which could stem from the ingestion of an apparently safe therapeutic agent, but perhaps more importantly it demonstrated that current methods of testing were inadequate. In future years the long-term benefits which have stemmed from the thalidomide disaster may even lead future generations to regard thalidomide as one of the most significant milestones in the field of pharmaceutical science. It led directly and immediately to a new appreciation of the testing which must be undertaken.

Coincident with the increased number of potentially toxic substances that are available, and the knowledge of the requirements for testing, has come a dramatic increase in the ability to transmit information rapidly around the world. With this increased information there has been a greater public knowledge of the problems which can arise from therapeutic substances. Pressure groups of concerned people have also had the effect of heightening this awareness. Unfortunately the increased awareness has not always been associated with increasing understanding of the fundamental nature of either the risk-benefit relationship or of the validity of the testing methods. Hence the discussion is not always fruitful.

Nevertheless the problem of toxicity of substances used in therapy exists, and will certainly not disappear. It therefore behoves those who are concerned with the testing of new pharmaceutical agents, and those who use them, to consider how best the current problems can be overcome. This book is concerned with precisely this area, and the present chapter therefore reviews the current situation and the existing problems, and attempts to forecast ways in which some of these problems may be solved before the turn of the 20th century.

THE SOCIAL SITUATION

In the Introduction to this book attention was drawn to the changing age pattern of the population and the influence that this would have on the gross national product. This changing age pattern also has direct effects on the pharmaceutical testing needs, quite apart from any economic effects that it may exert.

At the same time as the rate of population growth is declining in most industrially developed countries life expectancy is rising. This will significantly alter the age stucture of the population, and an increasing proportion of the population will fall into the elderly class. For example as was noted in the Introduction (Volume 1) "in the United Kingdom, whereas those over 65 formed 4.7% of the population at the turn of the century, they now (1985) form nearly 15%. Moreover the rise is due mainly to those that are very elderly and, by 1990, those over 75 are likely to form almost

6.5% of the total population".

Recent experience has demonstrated that toxic reactions are more common in old age. Indeed the withdrawal of most of those pharmaceutical products removed after introduction during the past few years[2], has resulted from the finding during clinical use that there is an unacceptable level of toxicity in the elderly where none had been predicted from clinical trial experience in a predominantly younger age group. This difference in toxicity risk may be due to different pharmacokinetic patterns, to different tissue sensitivity, or to the presence of other diseases or degenerations of tissues or organs.

Current animal testing methods are based upon the use of disease-free animals. Indeed over the past few years there has been an increasing tendency to use even pathogen-free animals to increase the sensitivity of animal studies. This use of carefully selected and tended animals is of great value in the prediction of significant toxic effects of the substance in the animals that are being used for testing. Moreover it may have validity for the determination of relevant issues in toxicity relating to young human beings. However it is far from ideal for prediction in the elderly. Indeed there may be benefits in the suggestion that toxicity studies in elderly animals and animals with a variety of inherent disorders should be an essential part of subacute toxicological study. Two difficulties, however, arise. First, if animals are being used which are either elderly or diseased then there is bound to be a greater difficulty over interpreting any observed apparent toxicity. Second, the range of recognized animal disorders is different from, and infinitely smaller than, the range of the important human disorders, particularly those afflicting the elderly. For example there are few animal models which are accepted as representing human atherosclerosis, yet this may be one of the important disorders which will affect the incidence of toxicity in the human elderly subject. Hence finding an equivalent animal model may be difficult.

The need for the development of suitable tests will be increased further by the search for pharmaceutical products which will deal with some of the disorders which are specific to the elderly, and particularly those diseases which lead to the greatest demand for the health care services. Hence at a time when recognition is coming that the present methods of testing do not cover the toxicological implications of the use of pharmaceutical substances in the elderly, there is a demand for an increasing number of substances active against disorders specific to that age group.

From what has been said it follows that the current methods of investigation are inadequate to study this group of substances. Four possible solutions would appear to exist:

1. Clinical studies should be more extensive in the elderly when there is the least chance that the substance concerned will be used in that age group.

2. Such clinical trials should also involve determination of the various metabolic and pharmacokinetic parameters. By the accumulation of a good data base for variations in the metabolic

and pharmacokinetic pattern with age, forecasting of possible difficulties will become more efficient.

3. Post-marketing surveillance must be improved. This whole question is examined in detail later (see page 252).

4. Since it is difficult to devise suitable animal models representing degenerations and diseases of the elderly, more reliance must be placed on the better basic understanding of the pathology involved. From such an understanding the prediction of likely adverse reactions should become feasible. Hence clinicians may be forewarned about possible problems on the basis of the available animal studies, coupled with a better knowledge of the pathological processes involved.

THE UNDERSTANDING OF THE RISK

One recent development which will influence the future is the better perception of risk-benefit and attempts at its quantification.

Diseases carry an inherent risk which can be expressed in terms of mortality and/or morbidity. All treatment also carries its own risk. The benefit of any treatment should therefore be expressed in terms of the balance between the improvement in the adverse effects of the disease and the risk of adverse effects of the treatment. This concept was developed excellently by Inman in Volume 1 (pages 43 - 62). Inman also gave an indication of the difference between the two risk levels which might be acceptable.

While this concept is gaining acceptance among clinical pharmacologists and physicians it is still not understood by the lay public, who appear to require a nil risk level from pharmacotherapy.

People respond to the hazards which they perceive and the probability of their occurrence. The perception is in part rational and in part dependent on subjective judgement[3]. Members of the public apply qualitative judgements to particular risks, e.g. carcinogenicity, and also expect a higher standard for occupational risks that are not seen as voluntary. In the field of therapeutics there are major differences between the level of risk that may be acceptable for pharmacotherapy (10^{-6}, see Volume 1, page 51) and surgery (10^1) for the same disorder.

Since the principle of toxicology is that it should assess risk before human exposure starts, it follows that factors which affect the assessment and acceptance of risk **in the minds of the lay public** are paramount in defining the extent and scope of toxicological study. It is the lay public, and particularly pressure groups in the lay public, who exert the major influence over the legislative activities of a government on safety, and hence the defined acceptable risk.

It therefore follows that over the next decade two important moves are necessary in this area:

1. Efforts must be made to achieve better education of the lay public over the whole matter of risk appreciation and under-

standing. This should not be left to one section of the interested medical community, but should be a shared respon-
sibility for all. Without adequate education an excessive and
unrealistic view of achievable safety of drugs is likely to
remain.

2. Quantification of all aspects of risk determination of diseases
and their therapy is an important area for further urgent
development.

NEW CHEMICAL CLASSES

Current methods of toxicological testing are based on a certain
amount of validation within the field of existing clinical usage and
exposure, whether this is deliberate or by accident.

The developments in chemistry referred to in the Introduction (Volume 1, page 9), and particularly in biotechnology, are
likely to result in an entirely new range of substances before the
end of the century. Unfortunately we have no means of knowing
whether the existing toxicological methods will be adequate to
determine unusual toxic effects which may occur from these new
chemical classes.

For example, thalidomide, which was subjected to the then
currently validated toxicological tests before being introduced to
the market, appeared to be a very safe compound. Clinical experience indicated that the current tests as applied to drugs were
inadequate to demonstrate this teratogenic effect. An effect such
as that exerted by thalidomide, be it specific organ toxicity,
teratogenicity or carcinogenicity, may occur with other compounds
in the future despite **current** methods of testing. The greater the
difference between the new chemical class and those that have been
validated, the greater the potential risk.

It follows that, while toxicological methods should involve the
use of validated techniques, both currently available and developed
in the future, the only final protection against tragedies arising
from a new type of toxic reaction is the epidemiological examination
of changes in mortality and morbidity. Such studies are, however,
difficult for, as in the case of the carcinogenic effect of smoking,
morbidity may only occur after prolonged exposure or possibly one
or two decades after such exposure. Hence one vital aspect of
development in toxicology is a first-class epidemiological monitoring
system. With the new computer-based data acquisition this should
be feasible.

Later in this chapter the question of extensive post-
marketing surveillance is considered in more detail.

ANIMAL TESTING METHODS

Current testing methods are based in the main upon acute, subacute and chronic toxicity studies in a variety of animal species.
Until recently acute toxicity studies formed a large component of
the overall testing procedure, but the relevance of the most widely

used form, the LD_{50} or "lethal dose 50", is now in great doubt, and its use is being considerably modified or even totally discarded[4,5].

The selection of the animal species which are used for the various studies is currently rarely based upon scientific logic. Thus for example until recently little effort has been made to match the test animals to the human subject on the basis of the metabolic and kinetic pattern of the substance to be tested, with the results that it is scarcely surprising that the predictive value of these tests has often been limited. For good reasons, therefore, the usefulness of much of the current routine toxicological testing has been sharply questioned[6].

Apart from the difficulties which exist over the definition of appropriate animal models there is a growing pressure from within society for the overall reduction of animal experimentation. This pressure ranges from the increasingly militant activities of anti-vivisection groups, which are dedicated to the total abolition of animal experiments, to those of the more responsible animal welfare organizations to refine, reduce and replace animal studies whenever this is possible (Volume 1, page 27; see also ref.7 below).

A typical example of the way that alternative tests can be developed and subsequently accepted internationally is shown in the reduction of the use of animals for the control of biological medicinal products (e.g. insulin). A representative meeting in London in 1985 considered and approved of many of these methods, and agreed to give further consideration to others[8].

LEGISLATION

Legal controls show marked variation between different areas and different countries. Even within a single country there is frequently a complicated set of laws often promulgated by different departments within the legislature.

International organizations, including the United Nations, the World Health Organization, and the European Economic Community, have attempted to ensure that gross national differences in legislation are reduced. While strenuous efforts are being made, much still remains to be done in this area. Future broad international agreement, however difficult, is an essential factor in the further development of toxicology.

THE CURRENT STATUS OF TESTING PROCEDURES

A detailed account of current methods of toxicity testing is outside the remit of this book. Several excellent accounts are available which relate both to general concepts[9-16]; to non-animal systems[9,17,18]; and to special areas of concern e.g. reproductive toxicology[19-21], carcinogenicity[22-24], immunotoxicity[25,26], among many others.

ECONOMIC ASPECTS OF PHARMACEUTICAL TOXICOLOGY

Current testing procedures are expensive, in terms both of time and money[27]. A major problem is the recoupment of the costs involved during the remaining period of the patent life. In most countries the patent life is measured from the date of first registration. The testing programme currently takes at least 10 years when any prolonged human exposure is anticipated. This effectively reduces the period of marketing within the original patent life to under one-half.

By some changes in toxicological methods, and by better programming, it may be possible to achieve some reduction in the length of time required for toxicological testing, but the reduction is unlikely to be substantial. The best possibility for appropriate financial return on research expenditure may come from a modification of patent law, to provide a more limited but defined number of years **after** development is complete.

RADICAL NEW APPROACHES

Modelling

A more rational approach to the whole question of testing for toxic manifestations of substances in general, and pharmaceutical drugs in particular, can come only when there is a better understanding of the fundamental reactions which are involved. This includes such aspects as:

1. metabolism and biotransformation of chemical classes and the influence on this of biochemical aberrations in the species and individual;

2. pharmacokinetic and pharmacodynamic differences both inter-species and intraspecies;

3. the effect of food and other environmental factors on cell, tissue and organ interaction with pharmaceutical substances;

4. the mechanisms and dynamics of receptor interactions, both those that lead to beneficial effects and those that produce adverse reactions;

5. genetic influences;

6. tissue, cell and subcellular mechanisms of toxicity.

As more of these factors become defined in quantitative form for a wide selection of therapeutic substances, and then validated by human experience, it should be possible to move toxicological testing forward

1. by better selection of animal models, route and regularity of dosing;

2. ultimately by the extensive representation of likely therapeutic and adverse effects by mathematical modelling on the basis of a reliable and extensive data base.

As one part of this process it will be desirable, if not essential, to undertake early human volunteer studies to determine the metabolic and pharmacokinetic parameters. Improvements in the techniques of chemical analysis, which make it possible to make determinations with low doses of the substances, make it possible to undertake such studies at an earlier stage than previously.

In these early volunteer studies, and indeed during the initial clinical trials, open, non-controlled use is in my opinion desirable, though both the good effects and the adverse reactions must subsequently be tested further in blind controlled trials.

DETERMINATION OF THE ALLERGENIC POTENTIAL

The prediction of toxic manifestations which occur regularly and commonly is already possible. Risk determination to this level is, however, inadequate and current medical and lay opinion demand a risk level of the order of 10^{-6} for acceptability of therapeutic substances (see Inman, in Volume 1, page 51).

One component of a level of toxicity of this grade must be some form of individual interaction. A proportion of these interactions are likely to arise from an allergenic response to the drug. Hence it is important that the allergenic potential of chemical substances and the factors that influence it should be defined.

The allergenic response is, however, a joint reaction between the substance and the host. With a low incidence of such reactions it is clear that part of the problem lies with the host. It would therefore be valuable if tests could be defined which would demonstrate which patient is likely to experience such immune-based adverse reactions.

POST-MARKETING SURVEILLANCE

Recent experience has demonstrated that even the best pre-marketing testing does not necessarily provide a safety level that is acceptable to the community at large[2]. In part it is inevitable that some substances which pass pre-marketing tests will fail when they are subjected to broad use. Pre-marketing testing rarely involves more than 10,000 patients yet, as Inman points out in Volume 1 (page 48), the use of 10,000 patients gives only a low confidence level of toxicity prediction. Thus for a study of 10,000 there is a 99% chance of recognizing toxicity at a level of 1 per 2000, compared with an unacceptable toxicity level of the order of one death per two million patients.

This means that even after the most scrupulous toxicological investigation and clinical study in a reasonable size cohort of the appropriate population (e.g. for sex and age) the introduction of a new product must be safeguarded by a process of close monitoring with adequate epidemiological control and surveillance. The number of cases of adverse reactions before a causal relationship is established will depend on the temporal relationship between the administration and the development of the adverse reaction. Thus, for example, Williams et al.[28] calculated that a stepwise introduction of thalidomide would have limited the number of victims to about 35 rather than the actual figure, which was in excess of 1000.

The length of time which will be required, and the number who will have to be studied during the post-marketing surveillance, will be determined by the incidence of the adverse reaction; the calculated acceptable risk level relative to the disorder which is being treated; and the interval between administration and the occurrence of the adverse reaction. For some adverse reactions these data are available; hence it will be relatively easy to define the period of the post-marketing surveillance.

The task of forecasting the period of the observation and the numbers involved for an entirely new or unpredicted toxicity will be difficult, if not impossible. This is particularly true, for example, for possible carcinogenic risks.

However despite the difficulties involved, well-controlled and well-monitored post-marketing surveillance must become a vital component of future risk determination for pharmaceutical substances. A detailed consideration of the techniques, pitfalls, etc., is outside the remit of this chapter, but has been considered in a recent multi-author text[1].

REFERENCES

1. Inman, WHW (ed.) (1980). Monitoring for Drug Safety. (Lancaster: MTP Press)
2. Dukes, G (1985). The Effects of Drug Regulation. (Lancaster: MTP Press)
3. Slovic, P, Fischhoff, B and Lichtenstein, S (1981). Perceived risk: psychological factors and social implications. Proc R Soc Lond, A376, 17-34
4. Anon (1984). Animals in testing; how the CPI is handling a hot issue. Chemical Week, 5 December, pp. 36-40
5. Brimblecombe, RW and Dayan, AD (1985). Preclinical Toxicity Testing: Pharmaceutical Medicine. (London: Edward Arnold)
6. Zbinden, G (1966). Animal toxicity studies: a critical evaluation. Appl Ther, 8, 128
7. Rowan, AN (1983). Alternatives: interaction between science and animal welfare. In Goldberg, AM (ed.) Product Safety Evaluation. (New York: Mary A Liebert), pp. 113-33
8. Conference Report (1985). Reduction of the use of animals in the development and control of biological products. Lancet, 2, 900-2
9. Balls, M, Riddell, RJ and Worden, AN (1983). Animals and Alternatives in Toxicity Testing. (London: Academic Press)
10. Tu, AT (1980). Survey of Contemporary Toxicology. (Chichester: John Wiley)
11. Plaa, GL and Duncan, WAM (1978). Proceedings of the First International Congress on Toxicology. (New York: Academic

Press)

12. Calabrese, EJ (1983). Principles of Animal Extrapolation. (New York: John Wiley)

13. Yoshida, H, Hiroshi, S, Hagihara, Y and Ebashi, S (1982). Advances in Pharmacology and Therapeutics, II. Volume 5: Toxicology and Experimental Models. (Oxford: Pergamon Press)

14. Hayes, AW (ed.) Methods in Toxicology. (New York: Raven Press)

15. Kaiser, HE and Elmar, H (1979). Species Specific Potential of Invertebrates for Toxicological Research. (Baltimore: University Park Press)

16. Timbrell, JA (1982). Principles of Biochemical Toxicology. (London: Taylor & Francis)

17. Symposium Report (1980). Isolated cell systems as a tool in toxicological research. Arch Toxicol, 44, 1-210

18. Goldberg, AM (ed.) (1983). Alternative Methods in Toxicology. (New York: Mary A Liebert)

19. Johnson, EM and Marshall, ME (1983). Teratogenesis and Reproductive Toxicology. (Berlin: Springer-Verlag)

20. Snell, K (1982). Developmental Toxicology. (London: Croom Helm)

21. Vouk, VB and Sheehan, PJ (1983). Methods for Assessing the Effects of Chemicals on Reproductive Functions. (New York: John Wiley)

22. De Serres, FJ and Ashby, J (eds) (1982). Evaluation of Short-Term Tests for Carcinogens: Progress in Mutation Research, Volume 1. (Amsterdam: Elsevier)

23. Arlett, CF and Parry, JM (eds) (1985). Comparative Genetic Toxicology: The Second UKEMS Collaborative Study. (London: Macmillan)

24. Ashby, J, De Serres, FJ, Draper, M, Ishidate, M, Margolin, BH, Matter, BE and Shelby, MD (eds) (1985). Evaluation of Short-Term Tests for Carcinogens: Report of the International Program on Chemical Safety Collaborative Study on In Vitro Assays. (Amsterdam: Elsevier)

25. Gibson, GG, Hubbard, R and Parke, DV (eds) (1983). Immunotoxicology. (London: Academic Press)

26. Dean, JH, Luster, MI, Bourman, GA and Lauer, LD (1982). Procedures available to examine the immunotoxicity of chemicals and drugs. Pharmacol Rev, 34, 137-48

27. Hartley, K and Maynard, A (1982). The Costs and Benefits of Regulating New Product Development in the UK Pharmaceutical Industry. (London: Office of Health Economics)

28. Williams, RT, Schumacher, H, Fabro, S and Smith, RL (1965). In Robson, JM, Sullivan, FM and Smith, RL (eds) Embryopathic Activity of Drugs. (London: Churchill), p. 167

11

Predictive Safety Evaluation: The Clinical Trial

N. W. SHEPHARD

A successful clinical trial is one that reaches the correct conclusion, not one that produces a positive result[1].

Man comes into contact with multiple substances, either environmentally, in food and drink, as medicines, as contaminants, by accident or by design. Safety evaluation is therefore relative to the characteristics of each substance, and to the circumstances in which it comes into contact with man. Side-effects acceptable for a medicine would be wholly unacceptable for a food colouring agent or herbicide. Predictive safety evaluation is therefore dependent upon what is an acceptable level of risk in relation to the benefit to society.

PREHUMAN STUDIES

The starting point for predictive safety evaluation in man is an examination of the available data including all prehuman exposure studies. The first question to be answered is how different can we expect human reaction to be from that found in animals? With the advent of better chemical analytical techniques a very early study of man can help determine the pharmacokinetic and metabolic pathways; and a reasonable forecast may be possible as to the metabolic disposition of the substance and its behaviour. Species differences for plasma half-lives and metabolic disposition of drugs are well recognized[2], so that comparing animal and early human results may yield valuable preliminary information about both the pharmacological and the toxicological pattern of behaviour.

The pharmacological and metabolic data may then be used to optimize future toxicological experiments, e.g. in the selection of application schedules and other modifications of procedures[3].

In the case of low incidence responses Plaa[4] suggested the existence of subpopulations with special sensitivities against certain drugs. Typical examples are sporadically occurring reactions such as cholestatic jaundice, hepatitis, agranulocytosis and collagen disease.

In prehuman studies we are seeking actual and possible effects upon biological systems, and to estimate the likelihood of the substances affecting man in a similar manner. For drugs the acceptable level of side-effects must be related to the disease being treated and to the clinical efficacy and duration of administration. For most other substances the question is "by what factor is the acceptable daily intake (ADI) related to the minimal side-effect-producing level?" Food additives, atmospheric contaminants and most other non-medicines must have a very considerable margin of safety.

Following upon this preliminary assessment, one must consider the toxic reactions which are unpredictable from animal experimentation. Mention has been made already of subgroups with special sensitivities, but early human experimental work must be concerned with both predictable and unpredictable, as well as special sensitivities.

A review of adverse reactions to drugs in man indicates that they are connected most frequently with functional disturbances of the central and autonomic nervous system[5]. An example is the frequency with which hypotension is observed in man but not seen in quadruped animals. Another example of an unpredicted effect in man was that of oculo-mucocutaneous syndrome associated with the administration of practolol; the real significance of this emerged only after very extensive careful clinical monitoring, following preliminary sporadic reporting[6].

Predictive safety evaluation in man is therefore divided into initial studies designed to show safety prior to first release for use, followed by a post-marketing programme. The former is now subject to governmental regulation in almost all parts of the world; the latter is in its infancy.

CLINICAL STUDIES

The earliest clinical studies in man involve small numbers of normal subjects studied in great depth, and include pharmacokinetic, metabolic and toxicological observations. Studies begin with very small single doses in the case of medicine, say 0.01% of the predicted therapeutic dose in man. They are increased by stages until the therapeutic range is reached. In the case of food additives a similar starting percentage of the forecast daily intake is used.

The subsequent development of early studies in normal subjects is very dependent upon the type of substance being investigated, and whether it is to be used as a medicine or comes into contact with man as a contaminant, e.g. agricultural sprays. At this stage the question of deliberate administration to normal subjects until side-effects are produced is debatable. It is based upon the logic of animal toxicological testing where massive unrealistic doses are routinely given in order to determine target organs and the type of pathology resulting. In man, however, our aim is to demonstrate safety within the context of likely exposure. Provided that testing is conducted with levels of exposure sufficiently high in relation to the use, then the deliberate induction of side-effects is hard to justify.

In the early stages of gaining experience in man, each experiment is designed to give sufficient basic information to enable the next stage of development to be embarked upon.

Whatever the substance being tested the early stages of development of experimental studies in man follow the same basic pathway, i.e.:

1. single ascending doses, given by mode(s) of administration or exposure in man;
2. multiple dosing over a short period, 1 or 2 days;
3. multiple dosing for longer periods.

Not only are we seeking to establish safety, but also pharmacokinetic behaviour, metabolic pathways and steady states. In addition any local, general or toxicological effects are sought.

The design of these clinical studies is to some extent dependent upon animal data, upon past experience with similar compounds, upon general toxicological principles and upon what is practical and reasonable to undertake.

There is no better time for the closest of medical observations than in the early stages of human exposure. Certainly the maximum opportunity should be made to gain as much clinical information as possible at this stage without impairing the basic aim of the study[7].

The initial studies are invariably conducted using small numbers of normal subjects, with the consequent limitations of such data. It is still far too common, however, for people to embark upon this work using an uncontrolled open design, with the subsequent great difficulty in interpreting any data which may deviate slightly from normal. It is my opinion that, whenever possible, all studies should be controlled. The failure to do this (usually related to economic excuses) often leads to the repetition of the study. The lingering doubt remains in everyone's mind that even when the problem is not reproduced under controlled conditions a hazard may still exist. One can safely predict that regulatory bodies are not going to become less critical during the foreseeable future, and the difficulties of interpreting data produced under uncontrolled conditions can be almost insurmountable in certain circumstances.

In large-scale studies this can be even more disastrous. Recently we have experienced the very considerable difficulty of clarifying the initial impressions given by the results of an uncontrolled study. After reviewing data produced in the original work no untreated comparison group was found. However, data produced had been subject to measurements and statistical analyses which were wholly unjustified, and it was necessary to set up a completely new study, with a control group and with randomized treatments and strict control of diet and environment (and of the physicians and scientists making the measurements). After additional expense in both money and time, a clear picture emerged of a very safe compound.

PROSPECTIVE STUDIES

Once the preliminary small-scale, but very detailed, work has been completed, it is necessary to embark upon the larger-scale studies that are aimed at giving sufficient information regarding safety to enable a compound to be used - either under special conditions in the case of certain medicines, or for general use. This does not necessarily mean that every possible side-effect has been determined, but that an acceptable degree of safety can be reasonably predicted. The major considerations are:

1. the type and design of the study(ies),
2. the sample size,
3. special considerations,
4. quality assurance.

THE TYPE AND DESIGN OF THE STUDY

It has already been stressed that uncontrolled studies contribute little more than being able to say at best that a number of subjects have received a substance with no apparent ill-effect and, in the case of a medicine, a percentage have improved or deteriorated and so on. At worst one can reveal changes, for example in clotting factors, which are utterly inexplicable and may or may not mean the substance is dangerous. Whatever the ultimate explanation, a carefully controlled study will avoid many of these difficulties. This particularly applies when large numbers of subjects are involved over long periods of time, which is essential at this stage of clinical evaluation.

Pocock[8] has described the many aspects of organizing and designing clinical trials. Although there are many subtleties of design and means of extracting statistically significant data from the minimal clinical information, very often the results are not clinically reassuring, and there can be no substitute for experience, i.e. numbers of carefully observed subjects.

SAMPLE SIZE

In any predictive study the sample size must always be as large as is practicable. It may be that it is simply not possible to study large numbers of people suffering from a particular disease, but for other than medicines there is really little excuse for not obtaining large-sized samples. Often the numbers of subjects are determined by the length of time or amount of money available resulting in an arbitrary number being chosen. Reviews of general medical publications and clinical trials have shown that many studies are too small to have a reasonable chance of detecting benefits or hazards[9-11].

The words "statistical significance" are wholly acceptable, but in predicitive clinical trials the object is to reduce an acceptable level of risk of obtaining a misleading result by making statistical significance and clinical importance coincide as nearly as possible.

For a medicine the primary requirement is for the physician to specify the acceptable level of safety in relation to the condition being treated; for other substances the acceptable level of incidence of any adverse effect (or, more specifically, which adverse effects) must be minuscule in relation to the level of exposure.

Before starting any study there must be a determination of the power of the study in order to produce a meaningful result. Several graphs for the calculation of sample size are available[12-14] and a simple nomogram is available for continuous variables[15]. The calculated size of a sample refers to subjects completing the study rather than those entering it, so that allowances should be made for likely drop-outs.

Trials carried out in too few subjects may fail to detect the effects being sought, added to which is the danger of false-positive findings. There have been several instances where conflicting results from a large number of small trials have led to great uncertainty about the benefit of particular treatments.

It may be reasonable to pool the results from several small trials and make a statistical analysis, but in general each study should be designed to be self-sufficient and to answer the questions being asked. A few large-scale multi-centre studies are always better than numerous small ones.

When devising studies it is common for us all to overestimate the number of subjects available and in clinical studies Munch's Third Law always applies: "estimates for patients eligible for study in a given clinic must be divided by ten to arrive at a true estimate"[16].

SPECIAL CONSIDERATIONS

It may be known that certain related chemicals have a particular effect upon some animal species, e.g. neurotoxicity, although the compound under investigation may show no such animal toxicity. It is always worthwhile considering what special investigations should be made and incorporated, not only into early work, but in the large-scale studies, e.g. ophthalmological tests, slit lamp examination, and phoria measurements. In the case of the sweetener, aspartame, special studies were made in relation to central nervous effects because of the presence of neurotransmitters. Moreover with all sweeteners the effect upon carbohydrate absorption, insulin production and the effects upon diabetics (both insulin- and non-insulin-dependent) should be studied carefully.

Formally devised studies may also be of value in assessing mutagenic effects. Bridges et al.[17] reviewed the evidence of the mutagenic effects of cigarette smoking. The best-documented effects which are considered genetic or closely related to genetic events are:

1. increase in numbers of morphologically abnormal sperm;
2. increased frequency of sister-chromatid exchanges in peripheral lymphocytes;
3. an increase in perinatal mortality amongst the children of

smoking fathers;
4.   an increase in the number of major congenital malformations amongst the children of smoking fathers.

These observations do not establish causality, and can be considered only to indicate a preliminary correlation between cigarette smoking and these events. It needs further confirmation.

A further example of special study is the relationship between vinylchloride and mutagenicity. There is an increase in fetal loss amongst workers exposed to vinylchloride, but no dose-effect correlation has been established, and it is known that vinylchloride produces chromosomal aberrations but does not produce dominant lethal effects in mice; nor does it produce the expected increase in congenital abnormalities one would expect with high fetal wastage.

It is encumbent upon future clinical assessments to provide answers not only in relation to general acceptability and tolerance, but to other special circumstances such as drug and food interaction, and behavioural changes with age, as well as with disease.

These are but a few examples of special considerations which must be made in relation to the predictive value of clinical studies. Each substance needs its own careful, scientific appraisal.

QUALITY ASSURANCE

Good laboratory practices (GLPs), standard operating procedures (SOPs), and very careful quality assurance programmes are well established in the laboratory. In clinical trials and practice the concept of quality assurance is only just starting to be established.

In normal volunteer studies quality assurance in subject selection, control of environment, diet and dosing are all attainable. The pressure of a quality assurance manager without prior notice, randomly checking on the progress and conduct of a study, has a salutary effect upon those carrying out the work.

Outside the confines of the clinical pharmacology unit, however, quality assurance in clinical studies is in its infancy, and is undoubtedly an area which will develop considerably over the next decade. The question of subject compliance has been recognized for many years, but even under hospital conditions there can be wide margins of variation never hinted at in reports.

A very simple example is the time of administration of medicines. In a series of observations made in a general hospital we discovered that this time could vary by as much as plus or minus 2 hours. Although this may not have been of clinical significance in the general treatment of patients, and depended upon the demands of the wards, in clinical research it was quite intolerable. Once this had been explained to the nursing staff, co-operation was exceedingly good.

It is very difficult to standardize procedures from one centre to another, but the development of this aspect of quality in clinical studies is essential, particularly since the immediate future undoubtedly will be in fewer, larger, and better controlled studies.

POST-MARKETING

Although in the future clinical studies will be aimed at answering the more demanding questions already being anticipated, once a substance has been released for general use, a means of post-marketing clinical observation is needed.

Post-marketing drug monitoring is still in its infancy. The many thoughts and practices about the problem have been well described[18]. Post-marketing clinical observations in other areas are very much dependent upon anecdotal reporting, and it is in this area that clinical study will have to develop. We have a fine tradition of epidemiological study in disease. The same care is needed to set up post-marketing studies, not only in relation to medicines, but in relation to food additives, agrochemicals and almost any environmental contaminant.

Exactly how this will be achieved is not clear, but it is certain that both industry and government can no longer be "opponents". Regulatory bodies need the support and encouragement of government, not the mutual antagonism which is still so common. Until these psychological and moral barriers are down I doubt whether much progress will be made in this direction, although society will eventually force it upon both parties.

In the future predicitive clinical evaluation will exploit the rapidly developing new techniques of biological and chemical assay. It will be asked to answer more demanding questions in relation to toxicity, to short- and long-term effects and to special circumstances.

The design of studies will need to provide the information society can reasonably expect before a product is released, and can reasonably expect after a product has become available.

The trend in most areas will be towards fewer studies involving large numbers of subjects combining statistical with clinical significance. They will be controlled studies and subject to very high standards of quality control.

Post-marketing clinical observations will form an important part in developing an overall balanced picture.

Society will accept risks it has chosen to take such as smoking and car driving - but it dislikes risks that are thrust upon it.

REFERENCES

1. Williams, CJ and Carter, SK (1978). Management of trials in the development of cancer chemotherapy. Br J Cancer, 37, 434-47

2. Baeder, C (1980). Non-human primates und ihre Bedeutung für die chronischen Toxizitätsstudien. In: Schneiders, B and Grossdanoff, P (eds) Zur Problamatik von Chronisehen Toxizitatsprufungen. (Berlin: AMI Berichte. Dietrich Reimer Verlag). pp. 29-32

3. Mitchell, JR and Jollow, DJ (1974). Metabolic activation of acetaminophen, furosemide and activation of acetaminophen, furosemide and isoniazid to hepatotoxic substances. In: Morselli, PI, Garattini, S and Cohen, SN. (eds) Drug Interac-

tions. (New York: Raven Press) pp. 65-79

4. Plaa, GL (1978). The problems of low-incidence response. In: Plaa, GL and Duncan, WAM (eds) Proc First Int Congr Toxicol. (New York, San Francisco and London: Academic Press) pp. 207-19

5. Zbinden, G (1966). Toxicology of new drugs. In: Damm, HC, Besch, PK and Goldwyn, AJ (eds) The Handbook of Biochemistry and Biophysics. (Cleveland and New York: The World Publishing Company) pp. 459-511

6. Leading article (1977). Hazards of non-practolol beta-blockers. Br Med J, 1, 39-77

7. Standard Operating Procedure (1986). Normal Subject Studies. (England, Medical Science Research)

8. Pocock, SJ (1984). Clinical Trials: A Practical Approach. (Chichester: John Wiley)

9. Hall, JC (1982). The other side of statistical significance: a review of type II errors in the Australian Medical Literature. Aust NZ J Med, 12, 7-9

10. Reed, JF and Slaichert, W (1981). Statistical proof in inconclusive "negative" trials. Arch Intern Med, 141, 1307-10

11. Freiman, JA, Chalmers, TC, Smith, H Jnr and Kuebler, RR (1978). The importance of both the type II error and sample size in the design and interpretation of the randomised controlled trial. N Engl J Med, 299, 690-4

12. Aleong, J and Bartlett, DE (1979). Improved graphs for calculating sample sizes when comparing two independent binomial distributions. Biometrics, 35, 875-81

13. Boag, JW, Haybittle, JL, Fowler, JF and Emery, EW (1971). The number of patients required in a clinical trial. Br J Radiol, 44, 122-5

14. Mould, RF (1979). Clinical trial design in cancer. Clin Radiol, 30, 371-81

15. Altman, DG (1982). How large a sample? In: Gore, SM and Altman, DG (eds) Statistics in Practice. pp. 6-8. (London: British Medical Association)

16. Kessler, A and Standley, CC (1980). International trials and tribulations. In: Turner, P (ed.) Proceedings of the First World Congress of Clinical Pharmacology and Therapeutics. (London: MacMillan) pp. 483-8

17. Bridges, BA, Clemmesen, S and Sugimura, T (1979). Mutagenic effects of cigarette smoking. Mutation Res, 65, 71-81

18. Inman, WHI (ed) (1980). Monitoring for Drug Safety. (Lancaster: MTP Press)

12

Artificial Sweeteners and the Control of Appetite: Implications for the Eating Disorders

J. E. BLUNDELL and A. J. HILL

Artificial sweeteners constitute an important class of food additives which are being used in ever-increasing amounts. The wide dissemination of these agents and their likely ingestion in large quantities by certain sub-groups of consumers makes it essential to consider the safety of artificial sweeteners not only with regard to their possible behavioural toxicity (induction of pathology) but with regard also to their impact on the natural physiological mechanisms regulating nutrient and fluid intake. This second type of action is unlikely to bring about observable physical damage but may lead to chronic readjustment (or maladjustment) of physiological regulation, in turn leading to abnormalities in patterns of eating and the expression of appetite. For this reason artificial sweeteners are here considered in relation to a socially important category of psychiatric disturbance - the eating disorders.

BACKGROUND TO EATING DISORDERS

For more than 50 years obesity has been a major health hazard in westernized civilized societies. In America it has been estimated that more than 35 million people may be regarded as suffering from mild obesity and approximately 2.5 million from severe overweight[1]. In the UK, Garrow[2] has estimated that approximately 25% of the population suffer from mild obesity (body mass index 30 or more). Although there seems to be a large biological component[3] in obesity it is not known whether the genetic potential becomes manifest through an increase in energy input (overeating) or a deficit in energy expenditure. Recent evidence suggests that fat people on the average do take in more calories than normal weight controls and consume larger meals[4]. Studies on animals clearly indicate an influence of nutritional factors on the development of obesity; this becomes clearly apparent when animals are fed highly refined, high fat diets of foods normally eaten by man[5,6]. In addition it has been alleged that a sizeable fraction of obese individuals show a craving for carbohydrates[7]. Certainly in part, then, obesity in-

263

volves aberrant levels of energy intake, patterns of consumption or nutrient selection.

Over the past 10 years there has been a marked increase in the other disorders of eating - anorexia nervosa and bulimia nervosa. The first of these disorders is clearly characterized, and has been known since the nineteenth century. Bulimia initially emerged as a sub-group of anorexia nervosa but was later identified as a separate condition by Russell[8]. In the following year it was officially recognized as a new eating disorder and appeared in the Diagnostic and Statistical Manual[9] produced by the American Psychiatric Association (DSM-III, 1980). This disorder has been termed bulimia (DSM-III), bulimia nervosa[8], bulimarexia[10] or dietary chaos syndrome[11]. The condition is characterized by powerful, intractable urges to eat, the morbid fear of becoming fat and the avoidance of fattening food together with the use of vomiting, purgatives or both[12]. It occurs largely in young adult women aged between 15 and 40. Together with the syndrome of binge eating its occurrence in the population is high. It seems that substantial numbers (over 50%) of overweight patients engage in binge eating on occasions[13]. Recent surveys of college populations have found a high incidence (13-67%) of self-reported binge eating in "normal" non-clinical samples[14-16]. In the UK Cooper and Fairburn[17] reported that 1.9% of women attending a family planning clinic showed the full diagnostic criteria for bulimia nervosa and a much larger proportion (26.4%) engaged in bingeing together with occasional vomiting (6.5%) or use of laxatives as a form of weight control. It is clear that eating disorders now constitute one of the most prevalent and disabling conditions afflicting young adults and children - particularly females. The disorder is not restricted to a change in eating habits but carries with it severe states of depression and anxiety. At the present time little is known for certain about the genesis or natural history of the eating disorders.

IMPORTANCE OF DIETING

The present era can be regarded as a time of crisis in which excessive attention is being directed toward the avoidance of obesity and the attainment of culturally defined idealized body shapes. The crisis arises because of a combination of factors: (a) the very high prevalance of obesity, (b) strong cultural disapproval of fatness and the exertion of social pressure on individuals (particularly women) to reduce plumpness or to avoid becoming fat, and (c) the lack of any safe, effective and reliable procedures for the treatment of obesity on the scale required[18]. This set of circumstances has produced two major consequences. First, many individuals (mainly women) devote excessive time to dietary control and slimming practices in an effort to achieve or to maintain a culturally acceptable low weight. The second, and linked consequence, is that many women have adopted desperate measures, including unregulated fasting, vomiting and the use of purges and laxatives. In certain places this has reached almost epidemic proportions[19]. Accordingly, the excessive concern about body shape and the awareness of fatness coupled with a lack of effective treatment had led to a massive increase in a class of eating disorders which are far more prevalent than previously believed[17]. Indeed it has been argued that there is a causal relationship between dieting and bulimia[20].

The tendency to diet can be conceptualized as the exercise of restraint, and this notion can be measured objectively by means of a short questionnaire[21,22]. One major consequence of restraint is that a cognitive control comes to dominate physiological regulatory processes. For example undereating normally promotes an increased motivation to eat and a tendency to overeat if food becomes readily available. In restrained individuals this motivational disposition is held in check but under particular circumstances, such as the occurrence of stress, the blockade of motivation can be dissipated. This inhibition of inhibition (or disinhibition) leads to the release of motivation and overeating (known as counter-regulatory overeating). Accordingly individuals who are restricting their food intake, by whatever strategy, exist in a chronic state of hunger which may range from mild to severe.

HUNGER, SATIATION AND SATIETY IN THE CONTROL OF EATING

It appears self-evident that our patterns of food consumption are related to cycles of hunger and satiation. However it is also clear that a state of hunger defined as energy depletion (or food restriction) is not a **necessary** condition for eating. Hunger may be prompted by the appearance of palatable food[23] and in animals marked overeating and obesity can be provoked merely by offering rats a highly palatable array of snack foods[5]. Moreover hunger cannot be said to be a **sufficient** condition for eating, since dieters and patients with anorexia nervosa experience strong feelings of hunger but the natural expression of this in eating is inhibited. However, these accounts draw attention to a severe problem facing many individuals. People who are undereating (by eating calorie-restricted foods, or by fasting for long periods) will experience hunger which, in the face of highly palatable and tempting foods, will be enhanced. Consequently, restrictors (or restrainers) will experience a strong urge to eat generated from more than one source. Hunger can be measured objectively on visual-analogue rating scales[24] and in experimental situations can be shown to correlate highly with the amount of food eaten[25].

Satiation is a term with a strict technical definition, and it refers to the process of terminating eating as a consequence of food ingestion[26,27]. This process develops and strengthens during the course of a meal and normally is composed of a number of elements. These include (a) a diminution in subjectively perceived hunger, (b) increase in feelings of stomach fullness, (c) decrease in the amount of food wished to be eaten (all of which can be objectively rated[24]) and (d) decrease in the perceived pleasantness of food. This last phenomenon is referred to as alliesthesia - literally changed sensation - and has been empirically defined by the French physiologist Michel Cabanac[28]. The time course of alliesthesia regarded as a change in the hedonic value (rated pleasantness) of a food or a test solution can be objectively monitored. Under normal circumstances, then, the phenomenon of satiation comprises co-ordinated temporal changes in the perceived hedonic value of food, the experienced degree of fullness and the intensity of hunger. Acting conjointly these elements constitute a psychobiological pool of information which brings eating to a halt - this process is termed satiation. Once a period of eating (meal or snack) has ended, then the further maintenance of inhibition over eating is referred to as the state of satiety. This state is composed of those elements which bring about satiation, and is associated with an increase in subjectively perceived sedation, together with diminished psychophysical indices of arousal. Satiety dissipates over time and gradually gives way to hunger.

The phenomenology of hunger, satiation and satiety can be clearly linked to physiological changes which accompany ingestion. For example changes in the perceived pleasantness of the taste of foods or sweet solutions (alliesthesia) are related to blood levels of blood glucose[29] which follows the consumption of a glucose or sugar load. In addition changes in perceived hunger are related to the number of calories consumed in a meal or snack. Although the situation is somewhat complex under normal circumstances, changes in perceived hunger and satiation are natural responses to the metabolic and sensory properties of foods. If our conscious sensations are to play any role in the regulation of energy intake then a systematic relationship of this type is a logical necessity. The capacity of foods to meet bodily needs must be reflected in conscious feelings of appetite which we apparently use to control the amount of food we ingest and the distribution of eating over time. It is therefore relevant to ask what would happen if the operation of this natural psychobiological mechanism is undermined in some way?

FOOD AND SLIMMING

One way in which individuals can personally intervene in their own psychobiological functioning is to consciously and deliberately restrict their own intake of calories. This can be done for political motives, as in the case of hunger strikers, or for conformity, as in the case of those people attempting to make their body shape conform to the cosmetic requirements of society. In both of these instances individuals must exert a direct control over their behaviour and repress or deny the feelings of hunger which signal their state of need. For example, there is good evidence that patients with anorexia nervosa experience strong feelings of hunger but manage to resist the powerful urge to eat.

In order to help these millions of individuals who are attempting to lose weight (or to avoid gaining it) an entire industry has developed to furnish slimming aids. Many of these aids are food products. The rationale is that, by eating foods which have bulk but contain fewer calories, individuals are relieved of the need to restrict the total amount of food consumed. In other words, individuals can appear to eat normally (usual bulk of food eaten) but they will actually consume fewer calories. How effective is this strategy?

As noted in the previous section the sensation of hunger is linked to the metabolic properties of foods, one aspect of which is the calorific content or energy density. Therefore if individuals are eating the same bulk of food but fewer calories they should experience more intense hunger. This hypothesis can be tested in a simple experiment. In the history of research on the control of food intake a number of investigations have assessed the capacity of individuals to monitor calories and to adjust intake in accordance with calorific needs. Many of these studies have used highly unusual feeding situations, including the use of liquid foods and sucking solutions from a hidden reservoir, etc. Recently we have examined the issue using real proprietary foods which are readily available to the public[30]. The foods were four frozen meals, two of which contained approximately 440 and two of which contained only 260 calories. When presented to the subjects the meals were indistinguishable in terms of bulk and palatability. The results of the study showed that after eating the low-calorie food subjects showed a higher post-meal level of hunger - this can be termed residual hunger. When given the opportunity to eat freely later in the day these subjects actually consumed more food. This study strongly suggests that people eating low-calorie foods will be left with strong feelings of hunger which, if not checked, will tend to promote additional eating. Consequently the problem facing many people using slimming products is not how to eat less food but how to deal with the hunger which arises from under-consumption of calories. It is in this context that it is important to examine the effects of sweetening agents which are intended to play a role in the control of calorie intake.

ROLE OF SWEETNESS IN EATING

Sweetness is a powerful psychobiological phenomenon which has both physiological and cultural significance, and it exerts strong effects on the pattern of food consumption. First, a preference for sweet-tasting substances is one innate disposition of many animals including man. Sweet-tasting substances are inherently pleasurable and can act as potent rewards. Consequently, on the basis of sensory qualities alone, the sweetness of a food will tend to promote its ingestion.

Moreover, there are good biological reasons for the existence of this phenomenon. In nature the sweet taste is almost invariably linked to high-calorie nutritionally useful commodities. Normally sweet-tasting foods can be readily consumed and are an important source of energy. Accordingly in naturally occurring food products there is a link between sweet taste and calorific properties. This association between the taste of a food and its metabolic value is important in the control of energy intake. One way in which organisms (including man) control episodes of eating is by predicting caloric value on the basis of taste (e.g. ref. 31). There is good evidence that the biological system is innately programmed to establish links between cues (taste sensations) and consequences (metabolic effects of food), and this constitutes a part of the biological wisdom of the body (e.g. ref. 32). The operation of this system allows organisms to anticipate the effects of food ingestion in advance of digestion and absorption of the products. The cephalic phase reflex is the term given to anticipatory responses which prepare the gastrointestinal system for the arrival of food. Such responses may be detected at various levels of the system including salivary secretion, gastric outflow and pancreatic secretion. In man the sight and smell of food are sufficiently potent stimuli to trigger cephalic phase insulin responses[33,34]. In rats the taste of saccharine can provoke a cephalic phase insulin response[35].

The universal reward value of sweet foods, together with the link between the sweet taste and energy value of foods, means that the phenomenon of sweetness occupies a central role in the control of consumption. However it is pertinent to ask what would happen if the sweet taste of a food could be uncoupled from its natural metabolic consequences?

Artificial sweeteners and the psychobiological system

The potent rewarding capacity of the sweet taste means that the consumption of foods can be increased by making them sweet. This can be readily demonstrated in rats, for example, by the addition of saccharine to the bland-tasting powdered chow. This fact has also been used by the food industry; increasing the palatability of a product by intensifying the sweetness will augment the attractiveness of a food and thereby tend to promote its consumption. Palatability is one of the most important dimensions controlling short-term intake in man.

However, when the palatability of low-calorie food is artificially raised by the addition of an intense sweetening agent then the natural link between sweetness and energy density is dissipated. The sweet taste can no longer be used as a predictor of metabolic value. This disengagement can lead to a disruption of a natural biological control system. Consequently it can be seen that the continued use of artificial sweetening agents could give rise to a number of consequences concerning eating. First, raising palatability will tend to enhance consumption. Second, the enhanced consumption of low-calorie foods will lead to a reservoir of residual hunger, i.e. people may eat considerable amounts but be left with a feeling of hunger. Third, sweeteners will almost certainly trigger cephalic phase responses in anticipation of energy input. Fourth, there is the likelihood of corrupting a natural biological regulatory system.

At the present time the family of artificial sweeteners is made up of saccharine, acesulphame-K, aspartame and certain lesser-known compounds such as stevioside and thaumatin. Aspartame is of particular interest because of its dipeptide composition. This feature may give rise to additional effects upon the control of food intake.

Aspartame and appetite: a case study

Aspartame is an intense sweetener with a potency of 200 times that of sucrose. It is composed of two amino acids - phenylalanine and aspartic acid - and its discovery was serendipitous. This particular composition means that aspartame (Candarel, Nutrasweet) may influence feeding control mechanisms in a variety of ways. For example phenylalanine is known to release cholecystokinin[48], a hormone released from the duodenum following food consumption. There is clear evidence that exogenous administration of cholecystokinin in both animals[36] and man[37] leads to a marked inhibition of food intake with a profile which resembles the natural development of satiation. Consequently, cholecystokinin may well be an endogenous anorectic substance. The release of this hormone by phenylalanine would therefore tend to suppress appetite and inhibit food consumption. On the other hand phenylalanine is a precursor of the catecholamine neurotransmitters dopamine and noradrenaline, and an increase in plasma levels of phenylalanine could lead to increased brain levels and to enhanced catecholamine synthesis. Indeed there is evidence from animal studies that the administration of aspartame is associated with large increases in whole-brain concentrations of phenylalanine and tyrosine[7,38]. Moreover, a further study has indicated that increases in the neurotransmitters noradrenaline and dopamine were observed in various brain regions after oral dosing of aspartame[39]. A dose-related increase in noradrenaline was found in the hypothalamus. This is the region where noradrenergic receptors are known to be crucially involved in the control of feeding patterns and nutrient selection[40]. Consequently, it can be deduced that, as a result of the chemical composition of aspartame on certain hormones and neurotransmitters, this agent could either increase or decrease food intake. These effects, together with those arising from the uncoupling of sweet taste and metabolic consequences, could generate a rather unusual profile of changes in the processes of hunger and satiation which normally control our patterns of eating.

These possibilities have been tested in a series of experiments in which the effects of aspartame were compared with the effects produced by energy-rich sweeteners such as glucose or sucrose. The experiments employed measures of behaviour and perception widely regarded as reflecting the intensity of satiation and satiety. For example changes in the perceived pleasantness of stimuli (alliesthesia) were combined with ratings of the motivation to eat and with preferences for particular foods.

In the first study 50 young adults (35 females, 15 males) of normal weght for height were tested. A between-subjects design was used and subjects received one of the following three loads.

A.   50 g glucose dissolved in 200 ml tap water (N=17);

B.   162 mg aspartame (nine tablets of Candarel) in 200 ml water (N=17);

C.   200 ml tap water (N=16).

Subjects made ratings of pleasantness and intensity of the sucrose solution on 100 mm visual analogue rating scales (providing a score of 0-100). Two booklets containing sufficient scales for the experiment were provided. One required subjects to rate the pleasantness of the sweet solution upon scales which were word-anchored by the phrases "extremely pleasant" and "extremely unpleasant". On the other subjects judged the intensity of the solution on scales ranging from "extremely weak" to "extremely strong". Ratings of **motivation to eat** were made on 100 mm visual analogue scales (word anchored at either end) in the following order. They were: (a) "How strong is your desire to eat?" (Very strong-Very weak); (b) "How hungry do you feel?" (As hungry as I have ever felt-Not at all hungry); (c) "How full do you feel?" (Very full-Not at all full) and (d) "How much food do you think you could eat?" (A large amount-Nothing at all). This last rating is called prospective consumption.

Subjects attended the laboratory immediately after lunch at 2 o'clock in the afternoon. They were instructed how to complete each of the assessments and were asked to make their first ratings of motivation to eat. They then collected a small plastic cup containing approximately 10 ml of the standard sucrose solution. They were told to take all of the tastant into their mouth and to keep it there for a few seconds, tasting it fully before spitting it out into a sink. Subjects immediately made ratings of the pleasantness and intensity of the taste, turning over each scale once completed to prevent future referral. These ratings were the baseline measurements. Subjects were then randomly assigned to one of the three load conditions (A, B or C) and 2 minutes after making their baseline judgements were required to consume the contents of their beaker within the period of a minute. Ten minutes after the load subjects again rated their motivation to eat, and sampled and rated the sucrose solution. Ratings of eating motivation were always completed prior to the rating of taste. This procedure was continued at 10-minute intervals for 1 hour. During this time subjects were asked not to discuss the experiment and not to smoke or eat until the completion of the study. Subjects were unaware that the tastants sampled at each 10-minute period were identical.

The result of consuming loads of glucose, aspartame and water on perceived pleasantness and intensity of a sweet taste are shown in Figure 12.1. There was a highly significant effect of the glucose load on ratings of pleasantness (F[6,96] = 5.952, p<0.01). On every occasion after the load the pleasantness of sucrose was significantly lower than baseline. Aspartame also significantly reduced the pleasantness of sucrose (F[6,96] = 2.741, p<0.05), although the extent of this change was about half of that experienced by the subjects in the glucose condition. Consuming an equal volume of water did not alter subjects' perception of pleasantness. Neither were there any effects of load upon ratings of intensity, i.e. altered perception of pleasantness was not due to changes in the perception of intensity.

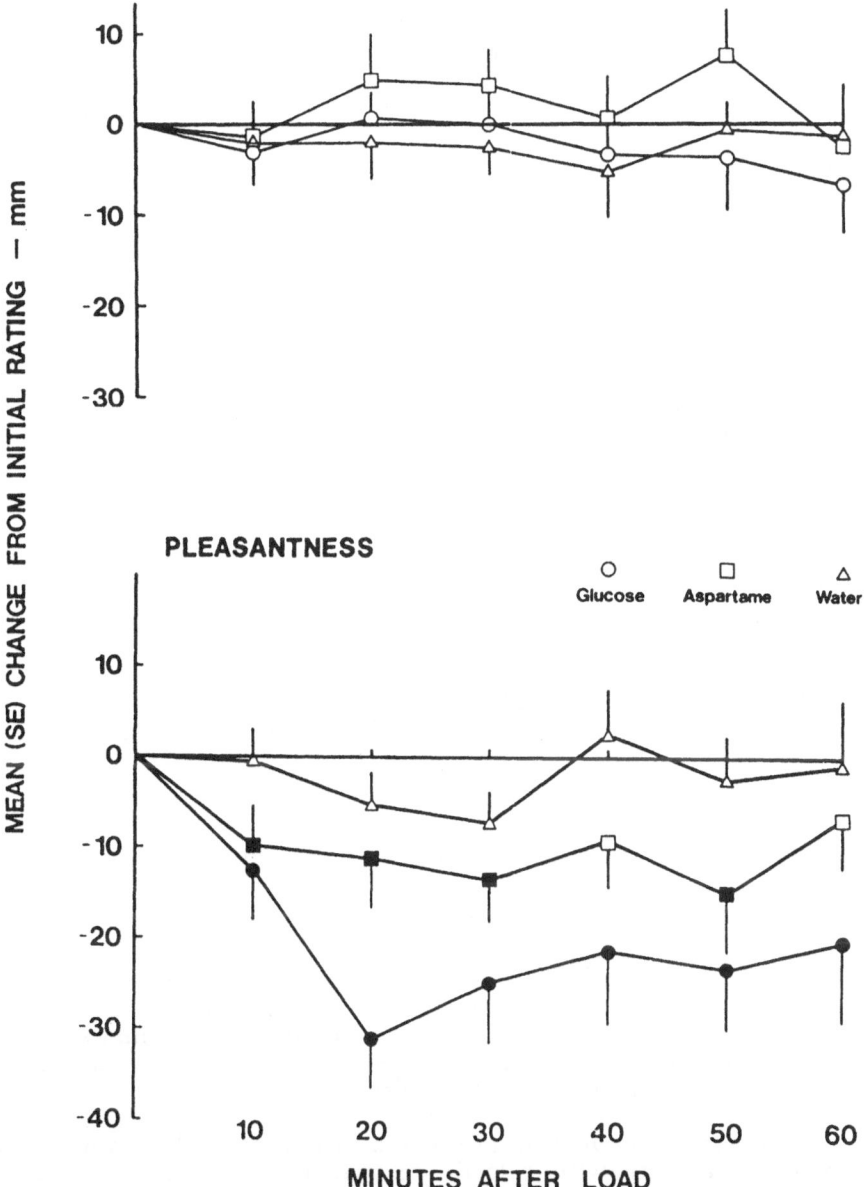

Figure 12.1 The effect of consuming glucose (circles), aspartame (squares) or water (triangles) upon the perceived intensity and pleasantness of sucrose at 10-minute intervals after the loads. Closed symbols indicate a significant change from baseline

Regarding the changes in motivation the treatments did not produce massive effects. This is because subjects had recently eaten and motivation to eat was relatively low. The data are shown in Figure 12.2. It can be seen that the changes produced by aspartame and glucose were invariably in opposite directions. The clearest separation occurred in ratings of prospective consumption where glucose reduced subjects' estimates of how much food they could eat (significant at 40 minutes), while aspartame increased this rating (significant at 50 minutes). Overall, there was a clear tendency for glucose to reduce ratings of hunger and appetite and to increase fullness, whereas aspartame acted in the opposite direction.

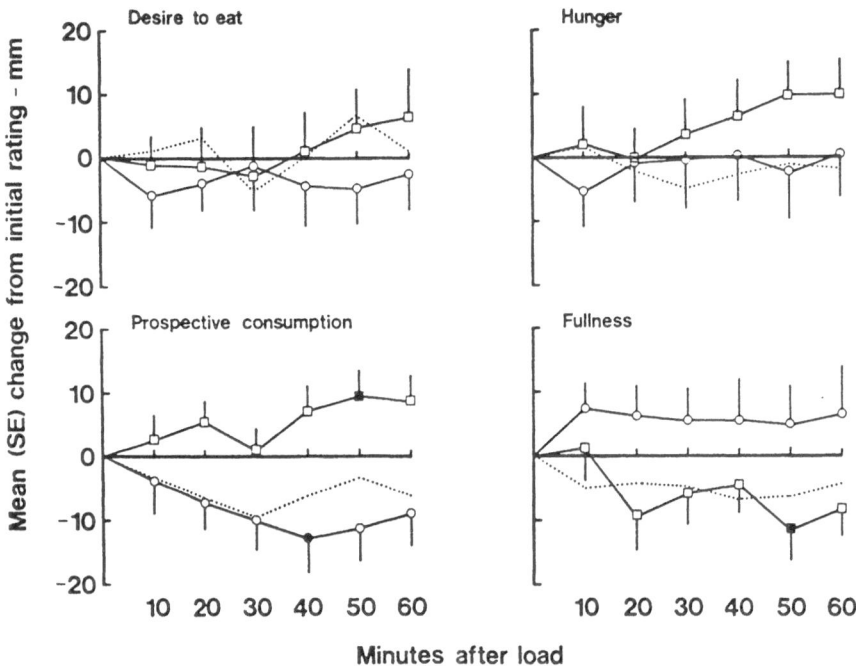

Figure 12.2 The effect of consuming glucose (circles), aspartame (squares) or water (dotted line) upon ratings of desire to eat, prospective consumption, hunger and fullness at 10-minute intervals after the loads. Statistically significant changes are indicated by closed symbols

Consequently in this study the oral glucose load which combined sweet taste with calorific properties produced a consistent effect upon the measures of satiation. Glucose markedly reduced the perceived pleasantness of sweet solutions, decreased measures of hunger and appetite and increased ratings of fullness. In contrast, aspartame gave rise to an ambiguous profile of effects. On one hand the aspartame load produced a moderate negative alliesthesia (decreased perceived pleasantness of sweetness) indicative of mild satiation, whilst on the other hand this agent tended to augment ratings of motivation (indicating a mild stimulation of appetite).

In a further study we have explored further the effects of aspartame and glucose on motivational measures in subjects who had been instructed to refrain from eating for 3 hours, and who therefore began the experiment in a hungry state. The results set out in Figure 12.3 indicate the changes in motivation which occurred at 30, 60 and 90 minutes after consuming the loads. This experiment used a within-subjects design so that the same subjects were tested under all three conditions (glucose, aspartame - concentrations as in the previous study - and water).

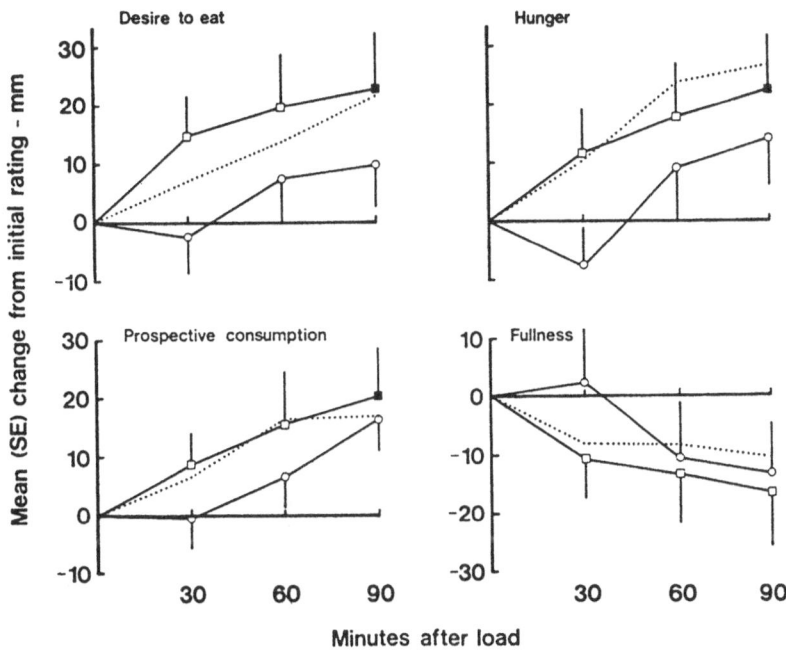

Figure 12.3 Effect of glucose (circles), aspartame (squares) or water (dotted line) upon motivational ratings 30, 60 and 90 minutes after the loads in subjects who had not eaten for 3 hours. Closed symbols indicate a significant change from baseline

Changes in ratings following the water load indicate that subjects became more hungry and less full over the 90-minute experimental period. This was entirely expected since these subjects were hungry at the start of the experiment. Over the first 30 minutes the glucose load reduced ratings of hunger and appetite and slightly increased feelings of fullness. Thereafter the glucose load markedly suppressed the motivation to eat compared with the control treatment (water load). In contrast aspartame did not suppress appetite or hunger at any interval; on the contrary aspartame tended to augment the rated motivation to eat and to lessen feelings of fullness.

Consequently in this study the non-calorific aspartame load failed to attenuate in any way the subjects' ratings of appetite, and at the end of the 90-minute test period subjects were left with a sizeable "residual hunger". From other experiments in which hunger ratings correlate well with food consumed (e.g. ref. 30) it can be deduced that this high level of residual hunger would give rise to increased food consumption.

Effects of aspartame and sucrose on appetite

In a further study in this series we have compared the effects of aspartame with those produced by the natural sweetening agent against which all artificial sweeteners are compared - namely sucrose. The general design of the study was similar to those described above. A within-subjects design was used and all subjects were female. They were tested following a 2-hour period of not eating. The four treatment conditions were as follows:

A.   50 g sucrose dissolved in 200 ml tap water;

B.   288 mg aspartame (16 tablets of candarel) in 200 ml water, calibrated so as to be of equal sweetness to the sucrose load;

C.   200 ml tap water;

D.   no ingestion

These treatments therefore had the following properties:

	Volume	Sweetness	Calories
A	Yes	Yes	Yes (188 kcal)
B	Yes	Yes	No (7 kcal - negligible)
C	Yes	No	No
D	No	No	No

The results of this experiment indicate that the sucrose load produced a consistent and synchronized effect on all measures of satiation. As predicted the sucrose load brought about a consistent decrease in ratings of pleasantness (i.e. moderate negative alliesthesia) together with a marked suppression of hunger and desire to eat and an increase in fullness. The effects for aspartame were quite different. Interestingly this high dose of aspartame (288 mg - twice the concentration used in our previous experiments) did not produce a stronger decrease in ratings of pleasantness - in fact only a rather weak negative alliesthesia was observed. This may indicate a rather unusual dose-response function for aspartame. (Indeed, in an unpublished study we have noted that this high concentration of aspartame produced more variable responses than the lower-strength solution - 162 mg in 200 ml.) For measures of motivation the effects of aspartame were similar to those for the water load and control condition. Over the course of the 60-minute test period aspartame gave rise to a significant increase (from baseline) in hunger and a decrease in fullness. Oddly aspartame produced one aberrant response - a significant decrease in rating of desire to eat at the 10-minute test point. This transient effect was reversed over the ensuing portion of the test period.

An interesting profile of changes emerged from the analysis of the food checklist responses. In keeping with the decrease in ratings of hunger and appetite the sucrose load gave rise to a small negative shift in the checking of food items (Figure 12.4). In contrast all other treatments gave rise to increases with the largest effect produced by aspartame. In other studies we have reported strong positive correlations between hunger, actual food consumption and checklist scores. Therefore these data suggest that this dose of aspartame is producing a mild facilitative effect on appetite.

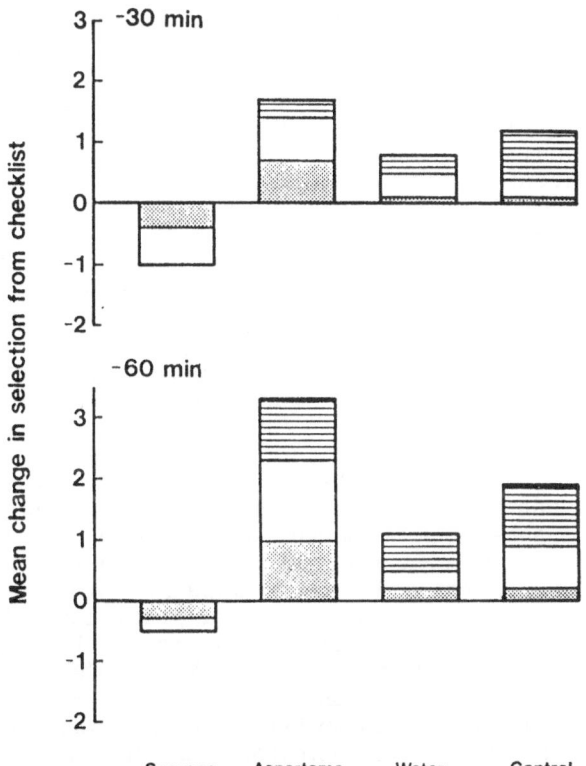

Figure 12.4 The effect of treatments on the selection of high-carbohydrate (stippled columns), high-fat (plain columns) and high-protein (graded columns) food items from the food preference checklist at 30 and 60 minutes after ingestion. The increase in selected items following aspartame is significant at 60 minutes (p<0.05)

Taken together the effects of sucrose demonstrated in this experiment are similar to those noted previously for glucose. A sweet and calorific load gave rise to a constellation of effects on measures of satiation which are consistent. In contrast aspartame, in this experiment, produced an ambiguous profile. Surprisingly, this high concentration of aspartame produced only a weak negative alliesthesia - indicating a very mild satiating effect. The pattern of effects for the motivational ratings showed the opposite effect - a slight facilitation of appetite but with one short-lived aberrant response. The checklist scores indicated a tendency to promote appetite.

IMPLICATIONS: UNCOUPLING SWEETNESS AND CALORIES

In all of the experiments described above subjects given oral loads of solutions high on sweetness and in calories displayed a consistent profile of responses. Measures of satiation, including hedonic ratings, hunger motivation scales and the food item checklist, all revealed a concerted pattern of effects. Consistent profiles were also displayed by treatments which were devoid of calories and sweetness. These conditions (water load or no ingestion) did not produce a decline in hedonic ratings (of the sucrose test solutions) and during the course of the testing period (60 minutes) appetitive motivation increased - subjects began to feel more hungry and less full. Consequently, when sweetness and calories co-vary consistent effects on satiation are disclosed. What happens when sweetness and calories are experimentally disengaged?

Artificial sweeteners provide an interesting experimental tool for investigating the critical factors (sensory or metabolic, sweetness or calories) which influence satiation. In the series of studies described here the intense sweetener aspartame has been compared with glucose, sucrose and control treatments. In contrast to those treatments in which sweetness and calories were linked, aspartame generally gave rise to a mixed profile of effects - some measures of satiation showing a moderate downward response and others showing no effect or being facilitated. Usually aspartame produced a decline in hedonic ratings (of sucrose test solution) but did not reduce, and sometimes enhanced, other motivational measures. Interestingly, a high concentration of aspartame did not strengthen the alliesthesia effect - indeed it appeared weaker. This feature requires further investigation but suggests that the effects of aspartame may vary in an unpredictable way with the dose applied. This may be particularly important in view of the additional effects on appetite control mechanisms which may be brought into play by the particular chemical composition of the aspartame molecule.

Consequently, in experimental investigations in the laboratory aspartame has been demonstrated to display irregular effects on measures of appetite control. What are the implications of this for artificial sweeteners in general use? First, for people consuming dietary products containing artificial sweeteners it can be predicted that the lowering of calorie intake would fail to bring about a normal depression of motivation. This would leave people with a residual hunger, i.e. a tendency to eat more if given the opportunity. Second, the intense sweeteners appear to display ambiguous effects on factors reflecting the operation of satiation (the process which stops eating). This suggests that the appetite control mechanisms will be activated in possibly conflicting ways, with some systems being turned down whilst other remain active. This confusion of psychobiological information cannot help the development of good control over eating. Third, there is evidence that under some circumstances aspartame actually stimulated hunger. This response appears very variable and probably depends upon the dose, time after administration and the characteristics of a particular subject. However, it does mean that certain individuals could respond to aspartame by becoming more rather than less hungry.

At the present time very few data are available to indicate how aspartame affects actual consumption. In one study, in which oral loads of a caloric solution containing either aspartame or sucrose were given before a test meal of snack food items, subjects ate 26% more calories after the aspartame than after sucrose[41]. The statistical analysis did not indicate whether or not this difference was statistically significant. However the data do indicate a degree of compensation of the system for the loss of calories in the load. Unfortunately the design of this study was extremely complex and in view of the large number of interacting variables it is difficult to draw any firm conclusions about the action of aspartame. Another study has investigated the effects of consuming high-calorie (149 kcal) and low-calorie (20 kcal) jello. The low-calorie jello was sweetened with aspartame rather than sucrose[42]. No difference in hunger was observed between treatments, nor was there any detectable difference in the intake of a test snack of cheese and crackers 1 hour after ingestion of the jello. The interpretation of this, and similar studies, was that the satiating power of food resides entirely in the sensory properties - in this case in the sweet taste. It is argued that taste alone is sufficient to suppress appetite, pleasantness of food and feeling of gastric emptiness. These data are not in agreement with those presented in the previous section which indicated a powerful effect of uncoupling sensory and calorific properties of consumed materials. However studies with unusual food materials like jello probably induce more cognitive demands (i.e. subjective intuitions about the effect of ingestion) than do experiments with sweetened solutions. In this case some cognitively mediated factor or some physical action of the jello appears to have produced a massive depression in the ratings of hunger which is greater than that often observed in the literature following the administration of anorectic drugs. Until more is known about the composition of this 'anorectic' jello the results of this study will remain difficult to interpret.

More extensive studies have been conducted on a metabolic ward in which either normal-weight or obese subjects ate from a menu of normal food products including sucrose-sweetened drinks and desserts, or from a menu in which the sucrose content of the sweet items had been replaced by aspartame. Consequently, these sweet beverages, puddings and fruits were calorically dilute[43-46]. These four papers all cover reports of two studies. The results indicated that when subjects were switched from the sucrose to the aspartame products overall caloric intake fell. However, despite the elegant technical accomplishments in the use of calorically disguised sweet items, the biological system was not totally deceived and subjects showed a caloric compensation of about 40%. Therefore on the full aspartame regime the subjects did overeat, but not by a large enough margin to achieve full compensation for the lost calories.

However, a number of comments can be made about these very ingenious studies. First, given the elaborate deception, the degree of caloric compensation is quite impressive. In order to regain the lost calories through consumption of the sweet items alone the subjects would have been obliged to consume massive and unacceptable amounts. Since the subjects were obliged by the methodology to sustain a certain caloric deficit through the sweet items (by mandatory consumption) which are calorically dense (calories per weight) the degree of overeating required through the other food items to obtain perfect compensation was unrealistic. Second, there is evidence that the normal subjects used were an unrepresentative sample who may have been nutritionally unbalanced before entering the study. Certainly the first baseline intake of these subjects was remarkably high, and the quality and palatability of the food offered probably caused an artificial elevation of intake over the first few days. Consequently, these studies leave certain questions unresolved.

At the present time it seems important to extend investigations into the effects of artificial sweeteners - and aspartame in particular. Considering the extent to which these substances are used in nutritional products, relatively little is known about their effects on mechanisms controlling appetite. Almost nothing is known about the effects of continued high levels of intake in individuals who are already drastically restricting caloric intake and who may have a highly abnormal pattern of eating. The most vulnerable individuals probably exist in this category. It is worth noting that in a survey of artificial sweetener use on more than 1.2 million men and women carried out by the American Cancer Society, a preliminary report on more than 78,000 women aged 50-69 indicated that users of artificial sweeteners were more likely than non-users to gain weight[47]. The weight changes were small but statistically significant, and it will be interesting to discover whether similar changes occur in other age groups.

Study of the sensory aspects of food consumption indicates that sweetness is an extremely powerful biological phenomenon. Its role in the control of food consumption should not be underestimated, and interventions which uncouple sweetness from its natural calorific consequences are unlikely to be completely benign. The use of particular sweeteners such as aspartame with a biologically interesting chemical composition should be examined closely for any effects on the appetite control system. It is not sufficient to show that these agents are non-toxic; they may have unrecognized long-term effects through their capacity to undermine or corrupt the natural system of psychobiological interactions which normally control food intake and which help to regulate body weight.

REFERENCES

1. Van Itallie TB and Abraham S (1985). Some hazards of obesity and its treatment. In: Hirsch J and Van Itallie TB (eds). Recent Advances in Obesity Research: IV (London: Libby), pp. 1-19
2. Garrow J (1982). Does plumpness matter? Nutrit Bull, 7, 49-53
3. Stunkard AJ, Sorensen TIA, Hanis C, Teasdale TW, Chakraborty R, Schull WJ and Schulsinger F (1986). An adoption study of human obesity. N Engl J Med, 314, 193-8
4. Kulesza W (1982). Dietary intake in obese women. Appetite, 3, 61-8
5. Sclafani A (1978). Dietary obesity. In: Bray G (ed): Recent Advances in Obesity Research, II. (London: Newman) pp. 123-32
6. Sclafani A and Springer D (1976). Dietary obesity in adult rats: similarities to hypothalamic and human obesity syndromes. Physiol Behav, 17, 461-71
7. Wurtman RJ (1983). Neurochemical changes following high-dose aspartame with dietary carbohydrates. N Engl J Med, 309, 429-30
8. Russell GFM (1979). Bulimia nervosa: an ominous variant of anorexia nervosa. Br J Psychiatry, 9, 429-48
9. American Psychiatric Association (1980). Diagnostic and Statistical Manual of Mental Disorders, 3rd edn. (Washington, DC)
10. Boskind-Lodahl M (1976). Cinderella's stepsisters: a feminist perspective on anorexia nervosa and bulimia. J Women Culture & Society, 2, 342-56
11. Palmer RL (1979). The dietary chaos syndrome: a useful new term? Br J Med Psychol, 52, 187-90
12. Fairburn CG (1984). Bulimia: its epidemiology and management. In: Stunkard AJ and Stellar E (eds): Eating and its Disorders. (New York: Raven Press), pp. 235-58
13. Loro AD and Orleans CS (1981). Binge eating in obesity: preliminary findings and guidelines for behavioural analysis and treatment. Addict Behav, 6, 155-66
14. Halmi KA, Falk JR and Schwartz E (1981). Binge eating and vomiting: a survey of a college population. Psychol Med, 11, 697-706
15. Hawkins RC and Clement PF (1980). Development and construct validation of a self-report measure of being-eating tendencies. Addict Behav, 5, 219-26
16. Toon K (1985) Bulimia and anorexia in a university population. MSc thesis, University of Leeds
17. Cooper PJ and Fairburn CG (1983). Binge-eating and self-induced vomiting in the community: a preliminary study. Br J Psychiatry, 142, 139-44
18. Blundell JE (1984). Behaviour modification and exercise in the treatment of obesity. Postgrad Med J, 60, (Suppl. 3), 36-48
19. Wooley SC and Wooley OW (1984). Should obesity be treated at all? In: Stunkard AJ and Stellar E (eds): Eating and its

Disorders. (New York: Raven Press), pp 185-92

20. Polivy J and Herman CP (1985). Dieting and bingeing: a causal analysis. Am Psychol, 40, 193-201

21. Herman CP and Mack D (1975). Restrained and unrestrained eating. J Person, 43, 647-60

22. Stunkard AJ and Messick S (1985). The three-factor eating questionnaire to measure dietary restraint, disinhibition and hunger. J Psychosom Res, 29, 71-83

23. Hill AJ, Magson LD and Blundell JE (1984). Hunger and palatability: tracking ratings of subjective experience before, during and after the consumption of preferred and less preferred food. Appetite, 5, 361-71

24. Hill AJ and Blundell JE (1982/3). Nutrients and behaviour: research strategies for the investigation of taste characteristics, food preferences, hunger sensations and eating patterns in man. J Psychiat Res, 17, 203-12

25. Blundell JE and Hill AJ (1985). Analysis of hunger: interrelationships with palatability, nutrient composition and eating. In: Van Itallie TB and Hirsch J (eds). Recent Advances in Obesity Research IV. (London: Libby), pp. 118-29

26. Blundell JE (1979). Hunger, appetite and satiety - psychological constructs in search of identities. In: Turner M (ed). Nutrition and Lifestyles. (London: Applied Science Publishers), pp. 21-42

27. Smith GP (1982). Satiety and the problem of motivation. In: Pfaff DW (ed). The Physiological Mechanisms of Motivation. (New York: Springer-Verlag), pp. 133-43

28. Cabanac M (1971). The physiological role of pleasure. Science, 173, 1103-7

29. Cabanac M and Duclaux R (1970). Specificity of internal signals in producing satiety for taste stimuli. Nature, 227, 966

30. Hill AJ, Leathwood PJ and Blundell JE (1986). Some evidence for short-term caloric compensation in normal weight human subjects: effects of low and high energy meals on hunger, food preferences and food intake. Human Nutr: Appl Nutr, (In press)

31. Booth DA (1980). Acquired behaviour controlling energy intake and output. In: Stunkard AJ (ed). Obesity. (Philadelphia: Saunders), pp. 101-43

32. Garcia J, Hankins WG and Rusiniak KW (1974). Behavioural regulation of the milieu interne in man and rat. Science, 185, 824-31

33. Sjostrom L, Garellick G, Krotkievsky M and Luyckx A (1980). Peripheral insulin in response to the sight and smell of food. Metabolism, 29, 901-9

34. Simon C, Schlienger JL, Sapin R and Imler M (1986). Cephalic phase insulin secretion in relation to food presentation in normal and overweight subjects. Physiol Behav, 36, 465-9

35. Berthoud HR, Bereiter DA, Trimble ER, Seigel EG and Jeanrenaud B (1981). Cephalic phase, reflex insulin secretion. Diabetologia, 20, 393-401

36. Smith GP and Gibbs J (1979). Postprandial satiety. Prog Psychobiol Physiol Psychol, 8, 179-242

37. Kissileff HR, Pl-Sunyer FX, Thornton J and Smith GP (1981). C-terminal octapeptide of cholecystokin decreases food intake in man. Am J Clin Nutr, 34, 154-60

38. Fernstrom JD, Fernstrom MH and Gillis MA (1983). Acute effects of aspartame on large neutral amino acids and monoamines in rat brain. Life Sci, 32, 1651-8

39. Coulombe RA and Sharma RP (1986). Neurobiochemical alterations induced by the artificial sweetener aspartame (Nutrasweet). Toxicol Appl Pharmacol, 83, 79-85

40. Leibowitz SF and Shor-Posner G (1986). Monoamine meal patterns in the rat. In: Carruba MO and Blundell JE (eds): Psychopharmacology of Eating Disorders: Theorectical and Clinical Advances. (New York: Raven Press), pp. 29-50

41. Brala PM and Hager RL (1983). Effects of sweetness perception and caloric value of a preload on short term satiety. Physiol Behav, 30, 1-9

42. Rolls BJ, Hetherington M, Burley VJ and Duijvenvoorde PM (1986). Changing hedonic responses to foods during and after a meal. In: Kare MR and Brand JG (eds). Interaction of the Chemical Senses with Nutrition. (New York: Academic Press), pp. 247-68

43. Porikos KP, Booth G and Van Itallie TB (1977). Effect of covert nutritional dilution on the spontaneous food intake of obese individuals: a pilot study. Am J Clin Nutr, 30, 1638-44

44. Porikos KP (1981). Control of food intake in man: response to covert caloric dilution of a conventional and palatable diet. In: Cioffi LA et al. (eds). The Body Weight Regulatory System: Normal and Disturbed Mechanisms. (New York: Raven Press), pp. 83-87

45. Porikos KP, Hesser MF and Van Itallie TB (1982). Caloric regulation in normal-weight men maintained on a palatable diet of conventional foods. Physiol Behav, 29, 292-300

46. Porikos KP and Van Itallie TB (1984). Efficacy of low-calorie sweeteners in reducing food intake: studies with aspartame. In: Lewis D et al. (eds), Aspartame - Physiology and Biochemistry. (New York: Marcel Dekker), pp. 273-86

47. Stellman SD and Garfinkel L (1986). Artificial sweetener use and one-year weight change among women. Prev Med, 15, 195-202

48. Gibbs J, Falasco JD and McHugh PR (1976). Cholecystokinin-decreased food intake in Rhesus monkeys. Am J Physiol, 230, 15-18

13

Tobacco and Smoking Products*

A. N. WORDEN

The direct correlation of tobacco - certainly of cigarette - smoking with human morbidity is perhaps the most widely known and generally accepted example of environmental carcinogenesis. Other adverse health effects are also attributed to heavy and continued smoking habits, and even to what is designated passive smoking.

It is not the intention of the present chapter to challenge a correlation which, however, has relied upon epidemiological and clinical observations rather than upon toxicological evidence. In this respect, as Sir Richard Doll has emphasized, it is not unique: indeed only a few of the recognized environmental carcinogens have been predicted from animal studies. There would seem a need, however, to examine the situation in the light of current - and potential - methods.

The views that follow have been obtained from among those who have strived to evaluate the predictive effect of tobacco and other smoking materials. Contact with much of the experimental work on the so-called new-smoking materials was sufficient to convince any unbiased observer that adequate confirmation of carcinogenic - and other toxic - hazard was difficult to achieve and that therefore reliance upon existing methods for comparative predictive purposes seemed somewhat dubious. This did not prevent the conduct of much valuable work, although it failed to yield animal models that could find universal acceptance.

Tobacco used in commerce, primarily for the manufacture of smoking products, is either Nicotiana tabacum or Nicotiana rustica. N. tabacum is the major source of manufactured smoking products world-wide and is widely cultivated, mainly in China, the Americas, Africa, India, Southeast Asia and Europe. N. rustica, otherwise known as makhorka, is commercially less important but is

---

*Compiled from several, including industrial, sources.

283

nevertheless a significant source of employment and revenue in the manufacture of smoking products, mainly in Pakistan, Bangladesh and some areas of European Russia. From the standpoint of toxicology the most important difference between these two types of tobacco lies in the principal alkaloid contained in their leaves. Nicotine is the main alkaloid of N. tabacum, nornicotine that of N. rustica. In addition, tobacco contains minor quantities of many other alkaloids, most of which are 3-pyridyl derivatives. The pharmacology of nicotine differs considerably from that of nornicotine, the former being very much the more active.

For present purposes consideration will be given only to N. tabacum and, where appropriate, only to its main alkaloid, L-nicotine. In tobacco grown for commerce, nicotine occurs at a level roughly between 0.2 and 4.75% of the dry weight of the leaf lamina, and constitutes between 85 and 95% of the total alkaloids present in the leaf. The concentration of nicotine in tobacco grown commercially depends mainly upon the tobacco variety, cultural conditions, climate, latitude and the position of the leaf on the main stem of the plant.

Prior to use in manufacture it is necessary to subject the raw tobacco leaf, after harvesting, to a process of "curing". There are three broadly different tobacco curing processes which relate, in turn, to the type of smoking product for which the cured leaf is most suitable. These three curing processes reflect three progressive stages in the natural transformation of the leaf constituents in the course of senescence, respiration and fermentation.

In the so-called "flue-curing" process, ripe leaves are allowed to wilt at ambient temperature and high humidity in barns until the natural leaf starch is converted largely into mono- and disaccharides. The respiration is then halted by heat and desiccation to inhibit enzymes and bacterial ferments. Flue-cured tobacco is characteristically yellow-brown in colour, contains a significant proportion of reducing sugars (ca. 20% of the dry weight), with relatively little change to other leaf constituents including protein, alkaloids, structural polysaccharides and lignin. It pyrolyses to give a smoke aerosol with a pH value on the acid side of neutrality. Nicotine and other bases are therefore present in the aerosol largely as cations and not as free bases, with important consequences for the route and rate of absorption by the smoker and hence for the pharmacological response of the smoker to ingestion of the alkaloid. Flue-cured tobacco is used to manufacture the so-called "Virginia" cigarette, typical of the UK market, and is an important component of "blended" cigarettes, typical of the US market, and of pipe tobacco blends.

In the air-curing process the natural processes of senescence and respiration are allowed to continue in the harvested leaf at ambient temperature and moderate humidity until nearly all the natural starch and reducing sugars have been transformed. The cured leaf is typically brown in colour, substantially free from reducing sugars, but with other leaf constituents relatively little changed. It gives rise on pyrolysis to a smoke aerosol with a pH value in the neutral/acid range. Air-cured tobacco, known commercially as "Burley" tobacco, is generally derived from varieties of seed which differ from those particularly well-suited to the production of flue-cured leaf. It is widely used in the manufacture of the blended US-style cigarette (along with flue-cured tobacco), and in pipe-tobacco blends.

Fermented tobacco is used almost exclusively for the manufacture of cigars. It is prepared from varieties of seed that give leaf particularly well-suited to the process of fermentation and to the desired end-use. Compared with that of flue-cured and Burley tobaccos, the production of cigar tobaccos is more limited and specialized, and is undertaken in fewer geographical areas. After completion of the natural air-curing process the leaf is further subjected to natural or forced fermentation until the leaf protein is extensively degraded, with some alteration also to alkaloids and structural polysaccharides. The end-product is darkish brown and is characterized by the presence of ammonium salts, free amino acids and peptides, and some nicotine transformation products like myosmine. The pH value of the smoke aerosol is on the alkaline side of neutrality, alkaloids being therefore present mainly as free base. This again has important consequences for the route and rate of absorption by the smoker which, to a significant extent, distinguish the pharmacological effects of cigar smoking from those of cigarette smoking.

Other minor types of tobacco which are grown for use in manufacture, such as "Turkish" tobacco and latakia, are of limited significance in the present context.

The typical merchant or manufacturer of smoking products purchases the cured leaf on the open market. Thereafter it is further processed prior to use in manufacture, by cleaning, grading, redrying or conditioning (to adjust its moisture content), removal of lamina from the leaf midrib ("stemming") and then, depending upon its proposed use, subjected to some form of comminution such as "threshing" or "cutting".

In what now follows consideration is given to the problem of predictive toxicology only in the context of N. tabacum. There is no realistic basis upon which to discuss the topic in the context of N. rustica.

Tobacco is used in commerce principally for the manufacture of smoking products, the product for consideration being not the leaf itself but the aerosol that is formed by its destructive distillation. Other minor uses for tobacco in commerce are for the manufacture of snuff and chewing tobacco. In these instances the leaf itself is of course used by the consumer - snuff by nasal ingestion of the finely powdered leaf, in admixture with inorganic salts and flavours, and chewing tobacco by masticating the cut leaf in admixture with sugary syrups and flavours. These two latter aspects will not be discussed further because, although of special interest and importance for some defined populations, e.g. snuff-taking in African Bantu, they do not command the much wider general concern, world-wide, that arises from the reported health consequences of tobacco-smoking. Nor is there sufficient information available about them in the context of predictive toxicology.

Smoking products confront the toxicologist at the outset with problems which, though subtle, are particularly intricate and important. He has to consider how best to approach the subject in a situation in which he is deprived of some of the familiar landmarks for products such as medicines, food additives and agricultural and industrial chemicals. This difficulty stems from the nature of the evidence which reportedly links tobacco smoking and, above all, cigarette smoking, with many different diseases. This evidence derives overwhelmingly from epidemiological studies, the results of which reportedly show that a particular disease is statistically associated with smoking in the sense that the incidence of the disease is higher in smokers than in non-smokers, and that there is a dose/response relationship within populations of smokers themselves.

The toxicologist has to consider how far such evidence can be relied upon to justify the conclusion that there is a direct causal relationship between the act of ingesting tobacco smoke and the onset of changes that characterize a particular disease - or how far a reported statistical association might be fortuitous or might be the result of an unidentified causal relationship which relates only indirectly to smoking habits.

Accordingly, at the outset, he will need to ask, for each reported statistical association, such questions as: (1) How strong is the association? (2) Is there a clear dose/response relationship? (3) Is the association consistent and free from unexplained anomalies? (4) Can a non-causative explanation of the association reasonably be ruled out? (5) Is there evidence to support causality from another discipline?

The literature reveals that, among the many diseases reported to be associated with cigarette smoking, there remains a wide disparity in the degree to which epidemiological evidence can be held to afford a completely satisfactory response to this kind of scrutiny.

Despite the seemingly overwhelming evidence in terms of lung cancer, the toxicologist in many instances lacks the concrete evidence - particularly for diseases that appear to be multifactorial in causation - that would enable him to identify with confidence the pathological mechanism whereby exposure to tobacco smoke can be said with certainty to cause a particular disease, and thereby to be confident as to which constituents of tobacco or tobacco smoke are likely to be toxicologically significant for predictive purposes.

Secondary to this difficulty, but adding to it, is that tobacco itself is a variable plant product which is subject before use by man for smoking to a process of destructive distillation. The smoke thereby produced is an immeasurably complex mixture of organic compounds, in contrast to the position with, say, a medicine or a food additive where usually only a single compound or its derivatives is concerned. The opportunities for additive or synergistic interaction are of special significance in the context of tobacco smoke.

The toxicologist has the choice of selecting relatively simple, often arbitrary, chemical markers on the basis of little else but hunch, or of seeking empirical quantitative biological laboratory tests which are judged to simulate the appropriate human pathology and which show a dose-response relationship. The well-recognized problems of extrapolation are involved whether laboratory animal or in vitro methods are adopted.

Attention has generally been concentrated for predictive

purposes upon the following broad aspects of the toxicology of known constituents of tobacco and tobacco smoke.

1.   The pharmacological effects of smoking doses of L-nicotine and its transformation products, including for example:

(a)   The finding that the "macro" toxicology of larger doses of nicotine may not be relevant to the problem of tobacco use for smoking, in which an individual subjects himself only to intermittent pulsed doses of very small quantities of the alkaloid.

(b)   The neurochemical, neurophysiological and behavioural effects of the small doses of nicotine, mediated through changes in the levels of circulating catecholamines, indoleamines and acetylcholine; these include effects on blood pressure, heart rate, vasodilation and vasoconstriction; behavioural effects have been identified in both laboratory animals and man, subjected to standard procedures for predicting and detecting the efficacy of stimulant and depressant drugs.

(c)   The possible consequences of such effects for cardiovascular disease in which it has been postulated, for example, that effects on platelet stickiness resulting from release of catecholamines might be significant.

(d)   The need to distinguish carefully between the acute effects of the intermittent intake of smoking doses of nicotine on the healthy heart (or on the heart which has already been damaged from causes unconnected with smoking) and the possible role of such doses of nicotine in causing the chronic degenerative changes which lead to atherosclerosis.

(e)   The unresolved problem of the nature of nicotine "dependence"; doubt remains as to how far any such "dependence" is physiological rather than psychological; to the extent that while the "dependence" might be physiological it is generally agreed that it cannot be described as "addictive" in the strict psychopharmacological sense.

2.   Carbon monoxide is a significant component of tobacco smoke. The delivery per cigarette of the compound in mainstream smoke, and its percentage by volume therein, depend upon the amount of tobacco burned during the puffing process, and upon the subsequent degree of dilution of the smoke with air during its passage along the unburnt portion of the cigarette and the filter, which is in turn affected by the porosity of the cigarette paper and any "ventilation" of the filter section. It has been argued that carbon monoxide derived from smoking could be an added stress factor for individuals who are already compromised by coronary disease, for example through increasing carboxyhaemoglobin and carboxymyoglobin levels. There is little satisfactory experimental evidence that blood levels of carbon monoxide typical of those in cigarette smokers contribute directly to the

development of occlusive arterial vascular disease, or to elevated levels of serum cholesterol or lipoprotein.

3.   Tobacco smoke contains small amounts of numerous low-molecular weight organic compounds which are irritant or otherwise toxic at appropriate doses. These occur in both the gas phase and the particulate phase of the aerosol. Hydrogen cyanide, oxides of nitrogen, acrolein, and hydrogen sulphide are typical examples. It is postulated that such constituents might, for example, contribute to cilia-stasis, pulmonary emphysema and hypersecretion of mucus, with secondary consequences for indices of lung function such as FEV. There is, however, no satisfactory experimental dose/response evidence to enable the toxicologist to be certain which, if any, of these low-molecular weight compounds singly might have quantitative toxicological significance for respiratory disease in smokers; or to place them in any sort of rank order for predictive purposes. Still less is there any useful information about possible additive or synergistic interaction between them.

4.   Tobacco smoke contains numerous compounds which are known from tests with laboratory animals to be tumorigenic, co-carcinogenic or tumour-promoting. Such compounds occur very largely in the condensible or "tar" fraction of the particulate phase of the aerosol, and include polycyclic aromatic hydrocarbons, nitrosamines, aromatic amines and phenols. Heavy metals and ionizing radiation are also present in smoke in trace quantities. Moreover, tobacco smoke "tar" has been shown to be carcinogenic when applied to the skin of the laboratory mouse. There is, however, no consistent experimental evidence that tobacco smoke can produce bronchial carcinoma in laboratory animals which are repeatedly exposed to maximum tolerable concentrations of the smoke.

The toxicologist who seeks an objective basis upon which to predict increased "safety" or reduced "hazard" for tobacco products lacks the necessary quantitative experimental or clinical evidence to enable him to approach this task on the basis of the toxicology of any specific constituents of tobacco or tobacco smoke. Moreover, even if it were possible in the present state of knowledge to relate with confidence any particular pathological response to a corresponding component of tobacco or tobacco smoke, there would remain a further difficulty in the way of relating this knowledge to the human smoker. The dose of a smoke constituent that reaches a target organ in the smoker is determined not only by the concentration of that constituent in the smoke or of its precursor in the tobacco, but also to a very significant degree by the self-selected smoking habits of the smoker. Quite obviously, the number of cigarettes smoked per day by an individual is a macro-determinant, but the variables of the smoking habit itself can greatly influence the intake of a constituent per cigarette smoked[37]. Puff volume, puff frequency and butt length are all such variables; and a smoker will alter these, either consciously or unconsciously, to accord with circumstances. If cigarettes were

modified so as to reduce the notional delivery of one or more constituents judged to be "hazardous", any advantage which might
thereby be expected to accrue could be reduced, or even negated,
if the smoker were to alter his smoking habits. This problem is
clearly recognized by some health educators and advisory agencies.
Thus the 1983 Report of the US Surgeon General[1], which was concerned with the problem of smoking and cardiovascular disease, includes the following observation on this difficult aspect of predictive toxicology:

> Reduction of the harmful components delivered to the smoker
> has been another priority objective, aimed at those smokers
> who will not give up the habit. This task has resulted in the
> introduction of a variety of low- and ultra-low-yield
> cigarettes. Whether risks for cardiovascular diseases are
> truly reduced when these products are used remains to be
> demonstrated. Several recent studies have shown that
> smokers alter their smoking behaviour when they switch to
> low-yield cigarettes and can receive increased smoke con-
> stituents as they attempt to satisfy a nicotine demand. It is
> probable that promotion of ultra-low-yield products will not
> suffice, since compensatory mechanisms may be triggered by
> sensory needs for taste as well as for nicotine.

Account must also be taken of the fact that few, if indeed any, of
the diseases with which we are concerned in the context of smoking are reported to be statistically associated solely with smoking
itself. Many have multifactorial associations, with the consequent
problems of elucidating, if possible, the interactions of numerous
different risk factors. In the circumstances it is not surprising
that many anomalies in the epidemiological evidence continue to
remain unexplained, nor that there are marked gaps in the requisite supporting evidence from clinical and experimental disciplines
that the toxicologist needs to have for the purpose of his task.

Regulatory and advisory bodies have therefore been left with
no real alternative to adopting the broadest general principles in
offering guidance to the smoker on the significance of different
constituents of tobacco smoke or on desirable changes in smoking
habit should he choose to continue to smoke.

"Tar", nicotine and carbon monoxide deliveries of cigarette
brands are now regularly measured by official agencies under
standard laboratory smoking conditions but other smoke components
are not so commonly measured routinely. "Tar" is a convenient
term for the total anhydrous nicotine-free residue of the particulate matter in cigarette smoke that is recovered when mainstream
smoke is subjected to efficient particle-phase filtration or to
electrostatic precipitation. The numerical values of the three variables referred to are then often published regularly, tabulated in
brand rank order, or printed on cigarette packets. It is important
to recognize that the rank order of a group of cigarette brands
will normally differ according to whether the variable is "tar",
nicotine or carbon monoxide. Official agencies then frequently
divide a rank of cigarette brands at arbitrary intervals, designat-
ing the sub-groups with qualitative descriptions such as "low tar",
"middle tar" and "high tar".

Smokers are generally advised that a lower yield of "tar" is predictive of a lower potential risk of contracting lung cancer and that a lower yield of nicotine and of carbon monoxide is predictive of a lower potential risk of contracting cardiovascular disease. Neither of these advisory presumptions has yet been verified through rigorous prospective epidemiological studies and advisory bodies are not unanimous in their conclusions. Thus the 1983 Report of the US Surgeon General[1], already referred to, states that "It is unlikely that a 'safe cigarette' can be developed that will reduce cardiovascular risk".

The 1981 Report of the US Surgeon General[2], entitled "The Changing Cigarette", referred to the relative value of four different, but complementary, approaches to the problem of the predictive toxicology of tobacco products. These were constituent toxicology, bioassay systems, observational epidemiology, and the study of fundamental mechanisms of disease production. Reference has already been made to the problems encountered with observational epidemiology and to the scarcity of knowledge of fundamental mechanisms involved. With the approach through constituent toxicology there can be no disagreement with the assessment of the Report that the sheer magnitude of the task "simply means that it alone cannot solve the problem". There remains the approach through the use of bioassay systems.

In this approach the objective is to devise realistic systems, whether animal models, or tissue or cellular responses in vitro, which can be relied upon first to reflect in a reliable way an appropriate aspect of human pathology, and secondly, to be capable of affording a quantitative measure of dose/response. By this means, if practicable, a measure of the "specific toxicity" of tobacco smoke or tobacco smoke condensate could be made which would be relevant to a particular aspect of tobacco use. In other words, the "toxicity" of tobacco per unit volume of tobacco smoke, or per unit weight of tobacco smoke condensate, could be measured. Given the ability to do this, the way would then be open to compare one smoking product with another in a way which would be independent of the level of exposure or intake, so that, under conditions where levels of exposure are equal, a true measure of relative toxicity could be derived. The availability of such tests would also afford a means whereby a chemical fractionation of tobacco smoke or tobacco smoke condensate could be monitored so as to identify any constituents that might be responsible for a particular aspect of toxicity. Further, a means would be available to search for modified tobacco products, or tobacco substitutes, which might offer the prospect of an order of magnitude reduction in risk that would not be attainable simply by arbitrary reduction in delivery of unaltered components like "tar", nicotine and carbon monoxide.

In practice, it has to be accepted that no bioassay system is yet available which is wholly satisfactory for these purposes. The 1981 Report of the US Surgeon General[2] summarizes the position as follows:

The limitation of the method is that the estimate of risk is only as good as the bioassay system. Unless the system truly approximates the disease process of concern, changes in that system may not reflect risk of disease. A number of bioassay systems exist for the study of cigarette risk. Unfortunately, none of them can be said to exactly duplicate human disease. At the present time, estimates derived from these systems cannot stand alone, but must be interpreted in the light of information derived from other methods.

The more important bioassay systems which have been considered for relevant purposes are discussed below.

LUNG CANCER

The type of lung cancer which on epidemiological evidence is of prime importance is bronchial carcinoma. Exposure of rats or mice to cigarette smoke itself results in only a small incidence compared with that in unexposed controls, of respiratory tract tumours, and these are primarily pulmonary adenomas, not bronchial carcinomas[3-5]. The Syrian golden hamster develops invasive carcinoma of the larynx, not the lung, after long exposure to cigarette smoke; and this test has been used to compare different types of cigarettes[6-9]. The mouse-skin painting test has been extensively employed to enable estimates to be made of several aspects of the tumorigenicity (including co-carcinogenicity) of tobacco smoke condensate and its fractions. The method was first established on a firm quantitative comparative basis by the pioneering work of T.D. Day and his co-workers[10] and has been adopted by many others[11-14] and used for a variety of purposes[15-18], including the assessment of a tobacco substitute[19]. The response of the rat lung to tobacco smoke condensate, and to fractions derived from it, administered by intratracheal instillation, has been similarly used[20]. Laboratory tests regarded as being predictive of carcinogenic potential have also been employed, including tests for mutagenesis[21-22], for which the results have not been consistent[23], and the sebaceous gland suppression test[24]. Tests for the induction of microsomal oxidases, notably arylhydrocarbon hydroxylase have given conflicting results[25-27].

CHRONIC OBSTRUCTIVE LUNG DISEASE

For this group of diseases, including chronic bronchitis, bronchiolar inflammation and pulmonary emphysema, there are no satisfactory animal models for measuring the toxicity of cigarette smoke or its condensate. Attempts to produce emphysema-like changes in the lungs of laboratory animals exposed to cigarette smoke have given conflicting and largely negative results[4,6,7,28-30] although attempts have been made to measure ciliatoxic activity[31,32].

CARDIOVASCULAR DISEASE

Long-term inhalation studies with laboratory animals to date have not produced any evidence of pathological changes similar to those of human coronary heart disease, nor any bioassay suitable for predictive toxicology in this area[4,6-8,28,29].

A prerequisite for tests for "specific toxicity" is the availability of means to expose laboratory animals, tissue preparations or cell cultures to measured doses of tobacco smoke, generated and delivered in a way that mimics as closely as practicable the generation and intake of diluted mainstream cigarette smoke by the typical human smoker. The international standards for analytical laboratory smoking machines[33,34] have been employed in the design of several efficient machines suitable for bioassay.

Tests for "specific toxicity" have been widely used in order to discover how far it might be practicable to alter tobacco growing variables and tobacco products manufacturing variables so as to effect a reduction in some aspect of the biological activity of tobacco smoke or tobacco smoke condensate which might be relevant. It is not appropriate to review this lengthy topic in the present context, but the interested reader can usefully refer for further information to the extensive studies in the USA, carried out under the auspices of the US Public Health Service[15-18]. Such studies have had to take into account that the typical manufactured smoking product of commerce contains many substances in addition to tobacco itself. Some of these are obvious, including, for example, filters typically made with cellulose acetate designed to afford some degree of selective filtration of smoke constituents[35]; and cigarette paper with a lap adhesive and print to identify the brand. Others, less immediately obvious, include humectants, flavours, "expanded tobacco" and "reconstituted tobacco sheet" made from comminuted tobacco reformed into a continuous web by a casting or paper-making process. Reference to such materials is made in the 1981 Report of the US Surgeon General already cited[2]. The identity of many such non-tobacco components of smoking products is, understandably, subject to commercial secrecy. In the UK, however, the use of non-tobacco additives in smoking products is subject to voluntary control under the aegis of the Independent Scientific Committee on Smoking and Health, which is advisory to the Department of Health and Social Services and to the tobacco manufacturers. The latter have agreed to disclose to the Committee all non-tobacco components used in manufacture, and to accept the guidance of the Committee as to the advisability of their use and the levels at which they may be used. The guidelines approved by the Committee have been published[36].

The future of the predictive toxicology of tobacco and smoking products is subject to much uncertainty on account of the marked gaps in knowledge. It is important, from the standpoint of the health educator, that these deficiencies should be removed, or substantially reduced as quickly as possible. Notably, there is a need to account for the remaining anomalies in the reported statistical evidence that associates smoking with so many different diseases; to remedy the serious lack of knowledge of what basic mechanisms might be involved if these associations are to be interpreted in causative terms; and to link any such mechanisms with tobacco smoke constituents by means of rigorous dose/response studies in reliably predictive bioassay systems. Clearly there remains a need for much more fundamental research if these objectives are to be achieved.

ADDENDUM

The complex issues associated with smoking and health would seem to be well exemplified by the finding that there is a significant increase in oestradiol 2-hydroxylation in premenopausal women who have smoked at least 15 cigarettes/day. Urinary excretion of oestriol relative to oestrone is significantly decreased and the likely result is decreased availability of oestradiol at oestrogen target tissues[38]. This would seem to be linked with a protective effect of cigarette smoking on endometrial cancer[39] but with early menopause and an increased incidence of osteoporosis[40,41].

REFERENCES

1. The Health Consequences of Smoking (1983). A Report of the Surgeon General. US Department of Health and Human Services, Public Health Service. Office on Smoking and Health, Rockville, Maryland 20857

2. The Health Consequences of Smoking. The Changing Cigarette (1981). A Report of the Surgeon General. US Department of Health and Human Services, Public Health Service. Office on Smoking and Health

3. Dalbey, WE, Nettesheim, P, Griesemer, R, Caton, JE and Guerin, MR (1980). Chronic inhalation of cigarette smoke by F344 rats. J Nat Cancer Inst, 64(2), 383-8

4. Guerin, MR (1959). Bulletin de l'Association francaise pour l'Etude du Cancer, 46(2), 295-309

5. Harris, RJC, Negroni, G, Ludgate, S, Pick, CR, Chesterman, FC and Maidment, BJ (1974). Int J Cancer 14(1), 130-136

6. Bernfeld, P, Homburger, F, Soto, E and Pai, KJ (1979). Cigarette smoke inhalation studies in inbred Syrian golden hamsters. J Natl Cancer Inst, 63(3), 675-89

7. Dontenwill, W, Chevalier, H-J, Harke, H-P, Klimisch, H-J, Kuhnigk, C, Reckzeh, G and Schneider, B (1977). Krebsforsch Klin Onkol, 89(2), 153-80

8. Dontenwill, W, Chevalier, H-J, Harke, H-P, Lafrenz, U, Reckzeh, G and Schneider, B (1973). Investigation on the effects of chronic cigarette smoke inhalation in Syrian golden hamster. J Natl Cancer Inst, 51(6), 1781-1832

9. Dontenwill, WP (1974). In: Karbe, E and Park, JF (eds). International Symposium, Seattle. Experimental Lung Cancer: Carcinogenesis and Bioassays. pp. 332-59. (New York: Springer-Verlag)

10. Day, TD (1967). Carcinogenic action of cigarette smoke condensate on mouse skin: an attempt at a quantitative study. Br J Cancer, 21(1), 56-81

11. Wynder, EL and Hoffman, D (1967). Tobacco and Tobacco Smoke. Studies in Experimental Carcinogenesis. (New York: Academic Press)

12. Dontenwill, W, Chevalier, H-J, Harke, H-P, Klimisch, H-J, Reckzeh, G, Fleischmann, B and Keller, W (1977). Z Krebsforsch Klin Onkol 89(2), 145-51

13. Hoffman, D and Wynder, EL (1971). A study of tobacco carcinogenesis. XI Tumor initiators, tumor accelerators, and tumor promoting activity of condensate fractions. Cancer, 27(4), 848-64

14. Lee, PN, Rothwell, K and Whitehead, JK (1977). Fractionation of mouse skin carcinogens in cigarette smoke condensate. Br J Cancer, 35(6), 730-42

15. Gori, GB (ed) (1976). Toward Less Hazardous Cigarettes. The First Set of Experimental Cigarettes. US Department of Health, Education and Welfare, Public Health Service, National Institutes of Health, National Cancer Institute, Smoking and Health Program, Report No. 1

16. Gori, GB (ed) (1976). Toward Less Hazardous Cigarettes. The Second Set of Experimental Cigarettes. US Department of Health, Education and Welfare, Public Health Service, National Institutes of Health, National Cancer Institute, Smoking and Health Program, Report No. 2

17. Gori, GB (ed) (1977). Toward Less Hazardous Cigarettes. The Third Set of Experimental Cigarettes. US Department of Health, Education and Welfare, Public Health Service, National Institutes of Health, National Cancer Institute, Smoking and Health Program, Report No. 3

18. Gori, GB (ed) (1980). Toward Less Hazardous Cigarettes. The Fourth Set of Experimental Cigarettes. US Department of Health, Education and Welfare, Public Health Service, National Institutes of Health, National Cancer Institute, Smoking and Health Program, Report No. 4

19. Clapp, MJL, Conning, DM and Wilson, J (1977). Studies on the local and systemic carcinogenicity of topically applied smoke condensate from a substitute smoking material. Br J Cancer, 35(3), 329-41

20. Davis, BR, Whitehead, JK, Gill, ME, Lee, PN, Butterworth, AD and Roe, FJC (1975). Response of rat lung to tobacco smoke condensate of fractions derived from its administered repeatedly by intratracheal instillation. Br J Cancer, 31(4), 453-61

21. Hutton, JJ and Hackney, C (1975). Metabolism of cigarette smoke condensates by human and rat homogenates to form mutagens detectable by Salmonella typhimurium TA 1538. Cancer Res, 35(9), 2461-8

22. Mizusaki, S, Okamoto, H, Akiyama, A and Fukuhara, Y (1977). The relation between chemical constituents of tobacco and mutagenic activity of cigarette smoke condensate. Mutat Res, 48(3/4), 319-25

23. Tso, TC and Chaplin, JF (1977). US Department of Agriculture Technical Bulletin 1551

24. Bock, FG and Gori, GB (1978). Proceedings of the Sixty-Ninth Annual Meeting of the American Association for Cancer

Research, 19, 43

25. Akin, FJ and Benner, JF (1976). Induction of aryl hydro-carbon hydroxylase in rodent lung by cigarette smoke: a potential short term bioassay. Toxicol Appl Pharmacol 36(2), 331-7

26. Gielen, JE, Goujon, F, Sele, J and Van Cantfort, J (1979). Organ specificity of induction of activating and inactivating enzymes by cigarette smoke and cigarette smoke condensate. Arch Toxicol (Suppl 2), 239-51

27. Bilimoria, MH, Johnson, J, Hogg, JC and Witschi, HP (1977). Pulmonary aryl hydrocarbon hydroxylase: tobacco smoke in exposed guinea pigs. Toxicol Appl Pharmacol, 41(2), 433-40

28. McGill, HC, Jr, Rogers, WR, Wilbur, RL and Johnson, DE (1978). Cigarette smoking: baboon model demonstration of feasibility. Proc Soc Exp Biol Med, 157(4), 672-6

29. Le Bouffant, L, Martin, JC, Daniel, H, Henin, JP and Nor-mand, C (1980). Action of intensive cigarette smoke inhala-tions on the rat lung: role of particulate and gaseous cofac-tors. J Nat Cancer Inst, 64(2), 273-81

30. Nicholas, H, Davies, P, Sornberger, C and Huber, G (1977). Alterations in lung parenchyma following experimental chronic inhalation of tobacco smoke. Chest, 72(3), 409

31. Battista, SP (1976). In: Wynder, EL, Hoffmann, D and Gori, GB (eds) Proceedings of the Third World Conference on Smoking and Health, New York, 2-5 June, 1975. Volume I: Modifying the Risk for the Smoker. US Department of Health, Education and Welfare, Public Health Service, National In-stitutes of Health, National Cancer Institute, DHEW Publica-tion No. (NIH) 76-1221, pp. 517-34

32. Battista, SP (1980). In: Gori, GB and Bock, FG (eds) (1980). Banbury Report 3, A Safe Cigarette? pp. 51-62 (New York: Cold Spring Harbor Laboratory)

33. Brunnemann, KD, Hoffmann, D, Wynder, EL and Gori, GB (1976). Chemical Studies on Tobacco Smoke. XXXVII. In: Wynder, EL, Hoffmann, D and Gori, GB (Eds) Proceedings of the Third World Conference on Smoking and Health, New York, 2-5 June, 1975. Volume I: Modifying the Risk for the Smoker. US Department of Health, Education and Welfare, Public Health Service, National Institute of Health, National Cancer Institute, DHEW Publication No. (NIH) 76-1221, pp. 441-9

34. Pillsbury, HC, Bright, CC, O'Connor, KJ and Irish, FW (1969). J Assoc Offic Analyt Chem 52(3), 458-62

35. Morie, GP (1977). Proceedings of the American Chemical Society Symposium, 173rd. American Chemical Society Meet-ing, Agricultural and Food Chemistry Division, New Orleans, 1977. Recent Advances in the Chemical Composition of Tobacco and Tobacco Smoke, pp. 553-83

36. (1980). Report of the Independent Scientific Committee on Smoking and Health on Tobacco Additives, London: HMSO

37. Benowitz, NL, Jacob, P, Kozlowski, Lynne T and Yu, Lisa U (1986). Influence of smoking fewer cigarettes on exposure to tar, nicotine and carbon monoxide. N Engl J Med, 315, 1310

38. Michnovicz, JJ, Herschcopf, RJ, Naganuma, H, Bradlow, HL and Fishman, J (1986). Increased 2-hydroxylation of estradiol as a possible mechanism for the anti-estragenic effect of cigarette smoking. N Engl J Med, 315, 1305-9
39. Lesko, SM, Rosenberg, L, Kaufman, DW, Helmrich, SP, Miller, DR, Strom, B, Schottenfeld, D, Rosenshein, NB, Knapp, RC, Lewis, J, Shapiro, S (1985). Cigarette smoking and the risk of endometrial cancer. N Engl J Med, 313, 593-6
40. Baron, JA (1984). Smoking and estrogen-related disease. Am J Epidemiol, 119, 9-22
41. Williams, AR, Weiss, NS, Ure, CL, Ballard, J and Daling, JR (1982). Effect of weight, smoking, and estrogen use on the risk of hip and forearm fractures in postmenopausal women. Obstet Gynecol, 60, 694-9

14

New Challenges in the Safety Evaluation of Drugs and Biologics*

W. M. GALBRAITH

INTRODUCTION

The development of recombinant and hybridoma technologies has resulted in many new investigational drugs and biological products which previously would not have been possible to produce in adequate quantities for preclinical and clinical research or product marketing. Drugs and biologics of current interest include growth hormones, interferons, interleukins, hormone releasing factors, neuroactive peptides, reproductive hormones, vaccines, immunosuppressive factors, and tumour necrosis factor. At this time recombinant human insulin, recombinant methionyl human growth hormone and two recombinant interferon alpha products have been approved for administration to humans in the United States. With the discovery and characterization of previously unknown endogenous peptides there has been a realization that many of these compounds and their analogues might have application in the treatment and diagnosis of disease. Availability and expense of producing compounds represented major road blocks to preclinical and clinical research and development of many protein products in the past. This can now be overcome by the new technological methods.

THE RECOMBINANT PROCESS

With the availability of new products produced by the new technologies, the Food and Drug Administration (FDA) has had to evaluate the existing science and develop policies that would allow for the continued safe development of these products. For example,

*Presented in part at the 6th Annual Meeting American College of Toxicology, Washington, DC, November 1985, and the Fall 1985 Meeting of the Drug Safety Subsection - Eastern Region, US Pharmaceutical Manufacturers Association.

the FDA has taken the position that the process used to produce a human drug product will not be the major factor in determining preclinical testing needs. However, until more information is available, the FDA will request relevant preclinical and clinical testing of recombinant products even if the products are similar in other respects to currently marketed products. This position has been taken because of the concern that there may be novel contaminants in recombinant products, and there is the possibility that subtle changes which can occur in chemical structure may influence pharmacokinetics, pharmacodynamics and/or immunogenicity. As we gain increased experience with products manufactured with the new technology, less preclinical and clinical evaluation will likely be necessary for well-characterized molecular entities.

DRUGS AND BIOLOGICS

Biotechnology has resulted in a large increase in the diversity of clinical indications which agents classified as biologics may be used to treat. The majority of the new investigational therapeutic agents produced by biotechnology techniques are defined for regulatory purposes as biological products by the FDA's Center for Drugs and Biologics. The official definitions for drugs and biologics are found in the Federal Food, Drug, and Cosmetic Act and the Public Health Service Act, Biological Products. The classification of an agent as a drug or biologic is not determined solely on the basis of intended clinical use. At this time the majority of biotechnology derived agents not classified as biologics are endocrine and metabolic drugs. These drug products are regulated by the Office of Biologics Research and Review in the FDA Center for Drugs and Biologics. The regulatory implications resulting from the classification of an agent as a drug or biologics are found in the Acts (laws) and in Title 21 United States Code of Federal Regulations (USCFR), which contain regulations promulgated under the Acts.

PRECLINICAL GUIDELINES

In the past the preclinical evaluation required for endogenous substances, especially when used in the treatment of a deficiency, has primarily focused on demonstrating that physiological, biochemical and/or pharmacological properties of the product were similar to those of the natural endogenous substance, and that the formulation was safe. A more extensive preclinical evaluation was necessary if the intent was to administer the substance in excess of normal physiological requirements. The testing protocols were designed on the basis of knowledge of the specific pharmacological class of the product because diverse physiological processes, potentially affected by endogenous proteins, may require specific evaluations.

No single list of considerations or set of guidelines can adequately address all specific concerns for every pharmacological agent and proposed clinical indication. In addition, as a result of the rapid rate at which information is being generated about the mechanism of action and biological effects of new biotech. products, formal guidelines would undoubtedly be obsolete when finalized. In order to provide guidance for product developers, in addition to guidelines, the CDB utilizes "Points to Consider" documents. These documents are intended to make developers of new products aware of scientific areas of concern as they develop their applications, and to solicit ongoing comments from interested parties for use in the formulation of further policy discussions in the area. They are not intended to be a set of instructions or guidelines which, if followed, will ensure a product's approval. Currently available "Points to Consider" documents are listed in Table 14.1.

Table 14.1 CDB "Points to Consider" documents

---

(1)   Manufacture of Monoclonal Antibody Products for Human Use

(2)   Characterization of Cell Lines Used to Produce Biological Products

(3)   Production and Testing of Interferon Intended for Investigational Use in Humans

(4)   Manufacture of In Vitro Monoclonal Antibody Products Subject to Licensure

(5)   Production and Testing of New Drugs and Biologicals Produced by Recombinant DNA Technology

---

MONOCLONAL ANTIBODY PRODUCTS

Monoclonal antibody products intended for parenteral administration represent a significant portion of the new biotechnological agents currently under investigation. Monoclonal antibodies are homogeneous populations of immunoglobulin molecules having antibody-combining sites that bind uniformly to discrete antigenic determinants (epitopes). They may be prepared in concentrated form, and may exert highly potent effects. A major concern for these products is that the antigenic determinant (or structurally similar epitope) may be present on human cells or tissues other than the intended target tissue, resulting in undesirable cross-reactions. Accordingly, laboratory tests should be conducted to assess this possibility and, when cross-reactions are encountered, the resultant potential hazard and/or risk to potential recipients should be evaluated.

For monoclonal antibodies, when coupled to toxins, drugs, radionuclides or other xenobiotics, preclinical animal toxicity testing should normally be performed in at least one species, such as the dog or primate, in addition to the rodents. The route and frequency of administration should be similar to that proposed for clinical use. At least one dose studied should be equivalent to the highest anticipated human dose. At least two doses which are mulitiples of the high human dose equivalent should also be evaluated. Animals to be sacrificed for histopathological evaluation are killed 24 hours following the single dose, or final dose in multiple-dose treatment. An attempt should be made to determine the "highest non-toxic dose" and the dose which produces drug-induced pathological alterations. The protocol should usually include test animals that will be observed for 14 days following treatment. The methods for animal handling, clinical observations and laboratory testing including haematology, urinalysis, clinical biochemistry, and histopathology which should be considered can be found in various sources[1-5]. All preclinical safety studies used in support of product approval should be in compliance with FDA Good Laboratory Practices regulations (21 CFR 58).

In addition to toxicity testing, consideration should be given to studies of product distribution, metabolic fate, excretory routes and kinetics in a relevant animal model. A more extensive discussion may be found in the latest monoclonal antibody CDB "Points to Consider" document.

ENDOGENOUS HUMAN PROTEINS

The FDA has published General Guidelines for Animal Toxicity Studies for Drugs[4]. These guidelines were developed primarily for the preclinical evaluation of xenobiotics. Although many of the considerations discussed in the document apply to the preclinical evaluation of any drug or biologic, the guidelines do not specifically address issues pertinent to the evaluation of parenterally administered endogenous human protein products.

Endogenous human proteins represent a wide spectrum of agents that cannot be comprehensively reviewed in a single document. Nevertheless, an attempt will be made to outline basic considerations that must be addressed in order to develop adequate and useful preclinical data needed to minimize human experimentation, identify potential hazards in initial human clinical trials, and design scientifically sound clinical dosage regimens. Preclinical toxicological experiments are usually designed so that there is a greater probability of toxicity that that in the human studies. If these study results are to be meaningful the toxicologist must select an animal model which is relevant for man. Two species, usually a rodent and a non-rodent, are requested for preclinical evaluation of the various categories of pharmacological agents, most of which are xenobiotics, in the FDA General Guideline for the Preclinical Testing of Drugs. This is desirable because metabolic and receptor sensitivity differences may exist between one or more species and humans. The evaluation of more than one species increases the probability of detecting potential human toxicities. In addition, as a result of the diverse genetic make-up of the human population, no one species is representative or predictive for all humans. The major biochemical discoveries of the past 40 years support the conviction that there are more similarities than there are differences between various mammalian species. Despite these similarities the extrapolation of toxicological testing results to humans must be made with caution, and we must be continually aware that preclinical evaluation in one relevant animal model will provide much more valuable information than that from several unpredictive models.

The preclinical evaluation of hormones and the associated testing issues have greater similarity to those associated with the new endogenous proteins than those for xenobiotics. As a result, our past experiences in the preclinical evaluation of hormones is more relevant to evaluation of the potential mechanisms by which an endogenous protein may elicit toxicity.

Study of a series of growth hormones from various species with different amino acid sequences clearly shows that there is greater specificity for receptors in the species of origin and a subsequent greater biological response is induced[6]. In view of the species specificity of endogenous human proteins, it is important to select a species for preclinical toxicological evaluation that demonstrates the greatest sensitivity to the human protein. SELECT AN ANIMAL MODEL IN WHICH THE PHARMACOLOGICAL ACTIVITY OF THE PROTEIN CAN BE DEMONSTRATED TO BE THE SAME AS FOR HUMANS. For example, an "in vitro" anti-viral assay can be used to evaluate species sensitivity to human interferons. Other methods will be required for other agents.

It has been demonstrated that at greater than normal physiological concentrations, receptors other than primary target receptors can be induced by bioactive proteins. For example, human placental lactogen (HPL) shows weak growth stimulating effects in humans. The potency is approximately one-hundredth of the potency of pituitary GH. At increased physiological concentrations this hormone, or other structural analogues, may exert physiological effects, such as growth promotion, that are not significant at normal physiological concentrations. It is reasonable to expect, when non-target receptors which are not induced at normal physiological concentrations are induced following therapeutic doses, that the resulting effect may represent dose-limiting toxicity.

A second mechanism of toxicity may be the result of widespread simultaneous induction of physiological effects in various organ systems following administration of biologically potent endogenous proteins which are only produced in small concentrations with limited tissue exposure under normal physiological conditions. Some people refer to this systemic response from agents that normally only produce local effects as "exaggerated pharmacology".

Table 14.2 lists other potential mechanisms by which endogenous proteins may elicit toxicity.

Immunogenicity

Immunogenicity of a human protein in the test animal may represent a major and sometimes insurmountable obstacle to meaningful preclinical evaluation in other than acute studies. Immunogenicity has not been a major obstacle in the preclinical evaluation of xenobiotics which are of relatively low molecular weight in com-

301

parison to most human protein investigational agents.

Table 14.2 Potential mechanisms by which endogenous proteins may induce toxicity

---

(1) Induction of non-target receptor resulting in unwanted physiological effects

(2) Systemic exposure to a protein that is normally present only in small quantities at specific sites may not be well tolerated ("Exaggerated pharmacology")

(3) Antagonist-receptor may be blocked and unable to respond to normal stimulation

(4) Agent specific concerns that may be related to the therapeutic regimen, i.e. toxicity resulting from chronic receptor induction

---

It is firmly established that when proteins from one species are injected into another species, even if a closely related species, antibody formation may be readily induced. Prior to performing other than acute preclinical toxicology studies with human proteins it is advisable to determine if antibody which diminishes biological activity will be produced as a result of protein product administration in the test animal. When subchronic studies are performed test animals should be evaluated for neutralizing antibody formation. It is noteworthy that a heterogenic antibody response has been observed in humans receiving human proteins. This heterogenicity is probably in part related to genetic variability within the species. It follows that there may be a heterogenic response in pharmacological relevant testing models receiving a human protein, and this has been observed in primate models.

CLINICAL OBSERVATIONS

The uncertainty in predicting the results of safety studies in animals before any studies have been done requires that basic observations be selected to permit detection of a variety of changes in animals which then can be used to alert the clinician to the possibility of such changes occurring in clinical trials. Many attempts[1-4] have been made to list important observations which should be made in conducting a toxicology study, and no attempt will be made here to repeat what has been adequately done by others.

Our experience with protein products results in the conclusion that an increased emphasis should be placed on the evaluation of in-life physiological observations made during acute and subchronic preclinical studies. For example, many study protocols do not routinely include an evaluation of blood pressure. Appropriate methods evaluating body temperature and the cardiopulmonary system may be desirable on a routine basis in the preclinical evaluation of endogenous human peptides.

MUTAGENICITY AND REPRODUCTION

It is not the purpose of this discussion to outline specific preclinical testing requirements which will apply to all proteins and/or biotechnology products. It is appropriate to comment on areas requiring special emphasis or for which the preclinical testing approach may significantly differ from that for xenobiotics. Several of these items have already been discussed. Two others, mutagenicity and reproductive testing, require comment.

If mutagenicity testing is to be performed on a protein product, a mammalian cell system is recommended. Experiments are conducted over a range of dose concentrations to obtain dose-response data and determine if the product is cytotoxic or exerts cellular proliferative or antiproliferative effects at potential therapeutic concentrations. Research is needed in order to clarify the place of currently available in vitro screening tests in the safety evaluation of endogenous proteins.

The need to perform reproductive toxicity testing is related to the proposed clinical indication and the patient populations which may receive the agent. If an agent is to be used in women of child-bearing age, or in pregnant women with non-life-threatening disease, reproductive toxicity studies are probably needed. If there is concern that an agent may be an abortifacient, as is the case for the interferons[7], then a subhuman primate reproductive study may be needed.

DISCUSSION

A prudent approach in the preclinical evaluation of human endogenous protein products is for the developer to identify an animal model in which biological properties of the product are similar to those expected in humans, and in which development of neutralizing antibodies does not prohibit meaningful study. In other respects the basic approach and goals for toxicity studies of endogenous substances intended for administration at concentrations in excess of normal physiological concentrations differ little from those for the preclinical evaluation of xenobiotics. Table 14.3 contains a synopsis of areas meriting special emphasis.

As with all agents, the preclinical testing needed prior to clinical trials must be determined on the basis of the biological properties of the test substance. Unanticipated findings obtained on initial testing of a new product may indicate the desirability of performing additional studies. Preclinical safety evaluations should be approached with the intent of learning about the compounds under study, not just to demonstrate the lack of harmful effects.

A discussion of the preclinical safety evaluation of biotechnology-derived products would be inadequate without mention of concern regarding the extent to which purification processes can exclude the presence of viruses and DNA. There is still uneasiness among some people regarding theoretical problems which may be related to the use of overtly tumorigenic cells to produce many products. Those interested in these issues are referred to the proceedings of a recent FDA Workshop of Abnormal Cells, New Products and Risks[8]. It is noteworthy that the issue will probably remain a major topic of scientific discussion and evaluation for some time in the future, and additional expert panel reviews are being planned.

Table 14.3 Synopsis of areas of special emphasis in the preclinical evaluation of endogenous human proteins

---

(1)   Select a relevant animal model - the best animal models are species in which appropriate pharmacological activity of the drug can be demonstrated as the same for humans

(2)   If possible, the duration and route of administration should be similar to that proposed for human administration

(3)   Monitor blood pressure and body temperature in acute and subchronic studies

(4)   Use mammalian cells for in vitro testing - determine cytotoxic, cellular antiproliferative potential

(5)   A subhuman primate reproduction evaluation may be necessary for some endogenous human   proteins

(6)   Perform the general safety test and other evaluations specified in the USCFR.

CONCLUSION

Much of the difficulty in the preclinical and clinical evaluation of many of the new investigational biotechnology agents results from our lack of understanding of the fundamental biochemical and physiological processes which they mediate in humans and test animals. This is especially true for the biological response modifiers. We know relatively little of their function at normal physiological concentrations. It is difficult, therefore, to predict the effects they may have when administered at high concentrations in patients with disease.

At this time our ability to produce human endogenous proteins has advanced ahead of our understanding of the biological systems in which they are essential. Hopefully the increased availability of compounds for research and development will ultimately lead to an increased understanding of their roles in various biological processes, and eventually in new therapeutic agents.

REFERENCES

1. Toxicological Principles for the Safety Assessment of Direct Food Additives and Color Additives Used in Food. (US Food and Drug Administration, Bureau of Foods, 1982)
2. OECD Guidelines for Testing of Chemicals. (Paris: OECD Publications Office)
3. Page, N, Sawhney, D and Ryon, M (19?). Proceedings of the Workshop of Subchronic Toxicity Testing (NTIS printed copy: A05 microfiche A01)
4. D'Aguanno, W (1973). Drug toxicity evaluation - pre-clinical aspects. FDA Introduction to Total Drug Quality. (Washington, DC: US Government Printing Office)
5. Zbinden, G (1973). Progress in Toxicology. (Berlin: Springer-Verlag)
6. Lesniak, MA and Gordon, P (1976). Growth hormone receptors. In Hormone-receptor Interaction: Molecular Aspects. Levey, GS (ed). (New York: Marcel Dekker)
7. Trown, PW, Wills, RJ and Kamm, JJ (1986). The preclinical development of RoFeron-A. Cancer (In press)
8. Hopps, HE and Petricciani (1985). Abnormal Cells, New Products and Risk. (Gaithersburg, Maryland: Tissue Culture Association)

Index